COMPARATIVE PATHOBIOLOGY OF MAJOR AGE-RELATED DISEASES

Current Status and Research Frontiers

MODERN AGING RESEARCH

Series Editors

Richard C. Adelman
Jay Roberts

George T. Baker III
Vincent J. Cristofalo

Volume 1: Neural Regulatory Mechanisms During Aging, Richard C. Adelman, Jay Roberts, George T. Baker III, Steven I. Baskin, and Vincent J. Cristofalo, *Editors*

Volume 2: Aging and Human Visual Function, Robert Sekuler, Donald Kline, and Key Dismukes, *Editors*

Volume 3: Intervention in the Aging Process, William Regelson and F. Marott Sinex, *Editors*. Published in two volumes. Part A: Quantitation, Epidemiology, and Clinical Research. Part B: Basic Research and Preclinical Screening.

Volume 4: Comparative Pathobiology of Major Age-Related Diseases: Current Status and Research Frontiers, Dante G. Scarpelli and George Migaki, *Editors*

COMPARATIVE PATHOBIOLOGY OF MAJOR AGE-RELATED DISEASES

Current Status and Research Frontiers

Proceedings of a Symposium held at
the National Institutes of Health,
Bethesda, Maryland, April 25–26, 1983

Editors

Dante G. Scarpelli, MD, PhD
Professor and Chairman
Department of Pathology
Northwestern University
Medical School
Chicago, Illinois

George Migaki, DVM
Chief Pathologist
Registry of Comparative Pathology
Universities Associated for Research and Education in Pathology, Inc.
Armed Forces Institute of Pathology
Washington, DC

Alan R. Liss, Inc., New York

Address all Inquiries to the Publisher
Alan R. Liss, Inc., 150 Fifth Avenue, New York, NY 10011

Printed in the United States of America.

Library of Congress Cataloging in Publication Data

Main entry under title:

Comparative pathobiology of major age-related diseases.

Proceedings of a symposium held Apr. 25–26, 1983, at the National Institute of Health, Bethesda, Md.
Includes bibliographies and index.
1. Age factors in disease--Congresses. 2. Pathology, Comparative--Congresses. 3. Aging--Congresses. 4. Aged --Diseases--Animal models--Congresses. I. Scarpelli, Dante G., 1927- . II. Migaki, George. [DNLM: 1. Geriatrics--Congresses. 2. Aging--Congresses. 3. Mesoderm--Congresses. 5. Brain--Congresses. W1 MO117 v.4 / WT 100 C737 1983]
RB210.C66 1984 618.97'07 83-25570
ISBN 0-8451-2304-1

Contents

Contributors and Participants

Carmela Abraham, Ralph Lowell Laboratories, McLean Hospital, Harvard Medical School, Belmont, MA 02178 **[373]**

***Stanley H. Appel,** Department of Neurology, Baylor College of Medicine, Houston, TX 77030 **[411]**

Michael D. Applegate, Department of Physiology and Pharmacology, Bowman Gray School of Medicine, Wake Forest University, Winston-Salem, NC 27103 **[333]**

***Endre A. Balazs,** Department of Ophthalmology/Research Division, Columbia University, New York, NY 10032 **[129]**

***Eugene Bell,** Department of Biology, Massachusetts Institute of Technology, Cambridge, MA 02139 **[69]**

***Gerald S. Berenson,** Department of Medicine, Louisiana State University Medical Center, New Orleans, LA 70112 **[307]**

Maria C. Birchenall-Sparks, Department of Chemistry, Illinois State University, Normal, IL 61761 **[47]**

***David F. Bohr,** Department of Physiology, University of Michigan Medical School, Ann Arbor, MI 48109 **[251]**

Douglas M. Bowden, Regional Primate Research Center and Department of Psychiatry and Behavioral Sciences, University of Washington, Seattle, WA 98195 **[207]**

Carlo Brugnara, Department of Physiology and Biophysics, Harvard Medical School, Boston, MA 02115 **[235]**

***Mitzy Canessa,** Department of Physiology and Biophysics, Harvard Medical School, Boston, MA 02115 **[235]**

***Charles C. Capen,** Department of Pathobiology, College of Veterinary Medicine, Ohio State University, Columbus, OH 43210

Linda C. Cork, Division of Comparative Medicine and Department of Pathology, Johns Hopkins University School of Medicine, Baltimore, MD 21205 **[385]**

Donald L. Curry, Department of Physiological Sciences, Animal Resource Service, University of California, Davis, CA 95616 **[109]**

Edward R. Dalferes, Jr., Department of Medicine, Louisiana State University Medical Center, New Orleans, LA 70112 **[307]**

*Participants at Symposium on Comparative Pathobiology of Major Age-Related Diseases: Current Status and Research Frontiers.

The number in brackets following each contributor's name indicates the opening page of that author's article.

Mahlon R. DeLong, Departments of Neurology and Neuroscience, Johns Hopkins University School of Medicine, Baltimore City Hospitals, Baltimore, MD 21224 **[385]**

Janet L. Denlinger, Department of Ophthalmology/Research Division, Columbia University, New York, NY 10032 **[129]**

Caleb E. Finch, Department of Biological Sciences, University of Southern California, Los Angeles, CA 90089-0191 **[401]**

***Donald B. Hackel,** Department of Pathology, Duke University Medical Center, Durham, NC 27710

Alex L. Harris, Department of Physiology, University of Michigan Medical School, Ann Arbor, MI 48109 **[251]**

Ronald W. Hart, National Center for Toxicological Research, Jefferson, AR 72079 **[19]**

John C. Hedreen, Neuropathology Laboratory, Department of Pathology, Johns Hopkins University School of Medicine, Baltimore, MD 21205 **[385]**

***Charles F. Howard, Jr.,** Division of Metabolic and Immune Diseases, Oregon Regional Primate Research Center, Beaverton, OR 97006 **[289]**

Yasuo Ihara, Department of Neuropathology, Ralph Lowell Laboratories, McLean Hospital, Harvard Medical School, Belmont, MA 02178 **[373]**

***T.C. Jones,** New England Regional Primate Research Center, Harvard Medical School, Southborough, MA 01772

Arnold J. Kahn, Department of Osteobiology, Washington University School of Dental Medicine, St. Louis, MO 63110 **[189]**

Charles Kilo, Department of Internal Medicine, Washington University School of Medicine, St. Louis, MO 63110 **[269]**

***Donald W. King, Jr.,** Department of Pathology, University of Chicago School of Medicine, Chicago, IL 60637 **[3]**

Cheryl A. Kitt, Neuropathology Laboratory, Department of Pathology, Johns Hopkins University School of Medicine, Baltimore, MD 21205 **[385]**

Alan Kopin, Department of Physiology and Biophysics, Harvard Medical School, Boston, MA 02115 **[235]**

***Kenneth S. Kosik,** Departments of Neurology and Neuropathology, Ralph Lowell Laboratories, McLean Hospital, Harvard Medical School, Belmont, MA 02178 **[373]**

***Philip W. Landfield,** Department of Physiology and Pharmacology, Bowman Gray School of Medicine, Wake Forest University, Winston-Salem, NC 27103 **[333]**

***Barnet M. Levy,** Dental Science Institute, University of Texas Dental Branch, Houston, TX 77225 **[221]**

***Robert M. Lewis,** Department of Pathology, New York State College of Veterinary Medicine, Cornell University, Ithaca, NY 14853

Jan O. Marcusson, Department of Pathology, University of Ůmea School of Medicine, Ůmea, S-90187 Sweden **[401]**

Alan McCluskey, Ralph Lowell Laboratories, McLean Hospital, Harvard Medical School, Belmont, MA 02178 **[373]**

***Joseph Meites,** Department of Physiology, Neuroendocrine Research Laboratory, Michigan State University, East Lansing, MI 48824 **[89]**

*__George Migaki,__ Universities Associated for Research and Education in Pathology, Inc., Armed Forces Institute of Pathology, Washington, DC 20306 **[xi]**

Susan J. Mitchell, Department of Neurology, Johns Hopkins University School of Medicine, Baltimore City Hospitals, Baltimore, MD 21224 **[385]**

*__David G. Morgan,__ Gerontology Research Institute, University of Southern California, Los Angeles, CA 90089-0191 **[401]**

Thomas A. Pitler, Department of Physiology and Pharmacology, Bowman Gray School of Medicine, Wake Forest University, Winston-Salem, NC 27103 **[333]**

*__Lawrence A. Pottenger,__ Department of Surgery, Section of Orthopaedics, University of Chicago, Chicago, IL 60637 **[159]**

*__Donald L. Price,__ Neuropathology Laboratory, Departments of Pathology, Neurology, and Neuroscience, Johns Hopkins University School of Medicine, Baltimore, MD 21205 **[385]**

Donald L. Price, Jr., Neuropathology Laboratory, Departments of Pathology, Neurology, and Neuroscience, Johns Hopkins University School of Medicine, Baltimore, MD 21205 **[385]**

Bhandaru Radhakrishnamurthy, Departments of Medicine and Biochemistry, Louisiana State University Medical Center, New Orleans, LA 70112 **[307]**

Chaudri G. Rasool, Department of Neuropathology, Ralph Lowell Laboratories, McLean Hospital, Harvard Medical School, Belmont, MA 02178 **[373]**

*__Lawrence G. Raisz,__ Division of Endocrinology and Metabolism, Department of Medicine, University of Connecticut Health Center, Farmington, CT 06032 **[145]**

*__Eve P. Reaven,__ Geriatric Research, Education and Clinical Center, Veterans Administration Medical Center, Palo Alto, CA 94304 **[109]**

Gerald M. Reaven, Geriatric Research, Education and Clinical Center, Veterans Administration Medical Center, Palo Alto, CA 94304 **[109]**

*__Arlan Richardson,__ Department of Chemistry, Illinois State University, Normal, IL 61761 **[47]**

Michael S. Roberts, Department of Chemistry, Illinois State University, Normal, IL 61761 **[47]**

*__Dante G. Scarpelli,__ Department of Pathology, Northwestern University Medical School, Chicago, IL 60611 **[xi]**

Dennis J. Selkoe, Departments of Neuropathology and Neurology, Ralph Lowell Laboratories, McLean Hospital, Harvard Medical School, Belmont, MA 02178 **[373]**

James A. Severson, Department of Psychiatry, University of Southern California School of Medicine, Los Angeles, CA 90033 **[401]**

Chakravarthi Sharma, Department of Medicine, Louisiana State University Medical Center, New Orleans, LA 70112 **[307]**

Sathanur R. Srinivasan, Departments of Medicine and Biochemistry, Louisiana State University Medical Center, New Orleans, LA 70112 **[307]**

Robert G. Struble, Neuropathology Laboratory, Department of Pathology, Johns Hopkins University School of Medicine, Baltimore, MD 21205 **[385]**

*Steven L. Teitelbaum, Department of Pathology and Laboratory Medicine, The Jewish Hospital of St. Louis, Washington University School of Medicine, St. Louis, MO 63110 [189]

*Robert D. Terry, Department of Neuropathology, Albert Einstein College of Medicine, Bronx, NY 10461 [357]

*Angelo Turturro, National Center for Toxicological Research, Jefferson, AR 72079 [19]

*David C. Van Sickle, Department of Anatomy, School of Veterinary Medicine, Purdue University, West Lafayette, IN 47907 [175]

Parakat Vijayagopal, Department of Medicine, Louisiana State University Medical Center, New Orleans, LA 70112 [307]

R. Clinton Webb, Department of Physiology, University of Michigan Medical School, Ann Arbor, MI 48109 [251]

Peter J. Whitehouse, Departments of Neurology and Neuroscience, Johns Hopkins University School of Medicine, Baltimore, MD 21205 [385]

*Darrell D. Williams, Regional Primate Research Center, Primate Field Center, University of Washington, Medical Lake, WA 99022 [207]

*Joseph R. Williamson, Department of Pathology, Washington University School of Medicine, St. Louis, MO 63110 [269]

*Robert W. Wissler, Department of Pathology, University of Chicago School of Medicine, Chicago, IL 60637 [xiii]

Preface

Aging and its related diseases are a major problem of our society, and are responsible for a diminished quality of life for those in the autumn years. This symposium includes selected topics on the basic aspects of aging, and major age-related diseases involving the mesenchyme, and the brain. The diseases encompassed in the program are well known to all of us, and about which we know little, such as osteoarthritis, osteoporosis, periodontitis, essential hypertension, diabetes mellitus, atherosclerosis, and Alzheimer's and Parkinson's diseases. The focuses are at the level of cellular biology and biochemistry, and whenever possible, mechanism. Some of the contributions are thought-provoking theoretical considerations, others are solid documentations of basic functional defects that underlie diseases related to aging; all serve to add to our understanding.

We are indebted to the various benefactors who gave so generously to ensure the success of this undertaking; these include the Animal Resources Branch of the Division of Research Resources, the National Institutes of Health (Public Health Service Grant No. RR00301), Universities Associated for Research and Education in Pathology, Inc., the Armed Forces Institute of Pathology, and the following industrial organizations: Bristol-Myers Company, Burroughs Wellcome Company, Eli Lilly and Company, Merrell Dow Pharmaceuticals Inc., Sandoz, Inc., Schering Corporation, Smith Kline and French Laboratories, and The Upjohn Company. Appreciation is also due to Charmaine Goetz for careful retyping of the manuscripts, and to Susan Allen and Merryanna Swartz for proofreading.

D.G. Scarpelli, MD, PhD
G. Migaki, DVM

INTRODUCTION

Robert W. Wissler, Ph.D., M.D.

Department of Pathology, The University of Chicago, Chicago, IL 60637

It is my privilege and pleasure to open this special symposium on the Comparative Pathobiology of Major Age-Related Diseases: Current Status and Research Frontiers. This meeting had its inception a little over five years ago, when the scientific advisory committee of the Registry of Comparative Pathology was having one of its frequent brainstorming sessions. It was the consensus of that meeting that the time was approaching when a conference on some of the comparative pathobiologic aspects of aging should be convened. It was agreed that there was a developing need, _not only_ to survey the current state of knowledge regarding the aging process but also to assess the needs of the future, emphasizing the problems, challenges and opportunities for longevity studies in experimental animals.

It was evident then and it is even more clear at present that research on aging must become much more extensive if we as a society are going to make life worthwhile for the constantly increasing proportion of our population which is going to survive into their 70's, 80's, and 90's. It was also evident then and is even more clear now that research on those disease processes associated with aging in our population is benefitting immensely from vast improvement in laboratory animal care and from the modern revolution in pathobiology and molecular biology. Furthermore, it is clear that the major chronic age-related disease processes in which substantial progress is being made are those in which excellent animal models, some spontaneous and some induced, make it possible to perform controlled studies which allow one to work out and establish major aspects of pathogenesis and develop effective methods of intervention. Conversely, I think that those age-related chronic disease processes which do not as yet have adequate animal models, in general exhibit slower progress toward establishing satisfactory ways to prevent, retard or reverse the effects of the disease.

Excellent examples of diseases with outstanding experimental and comparative pathology models are hypertension, atherosclerosis, diabetes and cancer, and progress has been amazingly swift in these areas. Disease processes for which we are still searching for adequate animal models such as the relatively newly recognized and not well understood Alzheimer's disease as well as several other important diseases, many with a virus trigger and an autoimmune or immune-complex pathogenesis and which take their toll, and take the fun out of the "golden years" for many individuals, still pose immense challenges and offer great opportunities for enlightened research.

That indeed is one of the major reasons for the Registry of Comparative Pathology. This registry has made it one of its main purposes to bring together in a meaningful way the best science from veterinary medicine and from other basic pathobiological research efforts to join with the best elements of creative scholarship in human pathology, so that new interactions of these areas will produce combined research in a way that will increase our knowledge of human disease.

This is the 7th state-of-the-art conference which the Registry of Comparative Pathology has held, all of which emphasized projection of knowledge in new directions (Lingeman, Garner 1969; Ribelin, Migaki 1975; Nielsen et al 1979; Montali, Migaki 1980; Hackel 1980; Desnick et al 1982). All have been successful in calling attention to areas which the prepared mind could use to make new progress in the conquest of disease, using comparative pathology approaches.

Special mention must be made of the help provided by Dr. John E. Holman of the Animal Resources Branch in developing the arrangements for this meeting in Building 31 at the National Institutes of Health. We also acknowledge the highly competent work of John Bowers and his co-workers who have done such a masterful job in recording and transcribing the discussion so that it can be edited for publication while the participants are still here.

The major part of the planning of this conference was done by the Advisory Committee of the Registry of Comparative Pathology in several long meetings with lots of homework in between. This committee included Dr. Charles C. Capen, Dr. Donald B. Hackel, Dr. T. C. Jones, Dr. Robert M. Lewis and myself. But the leadership has come largely from two persons, from Dr. Dante G. Scarpelli, the current chairman of the Registry's Advisory Committee who, during much of the planning period, also served as president of the Board of Directors of Universities Associated for Research and Education in Pathology, Inc. and from Dr. Donald W. King, whom the committee chose as its special advisor, contributor and leader, because of his demonstrated interest and innovative activity in the field of research on aging. The committee also acknowledges the helpful advice it has had from Drs. Don C. Gibson, Richard L. Sprott and Edward L. Schneider of the National Institute on Aging, who have shown a deep interest in this meeting and the general area which it covers.

Fortunately, as you who have attended have seen and heard and now can read, the committee has chosen well, and obtained virtually all of its first choices for speakers. We are proud of the results of our labor. But the quality of the program depends largely on the experience, understanding and leadership of Dr. Scarpelli and Dr. King, and the advice and help of the Registry's Advisory Committee and the National Institute on Aging.

As many of you know, the major reason for the success of the many projects the Registry undertakes is its hard working and completely capable Chief Pathologist, Dr. George Migaki. He and his very helpful staff have had the major part in organizing and developing the detailed arrangements for this meeting and its several functions.

I trust that you will find this monograph both stimulating and informative as you read this account of the Comparative Pathobiology of Major Age-Related Diseases: Current Status and Research Frontiers.

REFERENCES

Desnick RJ, Patterson DF, Scarpelli DG (eds) (1982). "Animal Models of Inherited Metabolic Diseases." New York: A. R. Liss.

Hackel DB, (ed) (1980). "Needs for New Animal Models of Human Disease." Am J Pathol 101 (Suppl).

Lingeman CH, Garner FM (eds) (1969). "Comparative Morphology of Hematopoietic Neoplasms," (NCI Monograph 32), Bethesda, Maryland: National Cancer Institute.

Montali RJ, Migaki G (eds) (1980). "The Comparative Pathology of Zoo Animals." Washington, D.C.: Smithsonian Institution Press.

Nielsen SW, Migaki G, Scarpelli DG (eds) (1979). "Animals as Monitors of Environmental Pollutants." Washington, D.C.: National Academy of Sciences.

Ribelin WE, Migaki G (eds) (1975). "The Pathology of Fishes." Madison, Wisconsin: The University of Wisconsin Press.

I. BASIC ASPECTS OF AGING

Comparative Pathobiology of Major Age-Related Diseases: Current Status and Research Frontiers, pages 3–17

BIOLOGY OF AGING

Donald W. King, M.D.

The Richard T. Crane Professor of Pathology,
The University of Chicago, Chicago, IL 60637

The aging process is a physiological phenomenon which affects all individuals of all species. The process is accentuated and accelerated by injurious agents and finally terminated due to the increased susceptibility and decreased resistance associated with the aging processes. A definitive statement as to when aging starts is in dispute. Some suggest conception or at birth; others propose puberty (age 14) or cessation of growth (age 18). Studies show marked decline in several physiological functions at approximately age 40.

DISEASES AND LESIONS

All species have a fairly definite range of life spans (Table 1) (Sachar 1980). For man it is between 90 and 100 years. Although acute or chronic disease processes may cause an earlier death, protective immune, endocrine and genetic factors may result in individuals living to longer ages. One must be careful to distinguish between aging diseases, those which occur in 90 to 100% of the population, (osteoporosis and osteoarthritis), those which occur in a large percentage of the population (hypertensive heart disease) and those which occur with lesser frequency, (maturity-onset diabetes). Atherosclerosis has been noted to be both a lesion of little consequence (lipid infiltration in aorta at infancy) and a definitive disease at other ages (atherosclerotic heart disease). Vascular amyloid deposits are lesions associated with the general aging process yet may be classified as a separate disease entity (senile cardiomyopathy) (Table 2).

Table 1
Estimation of Life Span

Common Name	Recorded Maximum Life Span yr
Southern wallaroo	24.5
Little brown bat	24
White-handed gibbon	31.5
Sumatran orangutan	>50
Chimpanzee	>44.5
Lowland gorilla	>39.33
Hairy armadillo	18.83
American beaver	>20
House mouse	3.5
Pack rat	7
Black rat	4.67
Guinea pig	7.5
Finback whale	>80
Sperm whale	>65
Coyote	21.83
Polar bear	34.67
Jaguar	23
Bengal tiger	26.25
Gray seal	41
Asiatic elephant	70
Mongolian wild horse	34
European wild boar	19.5
Red deer	26.5
Giraffe	36.58

(Modified from Sachar, G.A.: Mammalian life histories: their evolution and molecular-genetic mechanisms. Adv. Pathobiol., *7*:21, 1980.)

Table 2
Diseases and Lesions Associated With Aging

Diseases of Aging	Diseases Associated with Aging	Lesions Associated with Aging
Osteoporosis	*Without specific pathogenesis*	*Cellular*
	Maturity onset diabetes	Lipofuscin
Osteoarthritis	Alzheimer's disease	Atrophy
	Parkinson's disease	Hyperplasia
	Neoplasia	Hypertrophy
	Emphysema	
	Hypertension	
	With known pathogenesis	*Extracellular*
	Septicemia	Arteriosclerosis
	Pneumonia (bacterial, viral)	Amyloid deposits
		Immune deposits
	Cirrhosis (hepatitis)	Fractures
	Nephritis	Intervertebral disc disease
	Myocardial or pulmonary infarct	Cataracts, presbyopia
		Increased cross-linkage of collagen
		Disorganized extracellular matrices
		Pulmonary thrombosis or embolism

Modified from King DW, Fenoglio CM, Lefkowitch JH (1983). "General Pathology: Principles and Dynamics." Philadelphia: Lea & Febiger.

ORGAN CHANGES DURING AGING

Aging lesions appear in the reproductive organs in the 40s, represented by decreased ova (from several hundred thousand to ten or fifteen thousand) and decreased spermatogenesis associated with atrophy of the testes (Adler et al 1978). The thymus steadily decreases in weight following puberty and prominent atrophy is noted in both epithelial and lymphoid elements with replacement by fat and concomitant loss of thymic hormones (Boyd 1932). The adrenal hormone, dehydroepiandrosterone, reaches its lowest level in the early 30's although the significance of this is unknown (Schwartz et al 1981). Many vessels in the body show significant changes including thickening of the basement membrane of the capillaries, intimal atherosclerotic lesions of the arteries and valvular defects of the veins. An accentuation of the pathological aging phenomena is seen in the 60 to 80 age group, particularly involving the vessels of the heart, central nervous system, kidney, and brain.

In addition to lesions associated with general aging phenomena, the appearance of tertiary end stage lesions resulting from definitive disease processes occurs in various organs. These include cirrhotic lesions of the liver (following viral, toxic or alcoholic insult), compensatory hypertrophy and failure of the heart (following hypertension, coronary sclerosis or viral infectious processes) and nephrosis (following infection, immune and vascular injury or exposure to environmental agents over a period of many years).

In the 40-60 age group three neoplasias predominate: carcinoma of the lung occurring in individuals with a heavy smoking history, carcinoma of the breast associated with hormonal imbalance of several years duration accentuated by the menopause, and carcinoma of the colon perhaps associated with chemical carcinogenetic agents over a long period of time (King et al 1982a). In the 80 to 100 age group there appears to be a plateau in the incidence of new neoplastic lesions with two exceptions (Brody 1978). The first is carcinoma of the prostate which often is occult in the 60's, is slow growing for many years and metastasizes late. The second tumor of the elderly is hyperplasia of the stem cells of the bone marrow, particularly of the lymphoid cell series, with the appearance of monoclonal gammopathies or actual neoplasm (chronic lymphocytic leukemia). These are comparatively benign longstanding diseases, and the individual often dies of other causes long before succumbing to leukemia or prostatic cancer. Table 3 shows examples of the spectrum of disease throughout life (King et al 1982b).

Table 3
Spectrum of Disease

Age	*Cause*
0–5	Allergy Infection Neoplasia (leukemia, Wilms', medulloblastoma, retinoblastoma)
5–15	Allergy Diabetes (juvenile) Infection Accidents
15–30	Allergy (asthma) Accidents (suicide) Venereal disease Endocrine (women) Acne
30–40	Complications of pregnancy Ulcer Hypertension Suicide Homicide
40–60	Heart disease (infarct, hypertension, rheumatic fever) Liver disease (cirrhosis) Kidney disease (glomerular nephritis) Neoplasia (lung, colon, breast, ovary)
60–80	Neoplasia (lung, colon, prostate) Cardiovascular disease
80–100	Neoplasia (leukemia, lymphoma, prostate) Dementia (Alzheimer's, Parkinson's) Osteoporosis, osteoarthritis Accidents (fractures) Infection Cardiovascular disease

(Modified from King, D.W.: Health problems. *In* Young Adulthood. Edited by J. Scanlon. New York, Academy for Educational Development, 1979.)

CELLULAR AND EXTRACELLULAR CHANGES

Lesions of aging are associated with all organ systems. Every organ shows some evidence of injury with replacement of tissue by collagen, fibroblasts or lipid cells, and often infiltration by chronic inflammatory cells. The major cellular lesions are atrophy, either absolute loss or decrease in size, with compensatory hyperplasia or hypertrophy. Atrophy is greatest in the brain and the heart, in which no division and replacement is possible. Some postmitotic cells (myocardial cells) undergo hypertrophy. Intermitotic cells including cells of the gastrointestinal tract, genitourinary tract, and skin undergo hyperplasia. Endocrine, liver and kidney tubule cells, representatives of reverting postmitotic cells, undergo both hyperplasia and hypertrophy. Hyperplasia, metaplasia or neoplasia, including adenomas, papillomas, polyps and cancer of the bronchi, bladder, colon, prostate, breast, thyroid, parathyroid, pituitary, and adrenal occur with increasing frequency in the aging population.

In the extracellular tissue we find disturbances of the extracellular matrix associated with structural changes in collagen, elastin, hyaluronic acid, proteoglycans, and glycoproteins (Balazs 1977). This results in increased numbers of hernias, diverticula, bursae, prolapses, and general deterioration of tendons, ligaments, and mesenchymal tissues. We have shown an increase in thickness of basement membranes in capillaries of the psoas muscle in both males and females with age unrelated to any disease process (Xi et al 1982) (Figure 1).

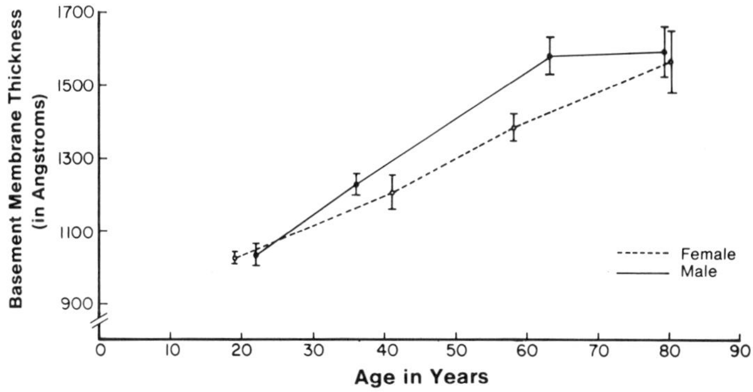

Fig. 1. Basement membrane thickness. Reproduced with permission from Xi YP et al (1982). Mech Ageing Dev 19:4, 1982.

The lesions of aging are atrophy, hyperplasia and hypertrophy of the cellular components, and structural disorganization of the extracellular components. Together they produce a variety of lesions (Figure 2). One of the most interesting lesions is amyloid. Glenner (1980) has classified amyloid into four principal types. Amyloid produced by plasma cells in multiple myeloma consists of light immunoglobulin chains. Amyloid deposited as a crystalloid protein in diabetes is proinsulin and in medullary carcinoma is calcitonin. Amyloid in senile cardiomyopathy has been suggested to be proalbumin. Amyloid secondary to chronic disease is a protein circulating in the serum (SA) and deposited in tissues as AA protein. This suggests that any crystalloid denatured protein may, under appropriate circumstances, form a B pleated sheet with staining characteristics of amyloid.

ETIOLOGY

Finally we come to a discussion of the cause or causes of aging and the factors which constitute the aging process. There is no single etiology, and the cause of death in many cases is unknown. Common demonstrable causes of death in

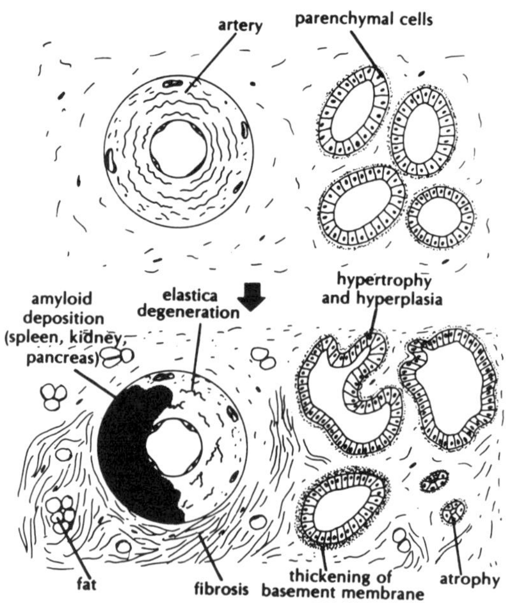

Fig. 2. Tissue changes in aging. Reproduced with permission from King DW, Fenoglio CM, Lefkowitch JH (1983). "General Pathology: Principles and Dynamics." Philadelphia: Lea & Febiger.

the aged are heart failure, stroke, neoplasia and infections. After the age of 80 even a small insult may cause death due to a lack of resistance while at age 20 a similar insult may be of little consequence (Table 4).

Table 4
Leading Causes of Death in the United States, 1976 and 1979

Rank	Cause of Death	Number of Deaths	Death Rate per 100,000 Population	% 1976 Total Deaths	% 1979 Total Deaths
	All causes	1,910,440	890.2	100.0	100.0
1	Diseases of heart	723,729	337.1	37.9	37.8
2	Cancer	377,312	175.8	19.9	20.6
3	Stroke	188,623	87.9	9.9	9.1
4	Accidents	100,761	46.9	5.3	5.5
5	Influenza and pneumonia	61,666	28.7	3.2	3.0
6	Diabetes mellitus	34,508	16.1	1.8	1.8
7	Cirrhosis of liver	31,453	14.7	1.6	1.6
8	Arteriosclerosis	29,366	13.7	1.5	1.5
9	Suicide	26,832	12.5	1.4	1.4
10	Diseases of infancy	24,809	11.6	1.3	1.1
11	Homicide	19,554	9.1	1.0	1.1
12	Emphysema	17,796	8.3	0.9	1.1
13	Congenital anomalies	13,002	6.1	0.7	0.7
14	Nephritis and nephrosis	8,541	4.0	0.4	0.5
15	Septicemia and pyemia	6,401	3.0	0.3	0.4
16	Other and ill-defined	246,087	114.7	12.9	12.8

US Census Figures

CONTROL SYSTEMS

Homeostatic control systems which appear to undergo marked physiological aging changes include the CNS, endocrine, neuroendocrine, and the immune systems. All are dependent on the basic genetic background of the individual. In addition, nutrition, geography, climate, and host environmental factors may accentuate, aggravate or markedly influence the homeostatic mechanism.

GENETIC

The genetic basis to aging is documented by wide ranging definitive life spans of various species (Sachar 1980) despite similar environments. A genetic relationship between cell doubling and maximum life span has been demonstrated by *in vitro* tissue culture systems (Table 5).

Table 5
Embryonic Fibroblasts

Species	*Range of Population Doublings for Cultured Normal Embryo Fibroblasts*	*Mean Maximum Life Span yr*
Galapagos tortoise	90–125	175 (?)
Man	40–60	110
Mink	30–35	10
Chicken	15–35	30 (?)
Mouse	14–28	3.5

(Adapted from Hayflick, L.: The cell biology of human aging. N. Engl. J. Med., *295*:1305, 1976.)

Programmed genetic aging is further exemplified experimentally by demonstration of less effective DNA repair in short lived species. Defective DNA repair is probably not linearly correlated with the life span (Hart, Setlow 1974) but there is a general correlative relationship between efficient DNA repair and the maximum life span. Our laboratory has shown that the same percentage of epithelial cells (approximately 60 to 80%) undergo DNA repair process in both young and old. However, the amount of tritiated thymidine isotope incorporated into DNA following injury, known as unscheduled DNA synthesis (UDS) and taken as representative of the extent of DNA repair is markedly diminished with increasing age (Nette et al 1983). This may be due to a variety of factors: basic genetic programming, lack of synthesis or increased destruction of repair enzymes, lack of substrates, transport problems or a marked increase in susceptibility and exposure to various environmental agents of disease over a long period of time.

CENTRAL NERVOUS SYSTEM

A second system markedly impaired with the aging process is the CNS. Areas of atrophy in the brain result in some 5-20% loss of weight but this loss is not uniform in all sections of the brain. Aging changes are partially based on changes in the blood vessels, including intimal atheroscleroses, medial amyloid deposits and an unknown degree of vessel damage associated with disturbances of transport in the blood brain barrier. There is also an intrinsic aging phenomenon of cellular degeneration with dropping out of cells, changes in Nissl substance, and the appearance of neurofibrillary tangles with amyloid deposits (Terry 1978). These changes characteristic of Alzheimer's disease are associated with decrease in choline acetyltransferase, an enzyme necessary for the conversion of choline to acetylcholine (Coyle et al 1981). In addition, there appears to be a decrease in the neurotransmitter dopamine. Changes associated with Alzheimer's disease are present to a variable degree in all individuals. Lesions associated with Alzheimer's, Parkinson's, or Pick's disease, diabetes, vascular disease, (aneurysm and shunts), and previous viral infection with consequent autoimmune phenomena all contribute to aging in the CNS.

ENDOCRINE

The endocrine system is similarly disturbed with the aging process. There are noted increasing relationships between the neuro and the endocrine system, well exemplified by somatostatin. This control hormone of the delta cells of the pancreas along with the insulin secreting beta cells and glucagon secreting alpha cells probably act synergistically to regulate blood and tissue glucose levels. Somatostatin also appears in peripheral nerve endings and in a wide variety of cells throughout the GI tract, lung and other organ systems. It is an example of a control hormone which is highly significant in the aging process (Fenoglio, King 1983) (Figure 3).

The blood levels of several hormones appear to be nearly normal in aged individuals. Adenomas, hyperplasias and atrophy in the thyroid, parathyroid, pituitary, adrenal, and pancreas, in addition to marked atrophy of the testes and ovary are structural counterparts of abnormal function. Synthesis, assembly and transport of hormones out of the cell and into the serum has not been well studied in the human. One phenomenon which has been studied is the number and distribution of target cell receptors. In maturity-onset diabetes, they appear to be decreased (Roth 1980).

We have performed morphometric studies of the cells producing GSH and prolactin in the pituitary, and found that there is a decrease in the number of total pituitary cells,

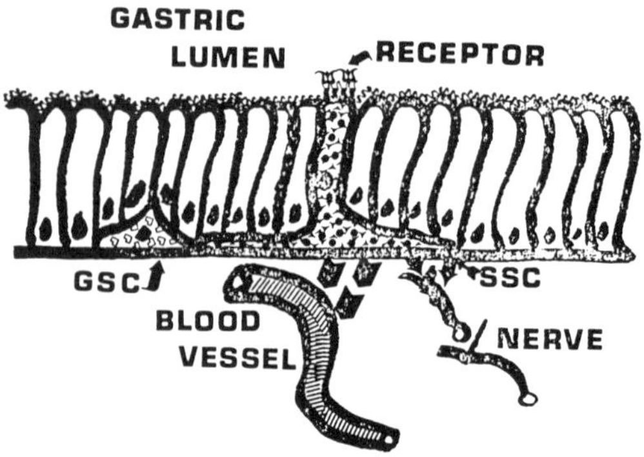

Fig. 3. Somatostatin. Reproduced with permission from Fenoglio C (1983). Hum Pathol 14:475.

as well as a decrease in the number of GSH and prolactin producing cells (Table 6) (Sun et al 1983). This decrease in the number of cells was not associated with a marked decrease in weight as the atrophied cells were replaced by fibrous stroma. Our studies on endocrine glands as well as our studies on DNA repair (Nette et al 1983) and thickened vascular basement membranes (Xi et al 1982) show that the most marked changes occur in the middle-aged group (40 - 60 years). This correlates well with previous physiological studies which showed a marked decline in these age groups (Shock 1977).

Table 6
Comparison of the Number of GH and PL Immunoreactive Cells

RELATIONSHIP TO AGE

Group	Number of of Cases	GH Immunostained Sections		PL Immunostained Sections	
		Number of GH Cells/mm^2	Number of Parenchymal Cells/mm^2	Number of PL Cells/mm^2	Number of Parenchymal Cells/mm^2
Young	13	30.88 ± 10.24	66.23 ± 9.34	5.74 ± 3.34	66.07 ± 7.23
Middle	6	21.09 ± 5.32	58.61 ± 7.57	4.52 ± 1.80	58.53 ± 10.12
Old	9	20.90 ± 8.90	57.01 ± 10.79	3.33 ± 2.78	56.67 ± 10.31

Reproduced with permission from Sun YK et al (1983). Hum Pathol (in press).

IMMUNE

Finally, we have studied the immune system and found, along with others, a decrease in helper T cells and an increase in suppressor T cells, serum immunoglobulin levels, immune complexes, and idiotypic autoantibodies associated with autoimmune disease (Suciu-Foca et al 1983). We have studied morphologically the decrease in follicles and germinal centers of several lymphoid organs and noted the involution of the thymus. We found focal hyper- and hypoplasia in the bone marrow. The lack of primary antibody response to new antigens contrasts with the increase in secondary antibody response (Table 7).

Table 7
Changes in the Immune System With Aging

Lymphocytes	No change in total number Decrease in B-cell maturation Increase in suppressor (T) cells Decrease in helper (T) cells
Complement	Deficient complement levels associated with age, neoplasia, and infection
Antibody	Lack of thymic-dependent antibody response Decrease in primary response to new antigens Increase in globulins associated with secondary response and autoimmunity (benign monoclonal gammopathies) Increase in idiotypic antibodies to receptors
Immune Complexes (Ag, Ab, C)	Presence in all obsolescent glomeruli Presence in many vessel injuries Presence in many tissues previously injured Presence as amyloid either as light chains or in complexes with other protein and carbohydrates
Tolerance	Decrease in natural and acquired tolerance
Lymphoid tissue	Involution of thymus Loss of thymic hormones Atrophy, hypertrophy of some lymph nodes Hyperplasia of selected lymphoid elements particularly in bone marrow Infiltration of lymphoid tissue in various organs (e.g., thyroid)

Reproduced with permission from King DW, Fenoglio CM, Lefkowitch JH (1983). "General Pathology: Principles and Dynamics." Philadelphia: Lea & Febiger.

There is increasing evidence of close interrelationships between the immune, endocrine and neural control systems. T cells are differentiated by thymic hormones secreted by epithelial cells of the thymus. Lymphocyte maturation is extremely sensitive to hormones such as the adrenal corticotrophins. Acetylcholine may increase lymphocyte toxicity and lymphokine secretion. In the local environment of most tissue all these factors must interact collectively.

SUMMARY

Genetic programming of cells along with endocrine, immune and neural control of cellular mechanisms interact to produce a systemic and local controlled environmental homeostasis. Once these control mechanisms are disturbed with age, the cells, tissues, organs and finally the organism become most vulnerable to injury and insult from a variety of environmental (physical, chemical, and infectious) agents. All individuals vary significantly in their structural characteristics and metabolic functional parameters but this variability markedly increases with age. Resistance to injury is decreased by a lifestyle of excess (involving alcohol, food, smoking), a lack of sleep and exercise, as well as over-exposure to a variety of occupational and psychological traumas. The maximum life span will probably continue to be in the present range. The extent of disease can be limited and the quality of life can be markedly improved during this period.

REFERENCES

Adler WH, Jones KH, Brock MA (1978). Aging and immune function. In Behnke JA, Finch CA, Moment GB (eds): "The Biology of Aging," New York: Plenum Press, p 221.

Balazs EA (1977). Intercellular matrix of connective tissue. In Finch CE, Hayflick L (eds): "Handbook of the Biology of Aging," New York: Van Nostrand Reinhold, p 222.

Boyd E (1932). The weight of the thymus gland in health and in disease. Am J Dis Child 43:1162.

Brody H (1978). Cell counts in cerebral cortex and brainstem. In Katzman R, Terry RD, Bick K (eds): "Alzheimer's Disease: Senile Dementia and Related Disorders," [Aging, Vol 7], New York: Raven, p 345.

Coyle JT, Whitehouse PJ, Price DL, Clark AW, DeLong MR (1981). Alzheimer's disease: Evidence for selective loss of cholinergic neurons in the nucleus basalis. Ann Neurol 3(2):122.

Fenoglio CM, King DW (1983). Somatostatin: An update. Hum Pathol 14:475.

Glenner GG (1980). Amyloid deposits and amyloidosis. The B-fibrilloses. N Engl J Med 302:1283.

Hart RW, Setlow RB (1974). Correlation between deoxyribonucleic acid excision repair and life span in a number of mammalian species. Proc Natl Acad Sci USA 71:2169.

Hayflick L (1976). The cell biology of human aging. N Engl J Med 295:1302.

King DW, Pushparaj N, O'Toole K (1982a). Morbidity and mortality in the aged. Hosp Pract 17:2.

King DW, Pushparaj N, O'Toole K, Gross EM (1982b). The value of human tissue in studies of aging. J Am Geriatr Soc 30:8.

Nette EG, Xi YP, Sun YK, Andrews AD and King DW (1983). A correlation between aging and DNA repair in human epidermal cells. Mech Ageing Dev (in press).

Roth GS (1980). Receptor changes and the control of hormone action during aging. Adv Pathobiol 7:228.

Sachar GA (1980). Mammalian life histories: Their evolution and molecular magnetic mechanisms. Adv Pathobiol 7:21.

Schwartz AG, Hard GC, Pashko LL, Abou-Gharbia M, Swern D (1981). Dehydroepiandrosterone: An anti-obesity and anti-carcinogenic agent. Nutr Cancer 3:46.

Shock NW (1977). System integration. In Finch CE, Hayflick L (eds): "Handbook of the Biology of Aging," New York: Van Nostrand Reinhold, p 639.

Suciu-Foca N, Reed E, Rohowsky C, Kung P, King DW (1983). Anti-idiotypic antibodies to anti-HLA receptors induced by pregnancy. Proc Natl Acad Sci USA 80:830.

Sun YK, Xi XP, Fenoglio CM, Pushparaj N, O'Toole KM, Kledzik GS, Nette GE, King DW (1983). The effect of age on the number of growth hormone immunoreactive and prolacting immunoreactive cells in the human pituitary. Hum Pathol (in press).

Terry RD (1978). Ultrastructural alterations in senile dementia. In Katzman R, Terry RD, Bick K (eds): Alzheimer's disease: Senile Dementia and Related Disorders," [Aging, Vol 7], New York: Raven, p 375.

Xi YP, Nette EG, King DW, Rosen M (1982). Age related changes in normal human basement membrane. Mech Ageing Dev 19:4.

DISCUSSION

DR. TURTURRO: You said that the subpopulations of the T cells are decreased. You named a variety of subpopulations but the total number stayed about the same. My question is, what cell subpopulations increase?

DR. KING: OKT3 and OKT11 subpopulations stay about the same. The subpopulations which change are 4 and 8, the inducer/helper and the suppressor/killer populations.

DR. TURTURRO: Do you think that those that increase have any sort of function?

DR. KING: I don't know.

DR. WISSLER: Well, this really has been an elegant presentation and I want to ask one question which I think is important when one is looking at autopsy findings in older individuals. How much of the observed effect in older people, particularly in the endocrine and lymphopoietic systems, is primary? How much would happen no matter what the nutrition of the aging person was? I ask this because in a very recent and elegant Lydia J. Roberts Memorial lecture by Hamish Munro sponsored by the University of Chicago Graduate Committee in Nutrition, Professor Munro indicated that many of the big questions about optimal nutrition for the aging person, especially protein nutrition, may hold the key to much of the aging phenomenon.

DR. KING: In the autopsy studies, we usually need four or five hours postmortem (we aren't lucky like Ben Trump who performs autopsies within ten minutes or so). We only evaluate substances which don't change drastically, e.g., collagen, and the morphology of structures which appear stable (e.g., lymph node follicles and germinal centers). All of our enzyme and DNA repair studies are done either on fresh surgical material or blood samples which we get within a few minutes. We found that synthesis, secretion, and other physiological and biochemical *in vitro* studies on autopsy tissue are not reliable but are easily done on blood and surgical pathologic specimens.

As far as the nutritional aspects are concerned, there is absolutely no question that one sees atrophy of the intestinal epithelium, a decrease in somatostatin cells and a decrease in follicles of the Peyer's patches with aging. How much is a result of the intrinsic aging phenomena and how much is brought on by nutritional imbalances or insults that have been carried on in the gastrointestinal tract over a period of 60 to 70 years is unknown. Questions remain on how one may stop or reverse the atrophy, or alter the hyperplasia and hypertrophy which appear as compensatory responses to the atrophy. How much is programmed intrinsically by the cell and how much is brought on by the environment? Every physiological aging phenomenon programmed into the cell is accentuated and accelerated by environmental insult; in that sense nutrition has a tremendous role to play.

DR. MAURER: The question I have concerns the use of the word "idiotype" in the T-cell system, i.e. antibodies against some antigen specific T-cell receptor determinant. We still do not know whether the T-cell receptor is an immunoglobulin. Until then, the problem of using idiotype in the T-cell anti-T-cell systems may be "pathological".

DR. KING: That is a nice term, "pathological". Idiotypes, in reference to T cells, have been accepted by referees in the journals of reputation despite the now convincing evidence that the T-cell receptor does not contain an immunoglobulin chain.

Comparative Pathobiology of Major Age-Related Diseases: Current Status and Research Frontiers, pages 19–45
Published 1984 Alan R. Liss, Inc., 150 Fifth Avenue, New York, NY 10011

DNA REPAIR MECHANISMS IN AGING

Angelo Turturro, Ph.D. and Ronald W. Hart, Ph.D.

Office of the Director and Director, National Center for Toxicological Research, Jefferson, AR 72079

The inheritance of a definite maximum achievable life span (MAL) by almost all metazoans (Comfort 1979), the central role of DNA in cellular development and the symptoms of "accelerated aging" seen in human diseases in which there is a known deficiency in the capacity to repair damage to the DNA (Williams, Dearfield 1981) are a few of the indicators of the importance of the genome in aging. The complex organization of cells into tissues and the interactions of these tissues in an organism are almost certainly important to understanding how specific pathologies associated with aging in a particular species arise. However, the inexorable loss of fixed postmitotic cells in many important cellular populations with time (see Table 1 for examples) and the gradual decline of functions associated with both non-replicating and replicating cells, as exemplified in Tables 2 and 3 respectively, suggest that aging derives its motive force from cellular phenomena. These cellular phenomena are probably the constraints within which evolution (Hart, Turturro 1981) and reproductive strategies (Robertson, Wexler 1962) work to determine life span.

Information flow in cells from the DNA is accomplished by a complex series of processes, which are subject to error at any point. Also complex are the mechanisms of replication, in which information must be transferred to a newly emerging cell. Defects in information flow can lead to loss of cellular function and/or death, while disturbances in replication can lead to mutation, cessation of reproduction and/or transformation.

Table 1
Loss of Fixed Postmitotic Cells in Aging

Brain	
Cerebral cortex	Brizzee 1975; Hall et al 1975; Vaughn, Vincent 1979
Visual cortex	Devaney, Johnson 1980
Hippocampus	Ball 1977; Landfield et al 1981
Cerebellum	Glick, Bondareff 1979
Locus ceruleus	Vijayashanker, Brody 1979
Substantia nigra	McGeer et al 1977
Putamen	Bugiani et al 1978
Kidney nephrons	Goldman 1976
Muscle fibers	Gutmann 1976; Hooper 1981

Table 2
Loss of Function in Non-Replicative Cells

Axoplasmic flow	McMartin, O'Connor 1979
Striatal dopamine receptors	Severson, Finch 1980; Marquis et al 1981
Forebrain cholinergic systems	Fibriger 1981
GABA transport	Wheeler 1982
Heart function	Lakatta, Yin 1982
Neuroendocrine function	Meites 1982
Neuromuscular function	Shock, Norris 1970; Hooper 1981
Renal function	Goldman 1976
Sensory-motor function	Krauter et al 1981

Table 3
Loss of Function in Replicative Cells

Aortic smooth muscle cloning efficiencies	Martin et al 1983
Nail and claw growth	Selmanowitz et al 1976
T-cell stimulation	Kay, Makinodan 1981
Antibody stimulation	Kay, Makinodan 1981
Prolonged transit time in crypts of the descending colon	Cameron 1972

Direct damage to the DNA molecule is one of the most important causes of defects in information flow and replication. Damage to the DNA template results from a number of processes (Painter 1982; Singer, Kusmierek 1982) as indicated in Figure 1, with the rate of spontaneous damage being particularly striking. Damage can take many forms and can induce changes at any level of DNA structure (Lipetz et al 1982). Examples of DNA damages include single-strand breaks (SSB), double-strand breaks (DSB), adduct formation, simple alkylation, hydration, cross-links, ring-openings, and intercalations (Schendel 1981; Singer, Kusmierek 1982).

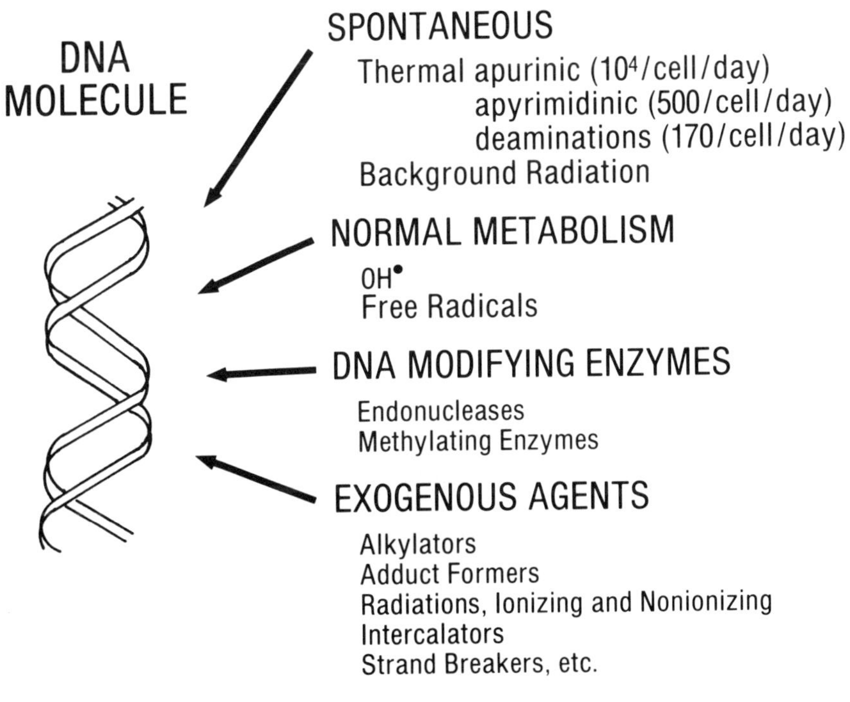

Fig. 1. Some mechanisms resulting in damage to the DNA.

There are a number of modulators of DNA damage. Hart et al (1980) have characterized four general categories, viz. metabolism, scavenging, repair, and expression (Figure 2), each of which can further be divided into subcategories based upon specific functions. Metabolism and scavenging are involved in the rate and amount of damage which attacks the genome. The damage which persists in the genome is determined by spontaneous decomposition, removal of damaged cells, and the activity of the DNA repair processes. The functional expression of DNA damage ranges from rendering the template incapable of being replicated to having no detectable effect. Some damages seem to exert their perturbation only when the DNA interacts with enzymes necessary for a specific activity, such as DNA alterations which cause base transitions during replication (mutation) (Singer, Kusmierek 1982).

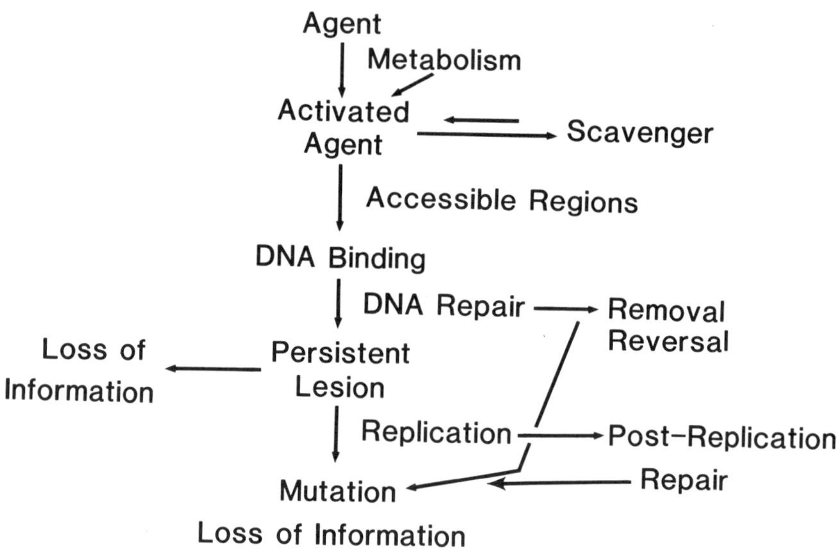

Fig. 2. Modulators of DNA damage.

Factors such as the physiological state of the cell, differentiation stage, etc., alter expression. For example, if a cell is contained in a tissue, and prevented from dividing, a damage which would have led to a base transition will not result in a mutation although it may have other consequences. Also, the longer cells can perform DNA repair prior to DNA replication, the less likely it is that a mutational or tranformational event will occur (Maher, McCormick 1979). A certain amount of damage in a rapidly dividing tissue may, therefore, be lethal, while the same amount in a slowly dividing tissue may have little effect.

DNA REPAIR

The term DNA repair subsumes a number of processes which modulate DNA damage. The special importance of DNA repair is implied by findings that 1) many of the processes of repair in mammalian cells are similar to those described in bacteria and thus assumed to be conserved during the course of evolution; and 2) all species examined thus far possess at least one form of DNA repair (Setlow 1980).

DNA repair can be considered as falling into three classes, reversal, removal and post-replicative "repair" as summarized in Table 4. Reversal includes those processes which act on the damage directly and eliminate any DNA alteration. Examples are: a) dealkylation of guanines alkylated at the O^6-position by a "transalkylase" that may or may not be reactivated. This directly removes an alkyl group introduced by an alkylating agent; b) (possibly) an insertase which places appropriate bases in apurinic/apyrimidinic (AP) sites induced by spontaneous thermal decomposition or as a result of glycosylase activity (see below); c) enzymatic photoreactivation of pyrimidine dimers, which monomerizes dimers.

Removal includes those processes which chop out an altered DNA base, cut the DNA backbone and remove damaged and non-damaged bases and then fill in the gap. Examples are: a) base excision repair, which involves excision of altered bases by a newly discovered class of enzymes, the DNA glycosylases. These enzymes, of which more than a dozen have thus far been discovered, seem to be somewhat damage-site specific in their action. Many of the substrates of these enzymes have been identified as being either the products resulting from UV irradiation of the DNA or of natural processes (e.g., spontaneous deamination) (Lindahl 1982), thereby suggesting that DNA repair processes have evolved to handle naturally occurring damages. Following the action of a DNA glycosylase, or at a spontaneous AP site, AP endonucleases can then excise a number of bases. In mammlian cells, the dominant AP endonuclease found is a class II enzyme (which cleaves DNA at the 5' end of a site)

Table 4
Mammalian DNA Repair Mechanisms

Reversal

1) Dealkylation utilizing a "transalkylase" (Bogden et al 1981).
2) AP site repair (direct repair of a removed base) (Livneh et al 1979), which is controversial for any system.
3) Photoreactivation (a light activated enzymatic mechanism specific for the breakage of the UV-induced covalent bond attaching two pyrimidines in a cyclobutane-type ring) (D'Ambrosio et al 1981), which is controversial for mammalian systems.

Removal

1) Base excision repair (a mechanism which permits the re-insertion of the proper base into the gap left by DNA glycosylases, which excise inappropriate moieties from the DNA as free base avoiding scission of the DNA back-bone [Livneh et al 1979] as well as a system similar to the bacterial one requiring strand scission [Verly, Paquette 1973]).
2) Nucleotide excision repair (a mechanism which removes bulky, noncoding lesions from the DNA in a manner similar to, but not identical with, bacterial nucleotide excision repair [Regan et al 1968]).
3) Strand scission repair (the process by which single and double strand breaks are rejoined with the addition of zero or few additional nucleotides through the action of a sealing enzyme) (Lett et al 1967).

Postreplicative "repair"

1) Replication bypass (the process which may function in mammalian cells as an alternative to recombination repair in which the bulky lesions are bypassed and the gap created filled) (Fujiwara, Tatsumi 1976).

with no associated exonuclease activity (Lindahl 1982). Subsequent polymerase activity by polymerase beta (although a role for polymerase alpha hasn't been totally excluded) (Miller, Chinault 1982) and ligase activity complete the process. The number of bases which are excised can vary, but have usually been considered less than 5 (Painter 1982). However, recent developments have put this assessment into jeopardy (Hanawalt et al 1982) and a controversy on this point now exists; b) nucleotide excision repair, which removes bulky DNA adducts and pyrimidine dimers. The backbone is cut in proximity of the lesion by an endonuclease and a number of bases excised. This process excises a region larger than base excision repair, 30-100 nucleotides, and has been termed "long patch" repair. However, the average patch size is much shorter than the "long patch repair" described in bacteria. And, unlike bacteria, the size heterogeneity is quite limited (Hanawalt et al 1982). The break is then repaired as in base excision repair. In *E. coli*, the system, termed *uvr*, involves the product of a number of genes. The seven complementation groups of XP (xeroderma pigmentosum), a clinical entity characterized by fibroblasts lacking this repair, suggests that the mammalian system is also complex. Interestingly, yeast seems to have the same number of complementation groups as mammalian cells, hinting that eukaryotic systems may have conserved the system; c) strand scission repair. SSB can result either from the above reactions or directly from the action of certain agents such as ionizing radiation. Given the mechanisms of the above excision repairs, repair of SSB may involve some of the same enzymes. DSB, which can result from similar processes that produce SSB (and have been shown to induce chromosome aberrations [Natarajan, Zwanenburg 1982]), are not repaired by any known mechanism, although there are indications that some DSB repair exists (Painter 1982).

Post-replicative "repair" involves replication over a defect in the DNA, permitting DNA replication in spite of damaged template. In this process, the damage is not removed, it is merely tolerated during replication. Other results of the damage may exist, but the damaged cell will soon produce many replicates with no damaged base, but with potentially mutated genomes. Replication bypass repair, in which bulky adducts are ignored in replication and a SSB is filled as noted above, is the system which most investigators think accomplish post-replication "repair" in mammalian cells.

In bacterial systems, DNA-DNA cross-links are removed using recombination repair (Cole et al 1976). Since no such system has been found in mammalian cells, the repair of these lesions is not understood. However, studies using mutant mammalian cells suggest that this repair involves the nucleotide excision repair system (Meyn et al 1982).

The above repair systems are considered constitutive, i.e., they are continually active within a given range, in mammals. However, in analogy with inducible bacterial repair systems, there is some evidence for inducible DNA repair, especially for reversal of O^6-methylguanine, though the existence of such a mechanism is still controversial in mammalian systems (Schendel 1981).

DNA REPAIR AND AGING

There are two major approaches to the study of DNA repair in aging: 1) evaluation of DNA repair during the life span of an organism, an example of the ontogenic approach, and 2) comparison of DNA repair between species with different MAL, which exemplifies the comparative evolutionary approach (Sacher, Hart 1978; Hart, Turturro 1983). In discussing these approaches, however, it should be emphasized that the extent of information available, other than that for UV excision repair and strand break repair, is meager within a species and, other than for UV excision repair, almost nonexistent between species. Also, very few tissues have been examined with comparable techniques. Thus, detailed analysis is very limited.

Evaluation of DNA Repair During the Life Span of an Organism

The effect of aging on DNA repair during the lifetime of an individual seems, at first glance, to be confusing due to conflicting data. *In vitro*, using cells derived from subjects at different ages, human fibroblasts have been shown to suffer no decline with age in the capacity either to perform unscheduled DNA synthesis (UDS) (Goldstein 1971; Hennis et al 1981) or colony formation (Hall et al 1982) after ultraviolet light (UV) induced damage. Indeed, there was even one report, using cells from two donors of different ages, that DNA repair increases with donor age of the fibroblasts (Dell'Orco, Anderson 1981). Since there is a natural range in UV-induced UDS in human fibroblasts from normal individuals taken from even the same age and sex (RW Hart, unpublished observations), too much significance should not be placed on the relative DNA repair in two separate cell lines derived under different conditions, in different laboratories by different methods.

There is also no decline in the ability to reactivate virus damaged by various agents in fibroblasts (Hall et al 1982). However, the statement by the authors that this indicates equal proficiency to perform repair of the damages produced by the various agents must be qualified since the proper comparison, to a repair deficient host, was not done. Virus reactivation, which can be accomplished by recombination in bacteria (Weigle 1953), may result from the same process in mammalian systems (Schendel 1981). Quantitative analysis of any mutagenesis, which is characteristic of Weigle-reactivation in bacteria, in newly formed virus was also not done. Repair in human keratinocytes (Liu et al 1982) was also found not to decline with age. Gensler (1981), using a suspension of lung, liver, or kidney cells saw no change in UV-induced UDS.

However, in human peripheral lymphocytes (Lambert et al 1979; Licastro et al 1982), rodent hepatocytes (A Richardson, personal communication) and rat lens epithelial cells (Treton, Courtois 1981), UV-induced UDS has been shown to decrease with age, although in the last case most of the decrease occurred during development. In lymphocytes (Turner et al 1982), beagle neurons (Wheeler, Lett 1974) or rabbit retina (Lett 1977), strand break repair following X-irradiation has no correlation with age.

The change with age in DNA repair induced by chemical insult also seems complicated. Repair stimulated by 4-nitroquinoline-1-oxide in the rat retinal ganglion is not a function of age (Ishikawa et al 1978), but the repairs induced by alkylation in rat mucosa (Kanagalingam, Balis 1975) or human fibroblasts (Fort, Cerutti 1981) seem to be. Interestingly, sensitivity to the effects of bleomycin, a DNA damaging agent which is thought to produce damages similar to X-irradiation (Painter 1982), is age-related in human lymphocytes (Seshadri et al 1979), suggesting that some part of the complicated process which converts bleomycin into X-ray-like damage is what is effected with age, not the simple repair of breaks.

Despite the seeming chaos, upon detailed analysis a consistent pattern can be seen to emerge. For UV excision repair, and bulky chemical adduct repair, those experiments which looked at cells grown from explants tended to show that DNA repair did not decline with life span of donor, while those experiments which used cells gathered in a fashion to reflect natural distribution, such as lymphocytes, tended to show decline with age. The exceptions to this used either 1) a population of cells that was constantly renewing itself, e.g., the retinal ganglion (also, the rats studied were less than two years old and, therefore, not truly old) (Ishikawa et al 1978); or 2) whole organ suspensions of different cell types which were released from normal organ replication inhibition by maceration (Gensler 1981). Since it was shown by Hart and Setlow (1976) that replication is an important factor in DNA repair (it tends to decrease with the turning off of DNA replication), then results showing no decline with age may be relevant only to the DNA repair capacity of a subpopulation of replicating cells in an aging tissue, i.e., the cells which emerge from the explant or are derived from a stem cell population during the middle of organism development.

Also, unlike the complicated UV or chemical excision repair systems which require a number of enzymes, strand break repair, which only requires a ligase and, perhaps, a polymerase, seems to be preserved in aging. This system is involved in 1) repair of the constant bombardment of spontaneous damage, so the cell would be swamped quickly without that repair; 2) constant functioning of the DNA. Therefore, cells with a substantial decline in strand break repair probably have limited survival, but cells with a decline in UV excision repair (and perhaps excision repair in general) probably have a much greater potential for survival.

Attempts at *in vivo* estimation of these parameters have been stymied by the lack of homologous experimental models for measuring DNA repair. This has led to paradigms with results which are difficult to interpret, such as one involving systemic injection of hydroxyurea (Niedermuller 1982) whose results are complicated by questions of effective local replication block and alterations of normal physiology after drug administration. Unfortunately, because of their great cost, definitive experiments quantitating adduct removal of DNA damaging agents in aging have not been done. Some work has been done (Likhachev et al 1981), but extensive interpretation is needed since the very effective spontaneous repair of N7-ethylguanine complicates understanding the observed change with age in the removal of this damage. However, careful analysis has been lacking (Eichhorn 1983). Quantitation of DNA repair *in vivo* will probably become much more common with the spread of the new techniques for measuring alkali-labile sites (Brash, Hart 1978) and DNA damage using antibodies

(Poirier 1981).

Comparison of DNA Repair Between Species with Different MAL

Information on DNA repair in species with different MAL using UV-stimulated damage is much more definitive. Hart and Setlow (1974) showed a log-linear correlation of UDS after UV in fibroblasts from a number of different species. A relationship was also found in two rodent species of differing MAL chosen for their similarity in most physiological variables (Sacher, Hart 1978). Unstimulated lymphocytes have also been shown to have a log-linear correlation with MAL for primates (KY Hall, personal communication). Francis et al (1981), using different species and a different technique, also reported a correlation, only they stated that a linear fit of total incorporated thymidine analogue with MAL represented the data more accurately. Some problems with this study were 1) the cells used were taken from animals at very different percentages of their MAL, with possible variance in, among other things, their rate of replication (it was not determined); 2) the material included different cell types; 3) inappropriate life spans were used for some species. DNA repair, as is shown above, can vary with age as well as replication potential.

To indicate the significance of these differences, the data of Francis et al (1981) was replotted, as shown in Figure 3. Figure 3A is the original data with the MAL as the ordinate. Figure 3B is the data plotted on a linear scale after removing species where the analysis was done on cells other than normal fibroblasts and correcting the life spans (as detailed in the figure legend). Figure 3C is the same data as in Figure 3B plotted on a log-linear scale. The data can be seen to appear to be linear on the log-linear axes.

While the work of Francis et al (1981) can be modified and replotted to compare to Hart and Setlow (1974), that of Kato et al (1980) cannot be. There are two critical problems with these data: 1) no internal control was used to provide a standard for variation in experimental conditions; and 2) no mechanism was used to arrest cell replication. First, for UDS autoradiography, an internal standard is essential to compare results from experiment to experiment. Grain counts can vary with emulsion preparation, emulsion thickness, breakdown of radioactive thymidine, etc. Variation can be quite large and

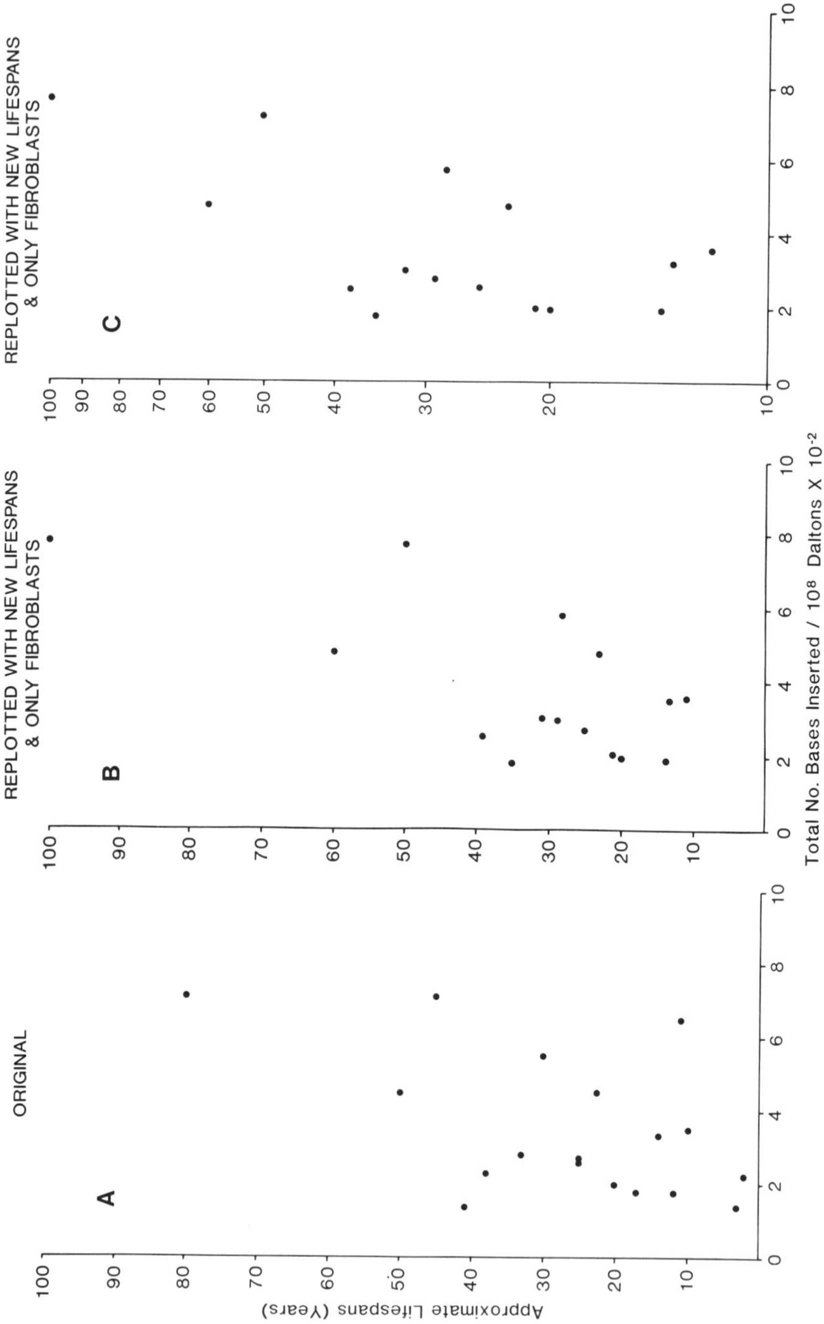

Fig. 3. (legend on page 13)

Fig. 3. (on page 12). Replotting of Francis et al 1981. A) The data as taken directly from that paper and replotted on axes similar to Hart and Setlow (1974). B) Data replotted after data from non-fibroblast cells were removed, and maximum life spans (in years) corrected as noted below, and plotted on linear axes.

Species	Francis	Corrected	Source
Man	80	> 100	Altman, Dittmer 1962
Elephant	50	60	Altman, Dittmer 1972
Gorilla	43	48	Jones 1982
Lion	25	29	Altman, Dittmer 1962
Ocelot	17	20	Jones 1982

C) Same data as in Figure 3B, plotted on log-linear axes. Note the linear appearance of the distribution.

---

is especially a problem in animals with the shorter life span where the total grain count is low. Second, the lack of an agent or process to arrest cell division will result in the counting of cells which are undergoing the initial stages of replication. This number and grain density will vary with the species tested, especially since optimal culture conditions for many species have not been well defined. The authors acknowledge this, and attempt to demonstrate that the presence of an agent which halts replication, hydroxyurea, will not affect the results. However, they vitiate their test by growing cells in media containing hydroxyurea for only one hour before challenging with UV, which is a much shorter time than used in standard UDS procedures (Hart, Setlow 1974). This leaves little time to either establish a block to replication or acclimate the cells to the material.

In addition to these critical defects there were a number of less serious, but troublesome, ones. They include: 1) The life spans used for a number of the animals were not correct--since a number of the species, especially the chiropterans (bats), have no generally accepted life span data, the authors used body size as a measure of life span, citing Sacher (1959) as a justification. The article cited discusses the use of brain weight and body weight as variables in determining life span, distinctly noting that body weight alone is insufficent. This article was later superceded by ones (Sacher 1976) which discuss the use of metabolism as a third variable which must be included, a variable which is a problem in bats and insectivores which go into torpor and hibernate. Thus, the use of the method in this article to estimate the life spans of bats and insectivores was unwarranted. Therefore, a number of species have questionable life spans. Interestingly, these data are the ones most deviating from a log-linear correlation. 2) Only one animal was used for each point--given the variation in UDS in a species, determining correlation from a single representative of a species is questionable and, given the availability of certain of the species, unnecessary. 3) Ignoring factors such as source of tissue, age of donor and passage--different tissues may have different DNA repair, age of donor is discussed above, and DNA repair has been shown to vary as a function of passage, especially in the early passages (Paffenholz 1978).

The critical problems, complicated by the minor ones, make this work, which is the only study which has shown no correlation between MAL and UV-stimulated UDS, too flawed to evaluate and compare to other published reports.

Interestingly, the work on correlation of MAL and repair is supplemented by the results of Paffenholz (1978), who, in a detailed study, showed a correlation between mean life span and UV-induced DNA repair for three inbred mouse strains. The data of Yagi (1982), although interpreted by the author as showing little difference between the three inbred mouse strains, is consistent with the above data since the longer-lived strains studied, C57Bl/10 and BALB/C, generally had a higher UV-stimulated UDS than the shorter lived C3H/He. Walford and Bergman (1979) found similar results in lymphocytes from two unrelated backgrounds of congenic strains of mouse for bleomycin sensitivity. The longest lived strains with similar genetic background had highest UV-stimulated UDS, although one relatively short lived congenic (B10.AKM) had a higher UDS than a strain which outlived it. Collier et al (1982), using the same B10 background found a short-lived congenic (B10.F) with the same amount of DNA repair as longer-lived strains in embryo cell suspension. The use of different cell types, again, complicates comparisons, especially since the data of Peleg et al (1976), suggest that embryonic repair varies with development.

The range of the life spans in an intraspecies comparison is so small, and the possibility that a strain can inherit some genetic defect causing it to be susceptible to some disease not related to DNA repair is so great (indeed, a number of strains were inbred with the express purpose of developing a model susceptible to a particular type of disease) that the use of strains in comparative work is fraught with peril. The strains usually did not go through a natural selection process which selected for fitness in the wild. Instead, they were selected for capacity to survive under captive breeding, which may not be correlated with DNA repair. Thus, although the possibility of a correlation of mean life span with DNA repair is interesting, caution should be used in interpretation.

There is some data that the correlation of MAL to UV excision repair does not hold for a number of cold-blooded vertebrates (Woodhead et al 1980; Regan et al 1982). It should be emphasized that the number of species tested are scanty (one box turtle and four fish) and, as usual, different tissues were used. Also, the data seem to indicate that the animals have little or no UV excision repair, not that there is general lack of correlation with MAL. This may indicate that something, perhaps in the culture conditions, is awry for measuring UV excision repair. Perhaps a study on the embryonic tissue of the different species will help determine the extent of UV excision repair, since this tissue has a high repair rate in mammals measured and this may be true in the lower vertebrates.

Since UV induced repair, although easy to stimulate and quantitate, is not the most appropriate model for most spontaneously induced damage, it is of interest that human liver cells were found to be 10 times as active in removing O^6-methylguanine as rodent liver cells (Pegg et al 1982), consistent with the increased capacity for this removal in human fibroblasts and lymphocytes compared to rodent cells. This suggests that the interactions of chemicals and DNA repair may be of interest to evaluate using the comparative evolutionary approach.

SIGNIFICANCE OF DNA REPAIR DIFFERENCES FOR AGING

The significance of the observed differences in DNA repair for the phenomena of aging is not straightforward. As noted above, measuring the response to UV-induced damage doesn't quantitate repair relevant to most spontaneously occurring DNA damage. The UV frequencies used to demonstrate UV excision repair are screened out by the ozone layer, and the upper levels of human skin are dead anyway. In the context of biological relevance of UV repair, it is interesting to consider the recent information concerning the incidence of various cancers seen in XP individuals, whose fibroblasts do not repair UV-induced damage. Although the relationship between cancer and DNA damage is also not a simple one, unrepaired DNA damage can be correlated to carcinogenesis (Hart et al 1977; Goth, Rajewsky 1974). While Cairns (1981) suggested that XP individuals have increased cancer incidences in only the skin and buccal cavity, i.e. at sites related to actinic exposure, Kraemer et al (1982), utilizing a larger number of individuals, has disagreed, suggesting that the cancer rate for a number of internal cancers is also elevated. These latter data are interesting, especially since XP individuals die at a relatively early age and probably do not have time to express cancers resulting from different times to tumor in different tissues. Therefore, epidemiological data may underestimate the potential incidence of internal cancers. Also XP has a number of characteristics of "accelerated" aging (Williams, Dearfield 1981). An increased incidence of internal tumors would definitely suggest that measuring the response to UV-induced damage, although measuring the effects of different UV frequencies than is present *in vivo*, is evaluating a very important biological process causally related to carcinogenesis and, perhaps, to aging.

One possible mechanism for a causal relationship is the relationship of UV-induced repair to the repair of bulky adduct chemical DNA damage. These damages may be significant to life span, especially since it has been shown by Pashko and Schwartz (1982) that the activity of the metabolic pathway which activates many different classes of chemicals to their DNA-binding form is inversely correlated with species MAL. It has been found that two strains of rat, Sprague-Dawley (S-D) and Long-Evans (L-E), have a 10-fold difference in their capacity for the removal of DMBA adducts (Sheikh et al 1981). This is brought into a proper context by considering that the amount of metabolic activation in the L-E is 10 times that in S-D, resulting in ten times the amount of adduct formation. The end result is that the accumulation of damage as a result of a certain dose of agent is comparable in the two strains. A conceptually consistent result is seen in non-dividing hepatocytes from donors of different ages, in which both the same metabolic activation system and DNA repair stimulated by UV both decline after 12 months of age in rodents (A Richardson, personal communication). It is not clear which part of the bulky adduct repair system is altered with age. However, for S-D and L-E, given the similarity of mean life span in the two strains, the general correlation of strain mean life span and UV-excision repair, and the similarity of the nucleotide excision repairs after the initial step, the probable source of the difference in repair is different capacity for removal by the damage specific enzyme. Thus, enzyme activities may coordinate so that only a certain amount of DNA damage to the genome can be allowed to persist and accumulate.

DNA DAMAGE ACCUMULATION

Evaluating the effect of DNA repair on DNA damage accumulation is difficult. DNA repair is only one of the modulators of DNA damage as noted above. Further, it is affected by physiological factors such as diet and hormonal status (Brash, Hart 1978). Chromatin structure, which is related to gene expression, appears to affect DNA repair (Lipetz et al 1982). Also, DNA repair itself will alter chromatin structure (Zolan et al 1982). Tissue differentiation, a consequence of gene expression, seems to cause significant differences in repair efficiencies (Sheikh et al 1981).

These factors may cause DNA repair not to completely restore the damaged genome, since DNA damage has been found to accumulate with age in all studies but one (Wani 1981). The rate of accumulation of DNA damage can not be quantitatively estimated with the present lack of data. It is of interest in this regard, though, for single-strand breaks, that mouse neurons (Price et al 1971) seem to accumulate the same relative amount of damage as beagle neurons (Wheeler, Lett 1974), only at approximately 6 times the rate. Therefore, the total accumulation is similar when normalized to MAL. Although SSB are repaired by a different pathway than DMBA damages in S-D, this result is consistent with the suggestion above that there seems to be a certain amount of DNA damage which is allowed to persist and accumulate. However, given the paucity of data much more work has to be done to put this conclusion on a sound footing.

Perhaps MAL or general DNA damage is entrained to UV excision repair in the placental mammals by a number of factors such as 1) UV damage is not dependent on metabolism;

2) temperature is fairly constant so the enzymatic systems are kept at approximately the same activity; 3) scavenging may remain fairly constant in various species, as demonstrated for the activity of an important scavenger, superoxide dismutase (Kellogg, Fridovich 1976); and 4) the placental mammal developmental sequence may be similar enough in various species that the fibroblasts and lymphocytes are at approximately the same differentiation stage during adult development.

DNA repair can be considered one of the factors which determines the amount of damage which is allowed to persist in the genome. This damage accumulates with age and seems to collect faster in animals with a shorter life span, perhaps, partially, as a result of a lower DNA repair capacity. DNA damage is associated with a number of pathologies associated with aging, e.g., carcinogenesis in replicating cells, or cytotoxicity in non-replicating ones. Evaluation of the effects of the different DNA damages and the factors which allow expression of that damage to produce biological effects, equivalent to a "promoter" in the multi-stage hypothesis of carcinogenesis, seems to be the pathway to take in elucidating the effects of DNA damage and repair, on aging.

REFERENCES

Altman PL, Dittmer DS (1962). "Growth." Washington, D.C.: Fed Am Soc Exp Biol, p 445.

Altman PL, Dittmer DS (1972). "Biology Data Book." Bethesda, Maryland: Fed Am Soc Exp Biol, p 229.

Ball MJ (1977). Neuronal loss, neuro-fibrillary tangles and granulovacuolar degeneration in the hippocampus with aging and dementia. Acta Neuropathol 37:111.

Bogden JM, Eastman A, Bresnick E (1981). A system in mouse liver for the repair of O^6-methylguanine lesions in methylated DNA. Nucleic Acids Res 9:3089.

Brash DE, Hart RW (1978). DNA damage and repair in vivo. J Environ Pathol Toxicol 2:79.

Brizzee KR (1975). Gross morphometric analyses and quantitative histology of the aging brain. In Ordy JM, Brizzee KR (eds): "Neurobiology of Aging," New York: Plenum Press, p 401.

Bugiani O, Salvarani S, Perdelli F, Mancredi GL, Leonardi A (1978). Nerve cell loss with aging in the putamen. Eur Neurol 17:286.

Cairns J (1981). The origin of human cancers. Nature 289:353.

Cameron IL (1972). Cell proliferation and renewal in aging mice. J Gerontol 27:162.

Cole RS, Levitan D, Sinden RR (1976). Removal of psoralen interstrand cross-links from DNA of Escherichia coli: Mechanism and genetic control. J Mol Biol 103:39.

Collier IE, Popp DM, Lee WH, Regan JD (1982). DNA repair in a congenic pair of mice with different longevities. Mech Ageing Dev 19:141.

Comfort A (1979). "The Biology of Senescence." 3rd edition. New York: Elsevier, p 86, 109.

D'Ambrosio SM, Whetstone JW, Slazinski L, Lowney E (1981). Photorepair of pyrimidine dimers in human skin in vivo. Photochem Photobiol 34:461.

Dell'Orco RT, Anderson LT (1981). Unscheduled DNA synthesis in human diploid cells of different donor ages. Cell Biol Int Rep 5:359.

Devaney KO, Johnson HA (1980). Neuron loss in the aging visual cortex of man. J Gerontol 35:836.

Eichhorn G (1983). Nucleic acid biochemistry and aging. In Rothstein M (ed): "Review of Biological Research in Aging," Vol 1, New York: A. R. Liss, p 295.

Fibriger HC (1981). Neurotransmitters during aging. In Schmike RT (ed): "Biological Mechanisms of Aging," (NIH Publication No. 81-2194), Bethesda, Maryland: National Institutes of Health, p 567.

Fort FL, Cerutti PA (1981). Altered DNA repair in fibroblasts from aged rats. Gerontol 27:306.

Francis AA, Lee WH, Regan JD (1981). The relationship of DNA excision repair of ultraviolet-induced lesions to the maximum life span of mammals. Mech Ageing Dev 16:181.

Fujiwara A, Tatsumi M (1976). Replication bypass repair of ultraviolet damage to DNA of mammalian cells: Caffeine sensitive and caffeine resistant mechanisms. Mutat Res 37:91.

Gensler HL (1981). The effect of hamster age on UV-induced unscheduled DNA synthesis in freshly isolated lung and kidney cells. Exp Gerontol 16:59.

Glick R, Bondareff W (1979). Loss of synapses in the cerebellar cortex of the senescent rat. J Gerontol 34:818.

Goldman R (1976). Aging of the excretory system: Kidney and bladder. In Finch CE, Hayflick L (eds): "Handbook of Aging," New York: Van Nostrand, p 409.

Goldstein S (1971). The role of DNA repair in aging of cultured fibroblasts from xeroderma pigmentosum and normals. Proc Soc Exp Biol Med 137:730.

Goth R, Rajewsky MF (1974). Persistence of O^6-ethylguanine in rat-brain DNA: Correlation with nervous system-specific carcinogenesis by ethylnitrosourea. Proc Natl Acad Sci USA 71:639.

Gutmann E (1976). Muscle. In Finch CE, Hayflick L (eds): "Handbook of Aging," New York: Van Nostrand, p 445.

Hall JD, Almy RE, Scherer KL (1982). DNA repair in cultured human fibroblasts does not decline with donor age. Exp Cell Res 139:351.

Hall TC, Miller AKH, Corsellis JAN (1975). Variations in the human Purkinje cell population according to age and sex. Neuropathol Appl Neurobiol 1:267.

Hanawalt PC, Cooper PK, Ganesan AK, Lloyd RS, Smith CA, Zolan ME (1982). Repair responses to DNA damage: Enzymatic pathways in E coli and human cells. J Cell Biochem 18:271.

Hart RW, Setlow RB (1974). Correlation between deoxyribonucleic acid excision repair and lifespan in a number of species. Proc Natl Acad Sci USA 71:2169.

Hart RW, Setlow RB (1976). DNA repair in late-passage human cells. Mech Ageing Dev 5:67.

Hart RW, Setlow RB, Woodhead AD (1977). Evidence that pyrimidine dimers in DNA can give rise to tumors. Proc Natl Acad Sci USA 74:5574.

Hart RW, Smith-Sonneborn J, Brash DE (1980). Aging in paramecia and man. In: "Conference on Structural Pathology in DNA and the Biology of Aging," Boppard, Germany: Boldt, p 65.

Hart RW, Turturro A (1981). Evolution and longevity-assurance processes. Naturwissenschaften 68:552.

Hart RW, Turturro A (1983). Species longevity as an indicator for extrapolation for toxicity data among placental mammals. J Am Coll Toxicol (in press).

Hennis HL III, Braid HL, Vincent RA Jr (1981). Unscheduled DNA synthesis in cells of different shape in fibroblast cultures from donors of various ages. Mech Ageing Dev 16:355.

Hooper ACB (1981). Length, diameter and number of ageing skeletal muscle fibres. Gerontol 27:121.

Ishikawa T, Takayama S, Kitagawa T (1978). DNA repair synthesis in rat ganglion cells treated with chemical carcinogens or ultraviolet light in vitro, with special reference to aging and repair level. JNCI 61:1101.

Jones ML (1982). Longevity of captive mammals. Zool Gart 52:113.

Kanagalingam K, Balis M (1975). In vivo repair of rat intestinal DNA damage by alkylating agents. Cancer 36:2364.

Kato H, Harada M, Tsuchiya K, Moriwaki K (1980). Absence of

correlation bewteen DNA repair in ultraviolet irradiated mammalian cells and life span of donor species. Jpn J Genet 55:99.

Kay MMB, Makinodan T (1981). Relationship between aging and the immune system. Prog Allergy 29:134.

Kellogg EW, Fridovich I (1976). Superoxide dismutase in the rat and mouse as a function of age and longevity. J Gerontol 31:405.

Kraemer KH, Lee MM, Scotto J (1982). Diseases of environmental-genetic interaction: Preliminary report on a retrospective study of neoplasia in 286 xeroderma pigmentosum patients. In Sugimura T, Kondo S, Takebe H (eds): "Environmental Mutagens and Carcinogens," New York: A. R. Liss, p 605.

Krauter EE, Wallace JE, Campbell BA (1981). Sensory-motor function in the aging rat. Behav Neurol Biol 31:367.

Lakatta EG, Yin FCP (1982). Myocardial aging: Functional alterations and related cellular mechanisms. Am J Physiol 242:H927.

Lambert B, Ringborg U, Skoog L (1979). Age-related decrease of ultraviolet light-induced DNA repair synthesis in human peripheral lymphocytes. Cancer Res 39:2792.

Landfield PW, Braun LD, Pitler TA, Lindsey JD, Lynch G (1981). Hippocampal aging in rats: A morphometric study of multiple variables in semithin sections. Neurobiol Aging 2:265.

Lett JT (1977). Cellular senescence and the capacity for rejoining DNA strand breaks. In Nichols W, Murphy D (eds): "DNA Repair Processes," Miami: Symposia Specialists, p 89.

Lett JT, Caldwell J, Dean CJ, Alexander P (1967). Rejoining of X-ray induced breaks in the DNA of leukaemia cells. Nature 214:790.

Licastro F, Franceschi C, Chiricolo M, Battelli MG, Tabacchi P, Cenci M, Barboni F, Pallenzona D (1982). DNA repair after gamma radiation and superoxide dismutase activity in lymphocytes from subjects of far advanced age. Carcinogenesis 3:45.

Likhachev AY, Anisimov VN, Ovsyannikov AI (1981). Alkylation of liver DNA purines in rats of different ages treated with diethylnitrosamine. Vopr Med Khim 27:349.

Lindahl T (1982). DNA repair enzymes. Annu Rev Biochem 51:61.

Lipetz PD, Galsky AG, Stephens RE (1982). Relationship of DNA tertiary and quaternary structure to carcinogenic processes. Adv Cancer Res 36:165.

Liu SC, Parsons CS, Hanawalt PC (1982). DNA repair response in human epidermal keratinocytes from donors of different age. J Invest Dermatol 79:330.

Livneh Z, Elad D, Sperling J (1979). Enzymatic insertion of purine bases into depurinated DNA in vitro. Proc Natl Acad Sci USA 76:1089.
Maher V, McCormick JJ (1979). DNA repair and carcinogenesis. In Grover PL (ed): "Chemical Carcinogens and DNA," Vol 1, Boca Raton, Florida: CRC Press, p 133.
Marquis JK, Lippa AS, Pelham RW (1981). Dopamine receptor alterations with aging in mouse and rat corpus striatum. Biochem Pharmacol 30:1876.
Martin GM, Ogden CE, Wight TN (1983). Comparative rates of decline in the primary cloning efficiencies of smooth muscle cells from the aging thoracic aorta of two murine species of contrasting maximum life span potentials. Am J Pathol 110:236.
McGeer PL, McGeer EG, Suzuki JS (1977). Aging and extra-pyramidal function. Arch Neurol 34:33.
McMartin DN, O'Connor JA Jr (1979). Effects of age on axo-plasmic transport of cholinesterase in rat sciatic nerves. Mech Ageing Dev 10:241.
Meites J (1982). Changes in neuroendocrine control of anterior pituitary function during aging. Neuroendocrinology 34:151.
Meyn RE, Jenkins SF, Thompson LH (1982). Defective removal of DNA cross-links in a repair deficient mutant of Chinese hamster cells. Cancer Res 42:3106.
Miller MR, Chinault DN (1982). Evidence that DNA polymerases α and β participate differentially in DNA repair synthesis induced by different agents. J Biol Chem 257:46.
Natarajan AT, Zwanenburg TSB (1982). Mechanisms for chromo-somal aberrations in mammalian cells. Mutat Res 95:1.
Niedermuller H (1982). Age dependency of DNA repair in rats after DNA damage by carcinogens. Mech Ageing Dev 19:259.
Paffenholz V (1978). Correlation between DNA repair of embryonic fibroblasts and different lifespan of 3 inbred mouse strains. Mech Ageing Dev 7:131.
Painter RB (1982). DNA repair. In Hsu TC (ed): "Cyto-genetic Assays of Environmental Mutagens," Totowa, New Jersey: Allanheld, Osmun, p 11.
Pashko L, Schwartz AG (1982). Inverse correlation between species life span and specific cytochrome P-448 content of cultured fibroblasts. J Gerontol 37:38.
Pegg AE, Roberfroid M, von Bahr C, Foote RS, Mitra S, Bresil H, Likhachev A, Montesano R (1982). Removal of O^6-methyl-guanine from DNA by human liver fractions. Proc Natl Acad Sci USA 79:5162.
Peleg L, Raz E, Ben-Ishai R (1976). Changing capacity for DNA excision repair in mouse embryonic cells in vitro. Exp

Cell Res 104:301.
Poirier MC (1981). Antibodies to carcinogen-DNA adducts. JNCI 67:515.
Price GB, Modak SP, Makinodan T (1971). Age-associated changes in the DNA of mouse tissues. Science 171:917.
Regan JD, Carrier WL, Samet C, Olla BL (1982). Photoreactivation in two closely related marine fishes having different longevities. Mech Ageing Dev 18:59.
Regan JD, Trosko JE, Carrier WL (1968). Evidence for excision of ultraviolet-induced pyrimidine dimers from the DNA of human cells in vitro. Biophys J 8:319.
Robertson OH, Wexler BC (1962). Histological changes in the tissues and organs of senile castrated kokanee salmon. Gen Comp Endocrinol 2:458.
Sacher GA (1959). Relation of lifespan to brain weight and body weight in mammals. In Wolstenholme GEW, O'Conner M (eds): "The Lifespan of Animals," [CIBA Foundation Colloquia on Ageing, Vol 5], London: Churchill, p 115.
Sacher GA (1976). Life table modification and life prolongation. In Finch CE, Hayflick L (eds): "Handbook of Aging," New York: Van Nostrand, p 582.
Sacher G, Hart RW (1978). Longevity, aging and comparative cellular and molecular biology of the house mouse, _Mus musculus_, and the white footed mouse, _Peromyscus leucopus_. Birth Defects 14:71.
Schendel P (1981). Inducible repair systems and their implications for toxicology. CRC Crit Rev Toxicol 8:311.
Selmanowitz VJ, Rizer RL, Orentreich N (1976). Aging of the skin and its appendages. In Finch CE, Hayflick L (eds): "Handbook of Aging," New York: Van Nostrand, p 496.
Seshadri R, Morley A, Trainor K, Sorrell J (1979). Sensitivity of human lymphocytes to bleomycin increases with age. Experientia 35:233.
Setlow RB (1980). DNA repair pathways. Basic Life Sci 15:45
Severson JA, Finch CE (1980). Reduced dopaminergic binding during aging in the rodent striatum. Brain Res 192:147.
Sheikh Y, Joyce NJ, Daniel FB, Oravec CT, Cazer FD, Raber J, Mhaskar D, Witiak DT, Hart RW, D'Amrosio SM (1981). Strain differences in organ selective DMBA-induced carcinogenecity: Comparative binding of dimethylbenz(a)-anthracene and its 2-fluoro analogue in Sprague-Dawley and Long-Evans rats. In Dennis AJ, Cooke WM (eds): "Polynuclear Aromatic Hydrocarbons," Columbus: Battelle, p 625.
Shock N, Norris AH (1970). Neuromuscular coordination as a factor in age changes in muscular exercise. Med Sports 4:92.

Singer B, Kusmierek JT (1982). Chemical mutagenesis. Annu Rev Biochem 52:655.

Treton JA, Courtois Y (1981). Evolution of the distribution, proliferation and ultraviolet repair capacity of rat lens epithelial cells as a function of maturation and aging. Mech Ageing Dev 15:251.

Turner DR, Griffith VC, Morley AA (1982). Ageing *in vivo* does not alter the kinetics of DNA strand break repair. Mech Ageing Dev 19:325.

Vaughn DW, Vincent JM (1979). Ultrastructure of neurons in the auditory cortex of ageing rats: A morphometric study. J Neurocytol 8:215.

Verly WG, Paquette Y (1973). An endonuclease for depurinated DNA in rat liver. Can J Biochem 51:1003.

Vijayashanker N, Brody H (1979). A quantitative study of the pigmented neurons in the locus coeruleus and subcoeruleus in man as related to aging. J Neuropathol Exp Neurol 38:490.

Walford RL, Bergman K (1979). Influence of genes associated with the main histocompatibility complex on deoxyribonucleic acid excision repair capacity and bleomycin sensitivity in mouse lymphocytes. Tissue Antigens 14:336.

Wani AA (1981). DNA damage due to spontaneous lability of nucleophilic agents. In Schimke RT (ed): "Biological Mechanisms of Aging," (NIH Publication No. 81-2194), Bethesda, Maryland: National Institutes of Health, p 211.

Weigle JJ (1953). Induction of mutation in a bacterial virus. Proc Natl Acad Sci USA 39:628.

Wheeler DD (1982). Aging of membrane transport mechanisms in the central nervous system. GABA transport in rat cortical synaptosomes. Exp Gerontol 17:71.

Wheeler KT, Lett JT (1974). On the possibility that DNA repair is related to age in non-dividing neurons. Proc Natl Acad Sci USA 71:1862.

Wilkens RJ, Hart RW (1974). Preferential DNA repair in human cells. Nature 247:35.

Williams JR, Dearfield KL (1981). Induction and repair of DNA/chromatin alterations. In Schmike RT (ed): "Biological Mechanisms of Aging," (NIH Publication No. 81-2194), Bethesda, Maryland: National Institutes of Health, p 245.

Woodhead AD, Setlow RB, Grist E (1980). DNA repair and longevity in three species of cold-blooded vertebrates. Exp Gerontol 15:301.

Yagi T (1982). DNA repair ability of cultured cells derived from mouse embryos in comparison with human cells. Mutat Res 96:89.

Zolan ME, Smith CA, Calvin NM, Hanawalt PC (1982). Rearrangement of mammalian chromosome structure following excision repair. Nature 299:462.

DISCUSSION

DR. LANDFIELD: I wanted to ask a question about the conceptual basis of this research. Is DNA repair being proposed as a basic, primary cause of aging at the cellular level, or is repair viewed as a secondary, modulatory phenomenon?

DR. TURTURRO: Aging is probably more a result of the cumulative effects of DNA damage. Repair is certainly a modulator of that. As I pointed out, UV excision repair seems to be entrained to the amount of DNA damage since other factors are fairly constant when compared in the placental mammals. However, when one attempts to compare placental mammals with nonplacental mammals, or poikilotherms, one is dealing with vastly different metabolic rates.

DR. LANDFIELD: I would agree with that viewpoint since any repair mechanism is unlikely to be perfect and DNA changes would therefore accumulate over time, even in the presence of a repair process. This suggests that time-dependent DNA changes might be an initial driving force and seems to argue for some sort of modulatory role of repair, if repair is involved in aging.

DR. BELL: In looking at the correlation between efficiency of DNA repair and an organism's life span, aren't there other factors that one might wish to consider? A mouse, for example, lives close to the ground under cover. In fact, even a gorilla lives under a canopy of foliage and, of course, is further protected by a furry coat, as is the mouse. Consequently, in man in contrast to these species, the efficiency of the mechanism of DNA repair may have evolved to a higher degree because humankind is basically hairless and the species exposes itself to the sun.

DR. FOX: Perhaps body temperature is involved.

DR. BELL: Body temperature is certainly another factor.

DR. TURTURRO: That is a very interesting point. First of all, a number of species that were referred to (Hall and

Hart, 1979) were different hairy primates so, presumably, their body temperatures would be quite similar.

Secondly, as I mentioned, UV excision repair does not measure something that is biologically relevant. UVA radiation, which we use for UV excision repair, is not a factor in species that live on earth. UVB seems to be the important factor. UVA, UVB, and UVC are different frequency ranges of ultraviolet light.

When metabolism is increased tenfold, adduct formation is also increased by a like amount as is recognition by specific damage nuclease.

When one studies species under comparable conditions, for instance, *Peromyscus leucopus* and *Mus musculus*, as was done by Hart and Sacher (1978), animals that are quite similar in terms of life style, habit, and size, and vary only in maximum achievable life span, one finds that they also vary in UV-induced DNA excision repair, perhaps for the reasons noted in our paper.

DR. MAURER: Possibly Dr. King has information on the following. Is there any way to correlate data from your studies on UV radiation repair excision damage, etc. and the experimental autoimmune model in the NZB mouse, or any other system where we know there is involvement of autoimmune disease? This may be in either the NZB mouse or the NZB/NZW F_1 mouse and the UV-DNA story you presented.

DR. TURTURRO: The problem with using a specific pathology is that you start getting into complex tissue interactions. What kills the NZB mouse may express itself differently in other species because of a different cell population which is at risk. For instance, Robertson has shown that in the Pacific salmon, the cells that seem to be at risk are those that control mineralocorticoid hormone elaboration. At the end of about 3 years of life, normal Pacific salmon show a surge of stress hormones as they swim upstream to reproduce. What one sees in these animals is pathology induced by sustained high levels of stress hormones.

If, on the other hand, the animals are castrated, this phenomenon is prevented, but at the end of eight or nine years one still encounters stress hormone-related-like tissue damage.

Dr. Walford's analysis of the autoimmune response, aging and the major histocompatability locus, I think, is a bit forced, and we discussed that in our paper, "Theory of Aging". There are a number of species that don't seem to have a major histocompatability locus and don't seem to have an immune system as we know it, and yet they still age. So, it is hard to make a general comparison for all systems. That is why, in our DNA repair studies, we tried to restrict our analysis to placental mammals.

Comparative Pathobiology of Major Age-Related Diseases:
Current Status and Research Frontiers, pages 47–68

THE POSSIBLE ROLE OF PROTEIN SYNTHESIS IN THE AGING PROCESS

Arlan Richardson, Ph.D., M. S. Roberts, B.S., and M. C. Birchenall-Sparks, Ph.D.

Department of Chemistry, Illinois State University, Normal, IL 61761

Because proteins play an essential role in the structure and function of all living cells, it is not surprising to find that changes in the synthesis of proteins can lead to a variety of pathological conditions. The effect of aging on protein synthesis has been studied extensively in a variety of organisms and tissues over the past two decades (Richardson 1981; Richardson, Birchenall-Sparks 1983). A decline in protein synthesis with increasing age has been observed in plants (Pillay 1977), fungi (Gottlieb 1975), insects (Baumann, Chen 1969; Levenbook, Krishna 1971; Webster, Webster 1979), nematodes (Sharma et al 1979), and a variety of tissues from mammals (Richardson 1981; Richardson, Birchenall-Sparks 1983). Young et al (1975) also showed that the rate of whole body protein synthesis in human subjects declined with increasing age.

The effect of aging on protein synthesis has been studied most in liver tissue from laboratory rodents. Studies prior to 1977 were contradictory; an increase, decrease, or no change in protein synthesis with increasing age were reported. Using suspensions of hepatocytes isolated from rats of various ages by collagenase perfusion, investigators were able to measure accurately rates of protein synthesis in a system that was comparable to the *in vivo* situation (Ricca et al 1978). Figure 1 shows a comparison of the relative rates of protein synthesis by hepatocytes isolated from male Fischer F344 (Coniglio et al 1979) or female WAG/Rij (van Bezooijen et al 1977) rats. During the first 24 months of age, a significant decrease in the rate of protein synthesis was observed. Although the

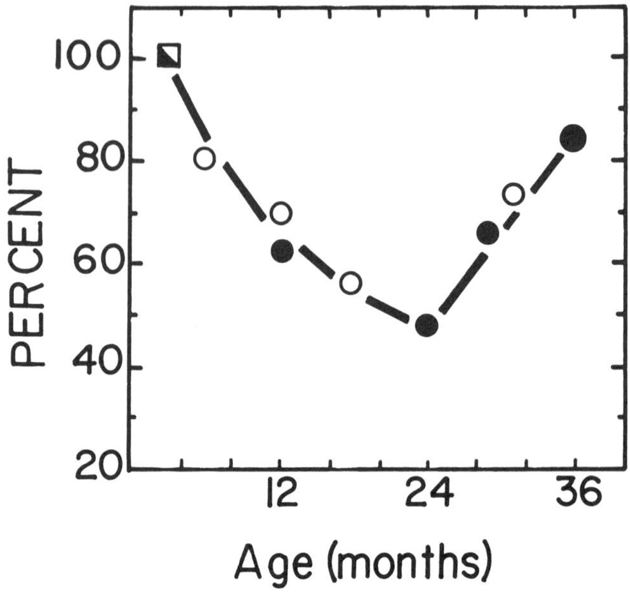

Fig. 1. The relative rates of protein synthesis by hepatocytes isolated from female WAG/Rij (●) and male Fischer F344 (○) rats. The rates of protein synthesis by hepatocytes from the two strains of rats were normalized by expressing each value as a percent of the rate of protein synthesis observed for 3-month-old rats. From Richardson (1981).

increase in protein synthesis in the very old rats was unexpected, several other investigators have subsequently observed that liver protein synthesis increases in very old rats (Bolla, Greenblatt 1982; van Bezooijen et al 1981).

A large amount of research has focused on the effect of aging on various components of the protein synthetic apparatus in liver. Layman et al (1976) observed a dramatic shift in ribosome aggregation with increasing age in the liver. This shift paralleled the decline in cell-free protein synthesis between 1 and 18 months of age. Claes-Reckinger et al (1982) recently confirmed this observation and showed that the increase in protein synthesis after 24 months of age (Figure 1) was paralleled by an increase in ribosome aggregation in the liver. An age-related decline in ribosome aggregation to mRNA has also been observed in the brain (Fando et al 1980), skeletal muscle (Britton, Sherman 1975; Srivastava 1969), lung (Mainwaring 1968), and prostate gland (Mainwaring 1968) of rodents as well as in _D. melanogaster_ (Webster et al 1981), nematodes, (Wallach, Gershon 1974), and fungi (Ricciardi et al 1974). Several investigators have studied the biological activity of liver ribosomes as a function of age. Kurtz (1975, 1978) showed that the translation of polyuridylate by rat liver ribosomes declined with age. However, aging had no effect on the fidelity of liver ribosomes to translate polyuridylate (Kurtz 1975, 1978; Mori et al 1979). Recently, Butzow et al (1981) observed that the accuracy of polyuridylate translation by liver ribosomes declined with age in the presence of the aminoglycoside paromomycin, which reduces the accuracy of protein synthesis.

The effect of aging on the aminoacylation of tRNA has been studied extensively (Mays 1981; Richardson 1981; Richardson, Birchenall-Sparks 1983). A gradual decline in the level of tRNA in the liver appears to occur with increasing age (Manjula, Sundari 1981; Neumeister, Webster 1981). In general, it appears that a gradual age-related decrease in the aminoacylation of most tRNA species occurs (Richardson, Birchenall-Sparks 1983). However, the effect of this decrease on protein synthesis is unclear. Recently, Foote and Stulberg (1980) showed that the fidelity of cell-free translation with tRNA isolated from the livers of adult and old mice was similar.

Only a few investigators have studied the effect of aging on the various protein factors involved in protein synthesis. Comolli et al (1979) reported that the activity of the ribosome dissociation factor from liver declined 80% between 1 and 180 days of age. Moldave et al (1979) measured the elongation factor activity (EF-1 and EF-2) of high salt extracts of liver ribosomes from 3- and 30-month-old rats. No significant change in the activity of EF-2 was observed. A 40% decrease was observed in the activity of EF-1, which catalyzes the binding of aminoacyl-tRNA to ribosomes. A decline in the activity of EF-1 has been reported for _D. melanogaster_ (Webster, Webster 1982) and nematodes (Bolla, Brot 1975). From cell-free studies, it appears that the elongation stage of protein synthesis is the step of protein synthesis primarily affected by the aging process. In addition, Coniglio et al (1979) showed that the ribosome half-transit time (the time required for the synthesis of an average half-length of a nascent polypeptide chain) by hepatocytes isolated from 4-month-old rats was 1.6-fold greater than for hepatocytes from 18-month-old rats. Therefore, the elongation rate of protein synthesis in whole cells also appears to decline with increasing age.

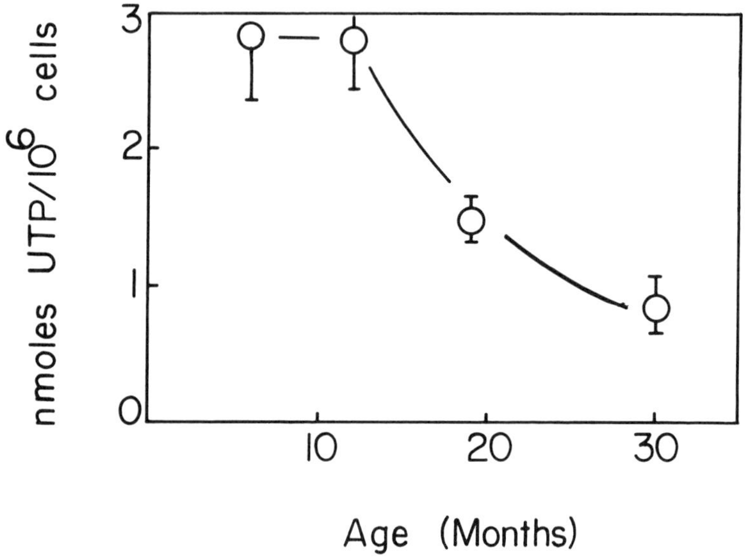

Fig. 2. The rate of poly(A)$^+$RNA synthesis by suspensions of hepatocytes. Each point represents the mean $\pm$ SEM of four animals. From Richardson et al (1983).

During the past three years, several investigators have studied the effect of aging on mRNA [poly(A)$^+$RNA] from liver. Moudgil et al (1979) reported that the percent of poly(A)$^+$RNA in polyribosomal RNA from the livers of adult and old rats was similar. In 1980, Moore et al found that the half-life of poly(A)$^+$RNA in the livers of 3- and 30-month-old rats increased from 3.6 to 15.2 hours. If the turnover of poly(A)$^+$RNA decreases while the poly (A)$^+$RNA content remains constant, one would expect that the rate of poly(A)$^+$RNA synthesis by the liver would decline with age. Recently, Richardson et al (1982) showed that the rate of poly(A)$^+$RNA synthesis by isolated hepatocytes decreased 60% between 12 and 30 months of age (Figure 2).

The effect of aging on the structure and biological activity of mRNA has only been studied during the past year. Bernd et al (1982) reported that the size of the poly(A)-segment on poly(A)$^+$RNA decreased with increasing age. Sparks et al (1981) recently showed the size of the poly(A)-segment of newly synthesized poly(A)$^+$RNA by hepatocytes was approximately 160 nucleotides. As shown in Figure 3, they found that the size of the poly(A)-segment on newly synthesized poly(A)$^+$RNA was the same for hepatocytes isolated from adult and old rats. Therefore, the effect of

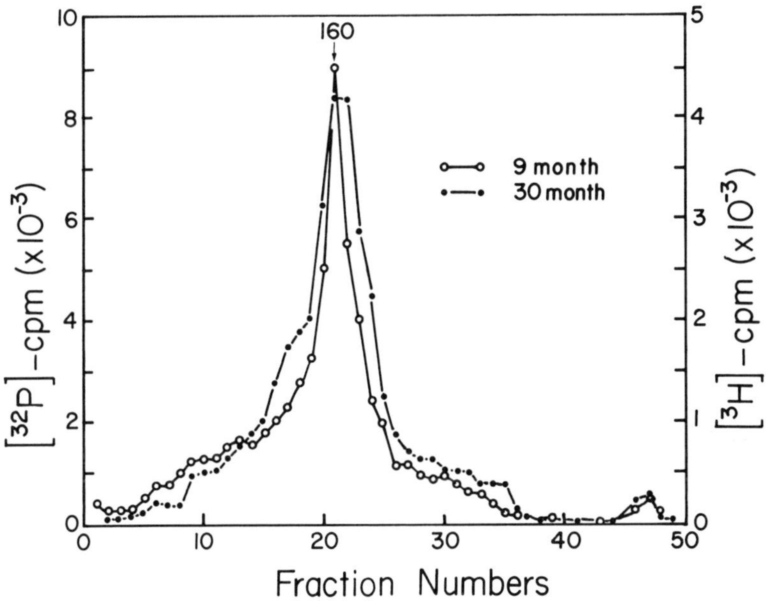

Fig. 3. The effect of age on the size of the poly(A)-segment of poly(A)$^+$RNA. Hepatocytes from 9- and 30-month-old rats were incubated with [^{3}H]-adenosine or [^{32}P]-phosphate. The poly(A)$^+$ isolated from the 9- and 30-month-old rats was combined, and the poly(A)-segment obtained by T_1 RNase digestion. The migration (left to right) of radioactivity on agarose-polyacrylamide gel electrophoresis is shown. The arrow indicates the migration of a poly(A) standard of 160 nucleotides.

aging on the poly(A)-segment of liver poly(A)$^{+}$RNA is not clear at the present time. The poly(A)-segment is believed to stabilize the mRNA; the shorter the poly(A)-segment, the more sensitive the mRNA is to degradation (Huez et al 1978).

Recently, Roberts et al (1983) compared the translational activity of poly(A)$^{+}$RNA isolated from 6- to 31-month-old rats. As shown in Figure 4, no age-related difference in the translational activity of the total poly(A)$^{+}$RNA extracted from rat liver was observed. However, age-related changes in the translational activity of specific mRNAs have been observed (Chatterjee et al 1981).

It is apparent from the discussion above that the protein synthetic activity of the liver changes significantly with increasing age. However, the age-related change in protein synthesis is not unique to the liver. As shown in Figure 5,

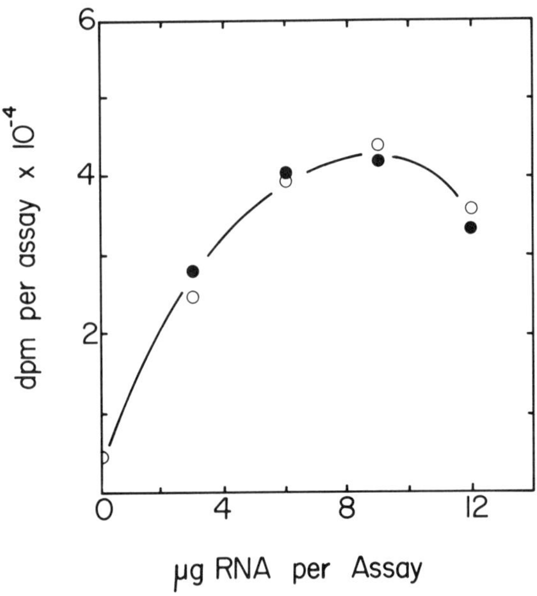

Fig. 4. The effect of age on the translational activity of liver mRNA. The ability of various concentrations of poly(A)$^{+}$RNA isolated from 6-(○) and 31-(●)month-old rats was determined in a wheat germ extract cell-free system. The poly(A)$^{+}$RNA was pooled from four rats for each age.

an age-related decline in protein synthesis is observed in a variety of tissues from Fischer F344 rats. In contrast to the liver (Figure 1), no increase in protein synthesis was observed in these tissues for very old rats. Therefore, it appears that the increase in protein synthesis in very old rodents is unique to the liver. An age-related decline in protein synthesis has been observed also in a variety of tissues from Sprague-Dawley rats (Richardson, Birchenall-Sparks 1983) and C57Bl/6J mice (Blazejowski, Webster 1983).

Although an age-related decline in protein synthesis appears to be a universal phenomenon, there is no informa-

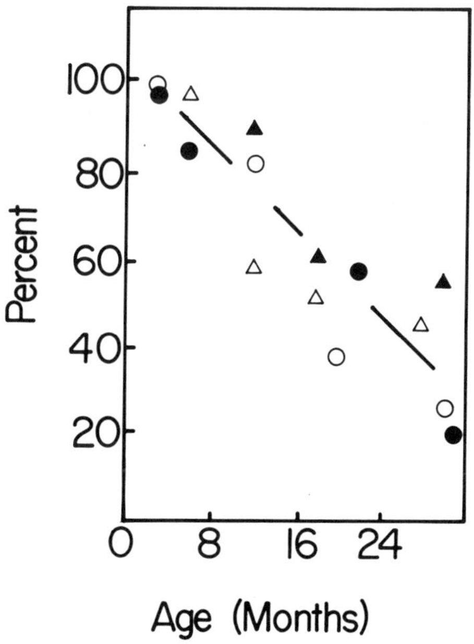

Fig. 5. The effect of age on the protein synthetic activities of various tissues from Fischer F344 rats. The data are expressed as a percent of that observed for 3- to 4-month-old rats for all tissues except the brain, which was expressed as a percent of that observed for 6-month-old rats. Brain (△) from Ekstrom et al (1980), kidney (●) from Hardwick et al (1981), testes (▲) from Liu et al (1978), and mitogen-induced spleen lymphocytes (○) from Cheung et al (1983).

tion currently available on the role protein synthesis may play in the aging process. Recently, our laboratory studied the effect of life-long dietary restriction on the age-related change in protein synthesis (Sparks et al 1983). Dietary restriction is the only strategy known to retard the aging process in homeotherms (Barrows, Kokkonen 1978). Using a restriction regimen that Yu et al (1982) showed increased the mean and maximum survival of male Fischer F344 rats over 45%, the rate of protein synthesis by hepatocytes isolated from rats fed ad libitum and a restricted diet were compared (Figure 6). As observed previously (Figure 1), a significant decrease in protein synthesis was observed between 2 and 19 months of age. However, the age-related

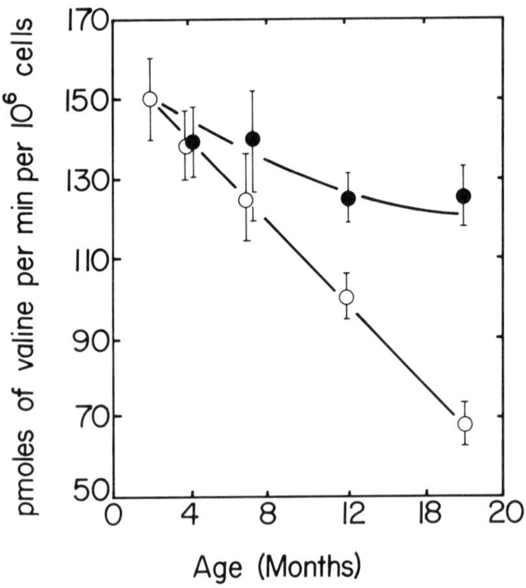

Fig. 6. The effect of dietary restriction on liver protein synthesis. The rate of protein synthesis was determined for hepatocytes isolated from male Fischer F344 rats fed ad libitum (○) or 60% of the diet consumed by the rats fed ad libitum (●). Each point represents the mean ± SEM of data from four to eleven animals. The age-related decline in the rate of protein synthesis by the rats fed ad libitum was significant at the P > 0.001 level; no significant change in the rate of protein synthesis by the rats fed the restricted diet was observed.

decline in the rate of protein synthesis by hepatocytes isolated from the rats fed the restricted diet was markedly retarded. Therefore, dietary restriction, which increases the life span of Fischer F344 rats, retards the age-related decline in protein synthesis by the liver.

The decline in protein synthesis with increasing age appears to be involved in the aging process because it is a universal phenomenon (Richardson 1981) and is retarded by dietary restriction (Sparks et al 1983). However, essentially no information currently exists on the physiological importance of the age-related decline in protein synthesis. It is clear that the decline in protein synthesis does not automatically lead to a decline in the protein content of a tissue. In general, the protein content of a tissue (Richardson, Cheung 1982) and the activities of most enzymes (Finch 1972) remain relatively constant with increasing age. Recently, Richardson and Cheung (1982) proposed that the decline in protein synthesis leads to a decline in protein turnover. The decline in protein turnover was the

Table 1

Studies Showing An Age-Related Decline in Protein Degradation and Turnover

Nematodes	
Soluble Proteins	Prasanna, Lane 1979; Reznick, Gershon 1979; Sharma et al 1979
Aldolase	Zeelon et al 1973; Reznick, Gershon 1979
Enolase	Sharma et al 1979
Triose Isomerase	Ghai, Lane 1981
Rodents	
Mouse Liver	
Ornithine Decarboxylase	Jacobus, Gershon 1980
Aldolase	Reznick et al 1981
Rat	
Liver Proteins	Lavie et al 1981
Heart Proteins	Meerson et al 1978; Crie et al 1981
Human Subjects	
Whole Body Proteins	Golden, Waterlow 1977; Uauy et al 1978
Muscle Protein	Uauy et al 1978

physiologically important consequence of the decline in protein synthesis. Several investigators have shown that protein degradation or turnover decreases with increasing age (Richardson, Cheung 1982; Rothstein 1983). A list of these studies is given in Table 1.

How is the decline in protein turnover physiologically important to an organism? Several lines of evidence indicate that the age-related appearance of altered enzymes is due to the decline in protein turnover (Rothstein 1983). However, not all proteins become altered with age; therefore, the physiological importance of the appearance of altered enzymes is uncertain. Richardson and Cheung (1982) proposed that the decline in protein turnover would lead to a decline in the responsiveness of an organism to stimuli; a general characteristic of all aging populations is the progressively impaired ability of an organism to respond to stimuli (Sartin et al 1980). Protein turnover has been shown to be an important factor in enzyme regulation, e.g., enzymes that have high turnover rates will respond more rapidly to changes in protein synthesis or degradation (Schimke 1970). Therefore, Richardson and Cheung (1982) predicted that a general decline in protein turnover with increasing age was an important factor in the age-related decline in the responsiveness of an organism to stimuli that involve gene induction.

SUMMARY

An age-related decline in protein synthesis appears to be a universal phenomenon. Protein synthesis has been observed to decline with age in organisms ranging from fungi and invertebrates to tissues from mammals, including humans. The effect of aging has been studied most extensively in the liver. The age-related change in protein synthesis is paralleled by a change in ribosome aggregation to mRNA. The elongation step of protein synthesis appears to be the step of protein synthesis primarily affected by the aging process. However, no age-related decline in the fidelity of protein synthesis occurs. Dietary restriction, which retards the aging process, retards the age-related decline in protein synthesis. It is proposed that the progressive decline in the ability of an organism to respond to change with increasing age arises, at least partially, from a decline in protein turnover, which arises from the age-related decline in protein synthesis.

ACKNOWLEDGEMENTS

The authors were supported by grants AG 01548 and AG 04091 awarded by the National Institute on Aging.

REFERENCES

Barrows CH, Kokkonen GC (1978). Diet and life extension in animal model systems. Age 1:131.

Baumann D, Chen PS (1969). Alterung und proteinsynthesis bei Drosophila melanogaster. Rev Suisse Zool 75:1051.

Bernd A, Batke E, Zahn RK, Muller WEG (1982). Age-dependent gene induction in quail oviduct. XV. Alterations of the poly(A)-associated protein pattern and of the poly(A) chain length of mRNA. Mech Ageing Dev 19:361.

Blazejowski CA, Webster GC (1983). Decreased rates of protein synthesis by cell-free preparations from different organs of aging mice. Mech Ageing Dev (in press).

Bolla RI, Brot N (1975). Age-dependent changes in enzymes involved in macromolecular synthesis in Turbatrix aceti. Arch Biochem Biophys 169:227.

Bolla RI, Greenblatt C (1982). Age-related changes in rat liver total protein and transferrin synthesis. Age 5:72.

Britton GW, Sherman FG (1975). Altered regulation of protein synthesis during aging as determined by in vitro ribosomal assays. Exp Gerontol 10:67.

Butzow JJ, McCool MG, Eickhorn GL (1981). Does the capacity of ribosomes to control translation fidelity change with age? Mech Ageing Dev 15:203.

Chatterjee B, Nath ST, Roy AK (1981). Differential regulation of the messenger RNA for three major senescence marker proteins in male rat liver. J Biol Chem 256:5939.

Cheung TH, Twu JS, Richardson A (1983). Mechanism of the age-related decline in lymphocyte proliferation: Role of IL-2 production and protein synthesis. Exp Gerontol (in press).

Claes-Rickinger N, Vandenhaute J, van Bezooijen CFA, Delcour J (1982). Functional properties of rat liver protein synthesizing machinery in relation to aging. Exp Gerontol 17:281.

Comolli R, Schubert A, Riboni L (1979). Changes in the activity and distribution of the ribosomal dissociation factor of rat liver during growth. Mech Ageing Dev 11:199.

Coniglio JJ, Liu DSH, Richardson A (1979). A comparison of protein synthesis by liver parenchymal cells isolated from Fischer F344 rats of various ages. Mech Ageing Dev 11:77

Crie JS, Millward DJ, Bates PC, Griffin EE, Wildenthal K (1981). Age-related alterations in cardiac protein turnover. J Mol Cell Cardiol 13:598.

Ekstrom R, Liu DSH, Richardson A (1980). Changes in brain protein synthesis during the life span of male Fischer rats. Gerontology 26:121.

Fando JL, Salinas M, Wasterlain CG (1980). Age-dependent changes in brain protein synthesis in the rat. Neurochem Res 5:373.

Finch CE (1972). Enzyme activities, gene function, and aging in mammals. Exp Gerontol 7:53.

Foote RS, Stulberg MP (1980). Efficiency and fidelity of cell-free protein synthesis by transfer RNA from aged mice. Mech Ageing Dev 13:93.

Ghai RD, Lane RS (1981). Synthesis of triose phosphate isomerase in senescent _Turbatrix aceti_. Fed Proc 40:1689.

Golden MHN, Waterlow JC (1977). Total protein synthesis in elderly people: A comparison of results with (^{15}N)-glycine and (^{14}C)-leucine. Clin Sci Mol Med 53:277.

Gottlieb D (1975). The aging process in the fungus _Rhizoctonia solani_. Phytophylatica 7:81.

Hardwick J, Hsieh WH, Liu DSH, Richardson A (1981). Cell-free protein synthesis by kidney from the aging female Fischer F344 rat. Biochim Biophys Acta 652:204.

Huez G, Marbix G, Gallwitz D, Weinberg E, Devos R, Hubert E, Cleuter Y (1978). Functional stabilization of HeLa cell histone messenger RNAs injected into _Xenopus_ oocytes by 3'-OH polyadenylation. Nature 271:572.

Jacobus S, Gershon D (1980). Age-related changes in inducible mouse liver enzymes: Ornithine decarboxylase and tyrosine aminotransferase. Mech Ageing Dev 12:311.

Kurtz DI (1975). The effect of aging on _in vitro_ fidelity of translation in mouse liver. Biochim Biophys Acta 407:479.

Kurtz DI (1978). A decrease in the number of active mouse liver ribosomes during aging. Exp Gerontol 13:397.

Lavie L, Reznick AZ, Gershon D (1981). Decreased protein and puromycinylpeptide degradation in livers of senescent mice. Biochem J 202:47.

Layman DK, Ricca GA, Richardson A (1976). The effect of age on protein synthesis and ribosome aggregation to messenger RNA in rat liver. Arch Biochem Biophys 173:246.

Levenbook L, Krishna I (1971). Effect of aging on amino acid turnover and rate of protein synthesis in the blowfly Phormia regina. J Insect Physiol 17:9.

Liu DSH, Ekstrom R, Spicer JW, Richardson A (1978). Age-related changes in protein, RNA, and DNA content and protein synthesis in rat testes. Exp Gerontol 13:197.

Mainwaring WIP (1968). Changes in the ribonucleic acid metabolism of aging mouse tissues with particular reference to the prostate gland. Biochem J 110:79.

Manjula, Sundari RM (1981). Variation in transfer ribonucleic acid population in liver of young, adult, and old female albino rats. Indian J Biochem 18:192.

Mays LL (1981). Posttranscriptional modifications of RNA in aging organisms. In Florini JR (ed): "Handbook of Biochemistry in Aging," Boca Raton, Florida: CRC Press, p 65.

Meerson FZ, Javich MP, Lerman MI (1978). Decrease in rate of RNA and protein synthesis and degradation in the myocardium under long-term compensatory hyperfunction and on aging. J Mol Cell Cardiol 10:145.

Moldave K, Harris J, Sabo W, Sadnik I (1979). Protein synthesis and aging: Studies with cell-free mammalian systems. Fed Proc 38:1979.

Moore RE, Goldsworthy TL, Pitot HC (1980). Turnover of 3'-polyadenylate-containing RNA in livers from aged, partially hepatectomized, neonatal, and Morris 5123C hepatoma-bearing rats. Cancer Res 40:1449.

Mori N, Mizuno D, Goto S (1979). Conservation of ribosomal fidelity during ageing. Mech Ageing Dev 10:379.

Moudgil PG, Cook, JR, Buetow DE (1979). The proportion of ribosomes active in protein synthesis and the content of polyribosomal poly(A)-containing RNA in adult and senescent rat livers. Gerontology 25:322.

Neumeister JA, Webster GC (1981). Changes in the levels and the rate of synthesis of transfer RNA in tissues of mice of different ages. Mech Ageing Dev 16:319.

Pillay DTN (1977). Protein synthesis in aging soybean cotyledons. Loss in translational capacity. Biochem Biophys Res Commun 79:796.

Prasanna HR, Lane RS (1979). Protein degradation in aged nematodes (Turbatrix aceti). Biochem Biophys Res Commun 86:552.

Reznick AZ, Gershon D (1979). The effect of age on the protein degradation system in the nematode Turbatrix aceti. Mech Ageing Dev 11:403.

Reznick AZ, Lavie L, Gershon HE, Gershon D (1981). Age-associated accumulation of altered FDP aldolase B in mice.

Conditions of detection and determination of aldolase half life in young and old animals. FEBS Lett 128:221.

Ricca GA, Liu DSH, Coniglio JJ, Richardson A (1978). Rates of protein synthesis by hepatocytes isolated from rats of various ages. J Cell Physiol 97:137.

Ricciardi RP, Holloman DW, Gottlieb D (1974). Age-dependent changes in fungi: Ribosomes and protein synthesis in Rhizoctonia solani mycelium. Arch Microbiol 95:325.

Richardson A (1981). The relationship between aging and protein synthesis. In Florini JR (ed): "Handbook of Biochemistry in Aging," Boca Raton, Florida: CRC Press, p 79.

Richardson A, Birchenall-Sparks MC (1983). Age-related changes in the synthesis and turnover of proteins. In Rothstein M (ed): "Biological Research in Aging," Vol 1, New York: A. R. Liss, p 255.

Richardson A, Birchenall-Sparks MC, Staecker JL (1983). Aging and transcription. In Rothstein M (ed): "Biological Research in Aging," Vol 1, New York: A. R. Liss, p 275.

Richardson A, Birchenall-Sparks M, Staecker JL, Hardwick JP, Liu DSH (1982). The transcription of various types of ribonucleic acids by hepatocytes isolated from rats of various ages. J Gerontol 37:666.

Richardson A, Cheung HT (1982). I. The relationship between age-related changes in gene expression, protein turnover, and the responsiveness of an organism to stimuli. Life Sci 31:605.

Roberts MS, Butler JA, Richardson A (1983). Age-related changes in gene expression in the liver. Fed Proc 42:751.

Rothstein M (1983). Enzymes, enzyme alteration, and protein turnover. In Rothstein M (ed): "Biological Research in Aging," Vol 1, New York: A. R. Liss, p 305.

Sartin J, Chaudhur M, Obenrader M, Adelman RC (1980). The role of hormones in changing adaptive mechanisms during aging. Fed Proc 39:3163.

Schimke RT, (1970). Regulation of protein degradation in mammalian tissues. In Munro HN (ed): "Mammalian Protein Metabolism," Vol IV, New York: Academic Press, p 178.

Sharma HK, Prasanna HR, Lane RS, Rothstein M (1979). The effect of age on enolase turnover in the free-living nematode, Turbatrix aceti. Arch Biochem Biophys 194:275.

Sparks MB, Ricketts WG, Rehwaldt CA, Cheung HT, Richardson A (1983). Effect of dietary restriction on gene expression. Fed Proc 42:1307.

Sparks MB, Roberts MS, Richardson A (1981). Characterization of the size of the poly(A) segments isolated from poly(A)$^+$RNA synthesized by hepatocytes from rats of different ages. Fed Proc 40:1572.

Srivastava U (1969). Polyribosome concentration of mouse skeletal muscle as a function of age. Arch Biochem Biophys 130:129.

Uauy R, Winterer JC, Bilmazes C, Haverberg LN, Scrimshaw NS, Munro HN, Young UR (1978). The changing pattern of whole body protein metabolism in aging humans. J Gerontol 33:663.

van Bezooijen CFA, Grell T, Knook D (1977). The effect of age on protein synthesis by isolated liver parenchymal cells. Mech Ageing Dev 6:293.

van Bezooijen CFA, Sakkee AN, Knook DL (1981). Sex and strain dependency of age-related changes in protein synthesis of isolated rat hepatocytes. Mech Ageing Dev 17:11.

Wallach Z, Gershon D (1974). Altered ribosomal particles in senescent nematodes. Mech Ageing Dev 3:225.

Webster GC, Webster SL (1979). Decreased protein synthesis by microsomes from aging *Drosophila melanogaster*. Exp Gerontol 14:343.

Webster GC, Webster SL (1982). Effects of age on the post-initiation stages of protein synthesis. Mech Ageing Dev 18:369.

Webster GC, Webster SL, Landis WA (1981). The effect of age on the initiation of protein synthesis in *Drosophila melanogaster*. Mech Ageing Dev 16:71.

Young VR, Steffee WP, Pencharz PB, Winterer JC, Scrimshaw NS (1975). Total human body protein synthesis in relation to protein requirements at various ages. Nature 253:192.

Yu BP, Masoro EJ, Murata I, Bertrand HA, Lynd FT (1982). Life span study of SPF Fischer 344 male rats fed *ad libitum* or restricted diets: Longevity, growth, lean body mass and disease. J Gerontol 37:130.

Zeelon P, Gershon H, Gershon D (1973). Inactive enzyme molecules in ageing organisms. Nematode fructose-1, 6-diphosphate aldolase. Biochemistry 12:1743.

DISCUSSION

DR. MEITES: I enjoyed your talk very much, Dr. Richardson, and I would like to report agreement with your results. Using rat diaphragm muscle, the classic system of Kostyo for studying the effects of growth hormone (GH) on protein synthesis, we recently found a significant decrease in the incorporation of [^{3}H]phenylalanine in old rats, after correcting for pool size. Furthermore, administration of GH increased protein synthesis in old rats, (Sonntag, Hylka, and Meites, unpublished). What puzzles me are your findings in the underfeeding experiments, which extend life span, but which you find prevent any decrease in protein synthesis.

Reducing food intake in the rat reduces GH secretion. I wonder whether you might have gotten different results had you studied a cell other than the hepatocyte.

Also, what would happen if you were to use cells from young animals and reduced their food intake? Would you find an increase in protein synthesis?

DR. RICHARDSON: What we have to define first is the type of system in which we have studied protein synthesis. You are right, protein synthesis in the liver is decreased by fasting. If you compare fasted to fed animals, it is well documented that protein synthesis is reduced by fasting. In our studies, the animals were fasted prior to the experiments measuring protein synthesis. Both the restricted and _ad libitum_ fed rats were allowed food intake for the same time interval. When one studies fasted and fed animals one is measuring the availability of amino acids for protein synthesis. In our study, we fasted the _ad libitum_ and restricted animals for the same length of time. Therefore, I think we have ruled out the problem of fasting versus feeding.

In addition, we studied several tissues. Although we have studied liver most thoroughly, we have also studied the kidney and lymphocytes. Restriction increased protein synthesis in all these tissues. I did not have sufficient time to show the data, but we have also studied protein synthesis in testes. In the testes we found, again, the protein synthetic activity is higher in restricted rats.

One interesting observation is that the cell-free protein synthetic activity of the brain appears not to be affected by dietary restriction.

DR. MEITES: What about starving young animals?

DR. RICHARDSON: I would predict that if you starved a young animal and compared it to a fed young animal you would find a difference. In other words, a starved animal would have lower liver protein synthesis.

DR. REAVEN: How long did you fast or underfeed your animals? Was this for a short period?

DR. RICHARDSON: It was lifelong.

DR. REAVEN: I thought that was the case and that is why Dr. Meites' question, although interesting, is a difficult one to answer when you are using a young animal. One can't really do the same experiment.

I have a second question. Would you say, based on what you just told us about fasting modulating the age-related decline in protein synthesis, that this phenomenon is not a true aging event?

DR. RICHARDSON: I think our study would suggest that the age-related decline in protein synthesis is related to the aging process because it is modified by dietary restriction. We don't have survival data on these rats because, unfortunately, we lost them all at 19 months of age. However, we were basically carrying out the same restriction procedure that Masoro used for Fischer F344 rats. This restriction procedure modifies the age-related decline in protein synthesis and, if you want to use the term, the aging process. The survival of the animals is modified significantly by this procedure. If you look at a variety of pathological conditions it appears that these, too, have been modified by this procedure.

DR. TEITELBAUM: Could you comment on what is known about the transcriptional events that are responsible for the decrease in mRNA synthesis, specifically as they relate to DNA methylation? Has that been looked at?

DR. RICHARDSON: I don't believe DNA methylation has been studied in detail as a function of age. There is a lot of information on total transcriptional activity of the liver which, incidentally, has been shown to decrease with age. When one studies total transcriptional activity, one is primarily looking at rRNA synthesis. Therefore, it was important that we looked specifically at messenger RNA (mRNA) synthesis which we found decreased with age. As far as regulation of transcription is concerned, the only studies that I am aware of have been done primarily from the standpoint of histone acetylation. Histone acetylation also appears to decrease with age, which would suggest that it may be involved in the decrease in transcription. In the case of DNA methylation, preliminary experiments suggest it, too, decreases with age. At the present time, we are in the process of cloning a variety of messenger RNAs from rat liver. We would like to use these with restriction enzymes to study whether or not changes in DNA methylation occur. We could also look at gene rearrangement with age.

DR. RAISZ: Dr. Richardson, that was an excellent talk. Pharmacologic studies have shown decreases in liver size both in some rats and in humans with age, so that the mass of protein can decrease. If you measure total smooth endoplasmic reticulum or some of the mixed function oxidases, their activity decreases. So, there is a loss of enzyme.

Another substance that changes with age which might relate to protein synthesis is somatomedin; it would be nice to measure that.

A third question relates to the problem of rapid early degradation as opposed to late degradation. You have been talking about the degradation of established proteins either secreted or in the cytosol. For collagen and a few other proteins there is a rapid early degradation phase as they come off the rough endoplasmic reticulum, that is, at the time of synthesis. It would be plausible that this might be a site for an age-related effect due to the increase in error frequency in protein synthesis and, therefore, an increase in this form of degradation, which we assume relates to error frequency. Have you looked at that?

DR. RICHARDSON: I can't comment on your latter two questions. We haven't looked at either protein degradation or somatomedin production. However, I can comment on the protein content of the liver. In male Fischer rats the liver weight actually increases with age. We do not see a decrease. An advantage of the isolated hepatocytes, which consist of parenchymal cells, is that we can measure the protein content of these cells. We find that the protein content increases from three to 12 months of age. The protein content of the parenchymal cells then remains constant with age, even though they are less active in protein synthesis.

You are correct about the mixed function oxidase system. We have also seen a decline in this particular system with age.

DR. RAISZ: Has this been seen in the Fischer rat as well?

DR. RICHARDSON: Yes, there are certain enzyme systems that change with age, i.e., decrease. However, there are certain proteins, e.g., albumin, whose synthesis increases with age. Liver protein synthesis appears to increase with age in very old rats. My feeling is that albumin synthesis may have a lot to do with the increase in protein synthesis in old animals. Albumin synthesis increases very dramatically between 12 and 24 months of age. The problem with the studies in this area, and I am criticizing our studies as well, is that we need to begin looking at the synthesis of specific proteins. We are beginning to do this using two-dimensional gel electrophoresis to study the synthesis of a large number of specific proteins. It is possible that the liver, in synthesizing more albumin, has to compensate and consequently the synthesis of other proteins will be depressed with increasing age.

DR. LEVY: You talked about what happens when you extend the age of the individual by restricted diet. Have you done anything with speeding up aging, let's say, by X-irradiation?

DR. RICHARDSON: No.

DR. WILLIAMSON: I enjoyed your presentation very much. I have two questions. One is, can you comment a little further on the mechanism whereby decreased dietary intake is thought to facilitate longevity, and, secondly, have the effects of dietary restriction been looked at in animals other than, say, the Fischer rat, in which the major cause of death is renal failure? What about animals in which the major cause of death is some other disease?

DR. RICHARDSON: I will answer your last question first. To my knowledge, the only study with Fischer rats was Masoro's study. Dietary restriction has increased the survival of a variety of rats, e.g., Sprague-Dawley, Wistar, etc., and mice as well. In a review, Barrows has cited studies in certain invertebrates, where dietary restriction also increases survival. A problem Cutler has pointed out, which I think is interesting, is whether dietary restriction has the same effect on longevity for animals that have a longer life span than rodents.

The mechanism of dietary restriction is not known. McCay initially proposed that dietary restriction increased longevity by delaying development. This belief has been generally accepted until the last two years. It was generally thought that if you didn't initiate the dietary restriction early in life you would not increase longevity. However, in the last year, Walford's laboratory showed that dietary restriction started at 12 months of age increased the survival of mice and decreased the incidence of tumors. Masoro's laboratory, using Fischer rats, was able to start the restriction regime at six months of age and increase longevity. One interesting point is that the average life expectancy of the rats started on dietary restriction at weaning was greater than those started at six months of age. In other words, it appears that the earlier you start the restriction, the greater the mean survival. However, it appears as though the maximum survival in rats that were started at weaning versus those that were started at six months is going to be about the same.

Exactly what dietary restriction is doing to increase survival is not known. It probably affects more than kidney pathology. In other rodents, in which you don't have the problem of renal failure, you still see an increase in survival.

DR. WISSLER: One brief question and a caveat. The question is, have you tried phytohemagglutinin (PHA) spleen cell stimulation in your cell-free system?

DR. RICHARDSON: No.

DR. WISSLER: I think it is quite possible that what you are measuring is fewer cells responding in the old animals, and that each cell might be responding as strongly as in the younger animals. In other words, protein synthesis per cell may be equal in the two ages.

DR. RICHARDSON: That is very possible.

DR. WISSLER: The caveat is that I have been interested in protein metabolism and synthesis for at least 40 years, and I have been interested in the studies which relate longevity to caloric and protein restriction. I think that the type you are describing today, in which total nutrition is only reduced to 60 percent, should not be regarded as an example of pseudohypophysectomy. This model represents getting back towards what is optimal nutrition for the rat--because the ad libitum chow-fed mature rat becomes obese and consumes too much of all food elements including protein. Under these circumstances the old rat, and especially the old male rat which dies in the third year, dies of an obstructive nephropathy which is probably connected with too much plasma protein passing through the glomeruli, too little being resorbed by the proximal tubules and ultimately obstruction of the collecting tubules. It is very similar to the type of renal disease seen in multiple myeloma. Hypertension, arteriolar changes and nephrosclerosis may occur along with a necrotizing arteritis. I think this is damage from far too much protein in the usual commercial rat chows, which are fine for growth but when fed ad libitum result in this type of renal disease and obesity.

DR. RICHARDSON: I think you are correct. In the past, nutritionists have determined the best diet as the diet that would give the most rapid growth. However, if you want the organism to live longer, it would appear that the maximal growth may not be a valid and important indicator.

One of the things I would like to mention with respect to the kidney is that we also looked at the excretion of protein in the restricted and ad libitum fed rats. Excretion of protein in the urine increases with increasing age, and we see that the animals that were fed the restricted diet excreted less protein.

There is one last comment I would like to make with respect to our restricted rats. We looked at the protein content of the hepatocytes from restricted and ad libitum fed rats. We observed a difference. On the basis of protein content, hepatocytes from restricted rats were significantly smaller. Other laboratories have also reported that the size of cells from tissues of restricted animals is smaller.

DR. SIMMONS: I would like to ask, particularly in regard to the neoplasms, were chemical contaminants in the diets measured or recorded? In other words, did you use diets that were PCB-free, PBB-free, or free of other suspected chemical carcinogens?

DR. RICHARDSON: We did not do studies on neoplasms. These were done by Walford's and Masoro's laboratories. I don't believe they have looked at this problem, but basically both groups of animals were fed essentially the same diet. Of course, the restricted rats would be consuming a smaller amount of any carcinogens that might be in the diet.

Comparative Pathobiology of Major Age-Related Diseases: Current Status and Research Frontiers, pages 69–87

CELLS MAY HAVE ESCAPED MORTALITY, THE PRICE PAID FOR FITNESS BY MULTICELLULAR ORGANISMS

Eugene Bell, Ph.D.

Department of Biology, Massachusetts Institute of Technology, 77 Massachusetts Ave., 16-820A, Cambridge, MA 02139

I wish to present a new perspective on the problem of organismic and cell aging. I suggest that some of the same gene products which insure youthful vigor and reproductive success in the multicellular individual may be responsible, throughout the individual's lifetime, for degenerative diseases and organismic as well as cell aging. This view is related to, but substantially different from the views of Medawar (1957) or Williams (1957) or Hamilton (1966) who postulated a class of genes called pleiotropic, having a favorable effect early in life, and a harmful one later. They consider genes of this class to be numerous, and hence aging which results from their expression as having many causes. My view is also different from that of Cutler (1976) who invokes genetic pleiotropy but unlike the foregoing authors he suggests that aging may be due to only a few pleiotropic genes. The new point I make is that some gene products incorporated into the genome because they enhanced reproductive capacity either directly, or indirectly by promoting fitness, act also to induce disease and undermine the individual throughout life, and not just late in life.

Haldane (1941) and Medawar (1957) have reasoned that evolution (natural selection) cannot remove harmful late acting genes since their effects are exerted after the period of reproductive activity. But I don't think it is a matter of late acting genes.

Early acting harmful genes might be retained if the disadvantages for species perpetuity of eliminating them are greater than those of keeping them. This may have been the strategy for optimizing reproductive vigor throughout evolution; hence there is good reason to believe that the genetic fabric of the multicellular individual is far from perfect. If harmful genes are retained because they primarily confer reproductive vigor, it is not surprising that a by-product of their long-term function might be gradual debilitation leading to self-destruction. Gene products such as certain growth factors, neurogenic substances, and hormones which perform necessary and desirable functions may also interact with non-target cells and tissues and promote degenerative changes as a side effect. Since their desirable effects may be indispensible, their cumulative adverse effects are tolerated by the individual at least until the conclusion of reproductive activity. It may not be easy for natural selection to eliminate genes which bolster reproductive capacity, regardless of how adversely they affect an organism in other respects, including the generation of disease and the promotion of aging.

I think that organismic aging then is a consequence of specialization and complexity. Products of differentiated clones impinge on cells of other clonal types to exert deleterious changes. These unplanned interactions, which I suggest lead to disease, may continue for years or decades before the individual or physician becomes aware of them and in this respect resemble the effects of carcinogens whose definitive action sometimes may not be manifest in humans for 3-4 decades. It is not a question then of pleiotropic genes, a vague concept to begin with, but of conventional gene products which take their cumulative toll from the outset. Consider the number of disease states attributable to single gene mutations, which persist in the gene pool. This alone suggests that organisms can and do tolerate degrees of self-destructiveness. Unlike single aberrent genes, the genes I speak of perform their specific functions perfectly; it is the side effects of their products which are damaging.

Given the mechanics of evolution, the probability that a multicellular organism would evolve with the perfection required for immortality is small, not because of the teleological arguments that immortality would lead to over-crowding and that genetic stasis would ensue, but because of the number of conditions each new gene added to an existing genome was required to satisfy.

How long it must have taken for a humoral factor such as

a hormone to be plugged into a system consisting of a great many cell types whose replicative activities and specific synthetic functions it could interact with and stimulate or perturb! Once inserted, the advantage of the hormone to the organism as reproductive machine may have been great, despite its consequences as an agent of organic disease and aging, hence the probability that a deletion mutation would yield a more successful genotype would be small.

It is true that extension of the reproductive period of the individual leading to increased numbers of offspring is advantageous, and changes favoring it would be selected for. However, retaining genes whose products were important for species propagation but were at the same time responsible for species-specific self-destructive phenomena would have been a strong counterforce severely limiting life span.

Hence the consequences of potential immortality for any multicellular organism may never have been tested. It has been pointed out that predation, disease, and environmental hazards may have been sufficient to insure mortality. Our view proposes that mortality was and is insured by the cell wars, that is, civil wars within multicellular organisms among cell types whose products slowly poison one another. Evidence to support the idea that civil wars are responsible for degenerative diseases of various kinds comes (Medawar 1957) from experiments which quantitatively perturb endocrine and neuronal secretions, (Williams 1957) from studies of self-destruct mechanisms and (Hamilton 1966) from the study of autoimmune phenomena.

The most dramatic perturbation of hormonal "balance" is brought about by ablation of a hormone source such as the hypophysis. Hypophysectomy in rats which are then given cortisone acetate confers as much as a 15-20% increase in life span (Everitt et al 1980, Everitt 1978). The treatment strikingly slows down a variety of aging processes, greatly reducing susceptibility to cancer, cardiovascular and renal disease and collagen cross-linking (Everitt 1976, Everitt et al 1968). These results are summarized in Table 1. A point of key importance is the correlation between the time that hypophysectomy is performed and the extent to which aging changes are ameliorated. Early removal bestows greater benefit, suggesting that even in the very young animal pathological changes have already begun (Everitt et al 1980). The protection bestowed by hypophysectomy against decline of immune competence is also remarkable (Bilder, Denckla 1977). Age-related changes are also muted in hypopituitary dwarf mice (Silberberg 1972). The neurohumors, released by neuronal

TABLE 1

Effects of Hypophysectomy in Rodents

Measure of Aging	Relative Age of Hypophysectomized Rat at 1000 Days of Age
Cross linking of collagen	500
Excretion of protein in urine	200
Wall thickness of thoracic aorta	100

Ref.: Everitt et al (1980)

Sign of Aging	Incidence In: Control	Hypoph.
Histological signs of renal disease	+	-
Hindleg paralysis at 1000 days	70%	0%
Tumors	64%	5%

Ref.: Everitt et al (1979)

	Control	Hypopituitary dwarf mice
Senile osteoarthrosis of the knee joint	+	-

Ref.: Silberberg (1972)

Immune Competence	Animal age	Control	Hypoph.
Xenograft (days required to reject)	450	13.8	6.5
Xenograft (days required to reject)	30	6.0	
Colloidal carbon clearance (Rate of clearance: V_{max} = mg/100 g/fat free body weight/min)	30	18.9	17.1
	450	2.5	15.5

Refs.: Bilder & Denkla (1977)

stimulation have also been shown to be fifth columnists. The accelerated development of atherogenesis in rats (that is, cardiovascular disease) can be brought about by hypothalamic stimulation or by stimulation of sympathetic nerves which serve the aorta (Gutstein et al 1978).

Evidence for the cell wars also comes from the extreme examples of organisms which undergo telescoped "aging" by self-destructing. The Pacific salmon and various species of octopus are examples. The life span of the salmon is three to four years. When the drive to spawn is triggered, a neuroendocrine cascade leads to rapid cardiovascular disease, renal failure, and skeletal deformations in the form of a humped back and hooked jaw (Robertson et al 1961; Wexler 1976). After the arduous battle upstream to the spawning grounds and ensuing reproductive activity, death occurs. The entire sequence can be blocked, however, as Robertson has shown (Robertson 1961), if the animals are castrated. Castration extends life three fold; however, administration of adrenocorticoids to immature animals induces the full spectrum of organic diseases (Robertson et al 1962). Similarly, the female octopus at breeding time ceases to eat, undergoes degenerative changes and dies soon after the brood becomes independent. If the optic gland, a neuroendocrine gland, is excised, life can be greatly extended (Wodinsky 1977).

Walford has pointed to the unmistakably positive correlation between aging and the occurrence of auto-antibodies in humans and mice (Walford 1974). In mice of the NZB strain a disorder likened to systemic lupus erythematosus, one of the most severe autoimmune diseases in humans, has been studied intensively. While these mice are normal for the first three months of life, soon afterward, they develop hemolytic anemia, circulating anti-DNA and anti-DNP antibodies, renal and cardiac lesions. Their T-cell functions, like allograft rejection and mitogenic response to phytohemagglutin, are also compromised. Walford has suggested that this disorder of autoimmunity is not unique to the autoimmune susceptible NZB strain, but that similar autoimmune phenomena are seen in long-lived strains. However, they arise at a time when the animal is slightly older. For example, anti-DNA and -DNP antibodies and anti-skeletal antibodies occur by 8 months in 33% of C57BL/6 mice (Linder et al 1972). Linder et al (1972) comment that similar changes probably occur in other strains and would be detected if sensitive methods were used. Even in its most minimal form autoimmune disease possibly common to all strains of mice may take its toll slowly throughout life and act as an undermining disorder. There is clearly a genetic predisposition in humans as well as in mice to autoimmune disease along with many other diseases such as cardiovascular, renal failure and arthritis.

I propose that the constellation of genetic factors whose expression leads to autoimmune disease was acquired in the course of evolution by various trade-offs which bestowed advantages important for species propagation but brought with them the conditions promoting autoimmune disease. I further suggest that other gene constellations which may be responsible for cardiovascular and other organic diseases were similarly acquired.

Genes of these "constellations" may have no relation to each other except that they act on a common target, which suffers because of some unplanned and untested effect exerted by them. The target may be the immune system or any cell, tissue or organ which as a result of the bombardment suffers systemic degradation.

I propose that aging genes as such do not exist but that species-specific genetic determinants are the chance results of the mechanics of evolution which select for reproductive vigor and accept with it the unplanned consequences to the individual, the cell wars, which result in mortality. Hence the genetic basis for species-specific aging may be considered trivial in a causal sense since the decline of the individual is due to species-specific systemic chaos brought about by long-term exposure to self-generated gene products which are harmful. The severity of the chaos may be an important determinant for species longevity. Nonetheless the same gene products are required throughout the life of the organism despite their degenerative consequences. It is this feature of multicellularity or organismic complexity, which has escaped the scalpel of evolution. We propose that it affects the organism even before birth through humoral factors generated in the embryo itself and through maternal factors which reach the embryo through the placenta.

A corollary of the generalization that organismic decline is due to civil wars among cell clones whose products poison one another is that cells as individuals may be immortal. Weismann (1891) considered aging a consequence of evolution and in particular a product of multicellularity. However, Weismann held that unicells, especially cells of the germ line, were immortal. We now raise the question: Are many cells of metazoans in addition to germ line cells potentially immortal? We know they are undermined to some degree by a process of poisoning intrinsic to the individual and by extrinsic influences such as radiation, diet, smoking and contaminants in air and water as well. They are certainly killed off when the organism dies! It is hard to know for how long cells can survive the organism they populate after their host dies. Hadorn's experiments (Hadorn 1966) suggest that imaginal disc cells of *Drosophilia* can be propagated indefinitely and can differentiate normally if put in a larval environment. Mouse teratocarcinoma cells can be propagated indefinitely *in vitro* but are "normal" in the sense that they can differentiate "terminally" into a variety of functional cell types under optimal conditions. Daniel's work with serial transfer of mouse mammary gland cells *in vivo* shows that cells can be kept alive for a period at least two or three times longer than the maximum life span of a mouse (Daniel 1977).

In addition, certain protozoans, amoebae in particular (Danielli, Muggleton 1959), and populations of tissue cells, usually transformed, appear to have indeterminate life spans.

Although WI-38 human diploid fibroblasts have been found to undergo what has been called senescence (Hayflick, Moorehead 1961) *in vitro*, a phenomenon attributed to an intrinsic genetic clock, recent work has given evidence that other types of cells are not limited in their proliferative potential *in vitro*. The limit of 50 $\pm$ 10 doublings continues to be extended as new hormonal and growth factors have been incorporated into cell culture media. In Coon's laboratory, cells cultured from the rat thyroid have undergone hundreds of doublings and remain karyotypically normal. They show no chromosomal changes detectible by quinocrine banding (Ambesi-Impiombato et al 1980), they synthesize thyroglobulin at a normal rate and remain morphologically differentiated. The approach has been that of isolating the cells in a low serum medium supplemented with a hormone cocktail. It is probable that other categories of cells may have indeterminate life spans under optimum conditions *in vitro*. With growth hormone supplementation, endothelial cells have been cultivated in at least three laboratories (Gospodarawicz et al 1976;

Folkman et al 1979; Romquin et al, in press) for hundreds of population doublings without evidence of slowing down. The true limits of the proliferative potential of stem cells are yet to be defined.

The tendency of fibroblasts to drift out of cycle using state of the art culture conditions may explain the present *in vitro* limits of fibroblast proliferative potential. The cell cycle heterogeneity (Merz, Ross 1973; Smith, Hayflick 1974; Martin et al 1974) of the system has made it difficult to compare, functionally, populations of low and high population doubling levels (PDL).

Finding that cells of high population doubling levels are different from cells of low population levels in certain metabolic or other properties may reflect the differential heterogeneity of each population. Phenotypic differences which emerge in the course of clonal growth of fibroblasts *in vitro* (Bell et al 1978) include doubling time, cell size, sister cell diversity with respect to cycling state, (that is, one sister may remain in cycle while the other leaves it) (Bell et al 1979b), cell velocity and loss of cytoplasmic fragments. A key difference between populations of low and high PDL is that the former contains a large number of cycling cells while the latter contains a small number (Cristofalo, Sharf 1973).

Recently, we discovered an experimental model in which this difference is eliminated (Figure 1). We have shown that fibroblasts of any PDL incorporated into a tissue equivalent matrix *in vitro* (Bell et al 1979a) are rapidly growth-regulated and remain out of cycle for as long as they are kept in the three-dimensional tissue equivalent lattice (Figure 2), but that this state is reversible (Sarber et al 1981). Following this observation, we reinvestigated the report that stimulation of the enzyme prolyl-hydroxylase by ascorbate is greatly reduced in cells of high PDL as compared with cells of low PDL when they are grown as monolayer (Chen et al 1977). We wished to know whether cycling state rather than PDL might determine the reduction of responsiveness to ascorbate of enzyme stimulation, since most high PDL cells are out of cycle while most low PDL cells are in cycle.

In the tissue equivalent lattice, both high and low PDL cells are equalized with respect to cycling state. In neither is prolyl-hydroxylase activity stimulated by ascorbate (Bell et al 1983) (Figure 3). The effect is strictly reversible. When cells are recovered from the tissue equivalent and plated

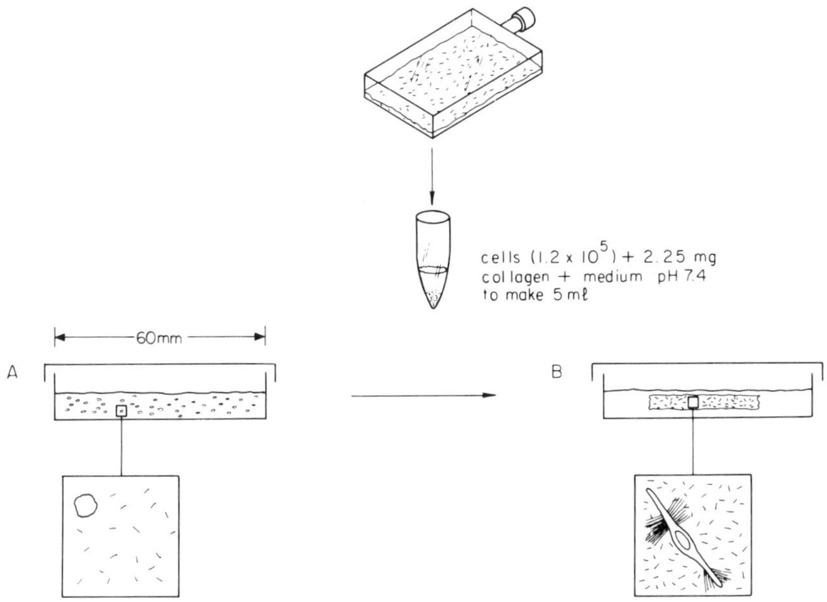

Fig. 1. Cultivated fibroblasts are combined with collagen, medium and 1.0 ml of fetal calf serum. Cells are added after the pH is raised to 7.4. (A) The mixture gels immediately, and cells still spherical after recovery from a culture flask are generally dispersed in it. (B) Cells elongate, compact and order the randomly distributed collagen fibrils. In the process, the entire lattice is contracted and fluid expressed from it. The tissue equivalent which forms, floats below the surface of the medium.

again as monolayer, they can again respond to ascorbate, low PDL cells being twice as responsive as high PDL cells. Similarly, the contractile capacity of low and high PDL cells in the same cycling state can be compared by measuring the rate and extent of contraction of tissue lattices in which cells are incorporated. Under conditions when cell division is blocked by colcemid (Figure 4) or Ara-C, fibroblasts of high PDL are at least as efficient as those of low PDL in

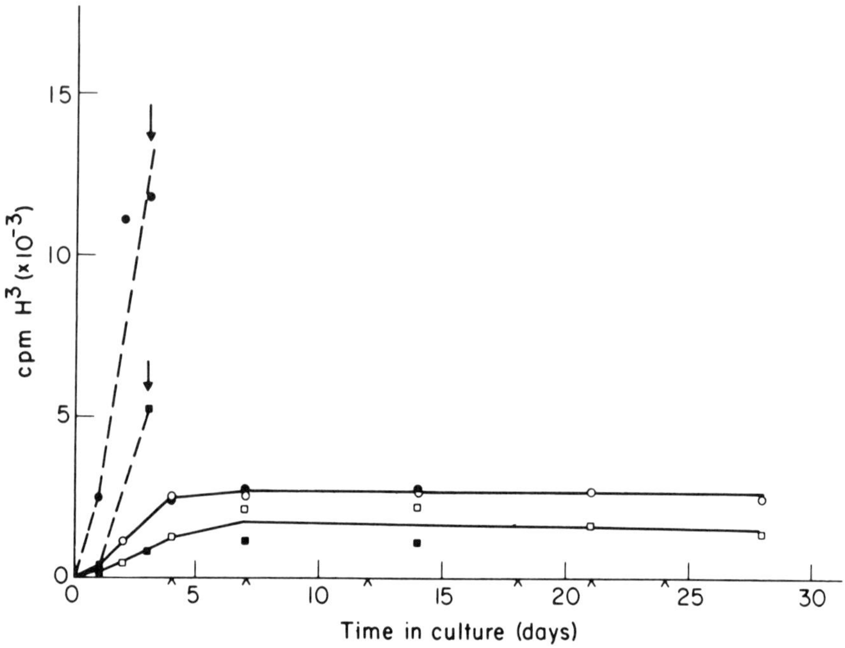

Fig. 2. Incorporation of [^{3}H]TdR into trichloroacetic acid precipitable material by IMR 90 cells of PDL 18(●), PDL 19 (o) and PDL 41 (□, ■) grown in 60 mm tissue culture dishes (---) and in collagen lattices (——). The cultures in the dishes appeared confluent at the time indicated by the arrows. In the experiments represented by the solid points, the medium was not changed throughout the incubation period; while for those experiments represented by the open points, the culture medium was changed as indicated by carets (^) along the lower axis.

carrying out contractile activities which are normally expressed in the repertoire of wound-healing activities of this cell type (Bell et al 1979a).

A case against a generalized failure of cell function has been made by Finch (1972) who tabulated those cellular functions including proliferative capacities which show no decline during aging. An important recent addition to this

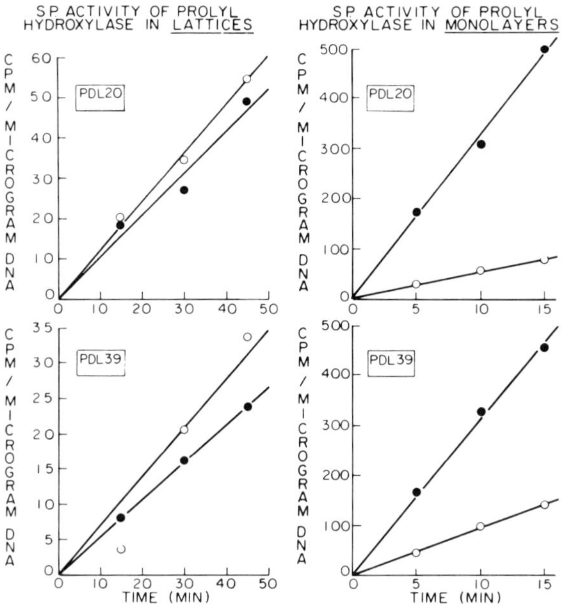

Fig. 3. Prolyl-hydroxylase activity in lattices made up with cells of low or high PDL (population doubling level) is unaffected by the addition of ascorbate. Enzyme activity is 6X stimulated in PDL 20 cells and 3X stimulated in PDL 39 cells. Open circles: without ascorbate; closed circles: with ascorbate. Unhydroxylated 4-L-[^{3}H]proline labeled collagen prepared and used as substrate for enzyme activity is expressed as CPM/mg DNA.

list is the report that DNA repair in human epidermal keratinocytes in individuals differing in age by 90 years is essentially the same (Liu et al 1982).

Too little information about the potential longevity of differentiated postmitotic cells is available. While it is known that some phenotypes, such as neurons, decrease in number as the organism ages, the phenomenon need not be interpreted as a sign of aging intrinsic to the cell; rather it may be one of attrition suffered by cells exposed to a hostile milieu. How long the life span of mitotic cells which persist to the end of the individual's life can be prolonged

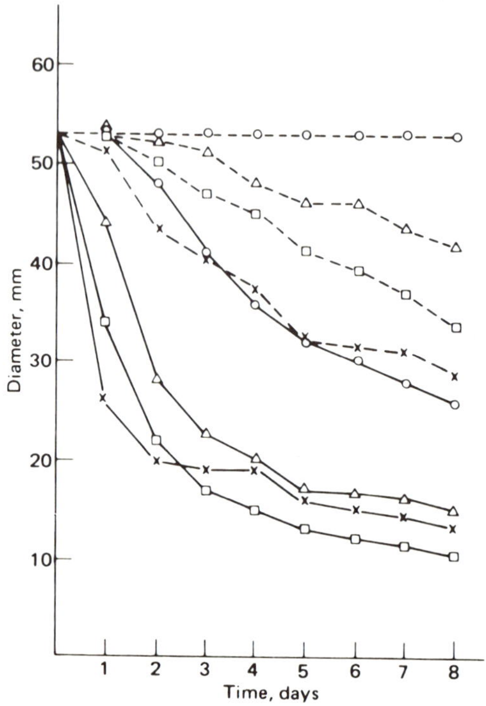

Fig. 4. Effect of colcemid at 0.36 μg/ml on protein lattice contraction by cells of different PDLs. ---, colcemid; ——, control; o, 5 x 10^4 19th PDL cells; △, 1.8 x 10^5 19th PDL cells; □, 2.7 x 10^5 19th PDL cells; x, 2.5 x 10^5 45th PDL cells. Protein C concentration was 570 μg/ml. Medium was changed on the 4th and 7th days.

is unanswered. Slow or non-growing mouse mammary gland cells have been subcultured for at least eight years by Daniel (Walford 1974). The issue is one of chronology of the cell as individual rather than progenitor and quite different from that of the life span of a strain or line of cells.

In summary, we do not think cells are genetically programmed to age. While some may degenerate and die as a consequence of unfavorable culture conditions *in vivo* as well as *in vitro*, many, particularly stem cell populations, may be immortal if optimum growth requirements are provided. In speculating on why dietary restrictions in rodents extend life span, I propose that reduced hormonal output which characterizes the metabolic state of the experimental animals creates a milieu more favorable for many cell types which inhabit the organism. In contrast to the cells which constitute it, the multicellular organism, because of its evolutionary history, is a victim of cell wars which are responsible for its mortality.

Instead of seeking an explanation for organismic aging in programmed cell severence and death, we see the tables turned and propose that the intrinsic immortality of cells is compromised in nature by the multicellular organism and in the laboratory (with some recent exceptions) by the limits of cell culture technology.

REFERENCES

Ambesi-Impiombato FS, Parks LAM, Coon HG (1980). Culture of hormone-dependent functional epithelial cells from rat thyroids. Proc Natl Acad Sci USA 77:3455.

Bell E, Ivarsson B, Merrill C (1979a). Production of tissue-like structure by contraction of collagen lattice by human fibroblasts of different proliferative potential in vitro. Proc Natl Acad Sci USA 76:1274.

Bell E, Marek LF, Levinstone DS, Merrill C, Sher S, Young IT, Eden M (1978). Loss of division potential in vitro: Aging or differentiation? Science 202:1158.

Bell E, Marek LF, Sher S, Merrill C, Levinstone D, Young I (1979b). Do diploid fibroblasts in culture age? Int Rev Cytol [Suppl 10]:1.

Bell E, Sher S, Hull B, Merrill C, Rosen S, Chamson A, Asselineau D, Dubertret L, Coulomb B, Lapiere C, Nusgens B, Neveux Y (1983). The reconstitution of living skin. J Invest Dermatol (in press).

Bilder GE, Denckla WD (1977). Restoration of ability to reject xenografts and clear carbon after hypophysectomy of adult rats. Mech Ageing Dev 6:153.

Chen KH, Evans CA, Gallop PM (1977). Prolyl and lysyl hydroxylase activation and cofactor specificity in young and senescent WI-38 fibroblast cultures. Biochem Biophys Res Comm 74:1631.

Cristofalo VJ, Sharf BB (1973). Cellular senescence and DNA synthesis: Thymidine incorporation as a measure of population age in human diploid cells. Exp Cell Res 76:419.

Cutler RG (1976). Nature of aging and life maintenance

processes. Interdiscipl Topics Gerontol 9:83.
Daniel CW (1977). Cell longevity: In vivo. In Finch CE, Hayflick L (eds): "Handbook of the Biology of Aging," New York: Van Nostrand Reinhold, p 122.
Danielli JF, Muggleton A (1959). Some alternative states of amoeba, with special reference to lifespan. Gerontology 3:76.
Everitt AV (1976). Hypophysectomy and aging in the rat. In Everitt AV, Burgess JA (eds): "Hypothalamus, Pituitary and Aging," Springfield, IL: C. C. Thomas, p 68.
Everitt AV (1978). Hypothalamic and pituitary determinants of life duration. Proc 50th Symp Jpn Assoc Med Sci, Hakone.
Everitt AV, Olsen GG, Burrows GR (1968). The effect of hypophysectomy on the aging of collagen fibers in the tail tendon of the rat. J Gerontol 23:333.
Everitt AV, Seedsman NJ, Jones F (1980). The effects of hypophysectomy and continuous food restriction, begun at age 70 and 400 days, on collagen aging, proteinuria, incidence of pathology and longevity in the male rat. Mech Ageing Dev 12:161.
Finch DE (1972). Enzyme activities, gene function and ageing in mammals (review). Exp Gerontol 7:53.
Folkman L, Haudenschild CC, Zetter BR (1979). Long term culture of capillary endothelial cells. Proc Natl Acad Sci USA 76:5217.
Gospodarawicz D, Moran J, Braun D, Birdwell C (1976). Clonal growth of bovine vascular endothelial cells: Fibroblast growth factor as a survival agent. Proc Natl Acad Sci USA 73:4120.
Gutstein WH, Harrison J, Parl F, Kiu G, Avitable M (1978). Neural factors contribute to atherogenesis. Science 199:449.
Hadorn E (1966). Dynamics of determination. In Locke RM (ed): "Major Problems in Developmental Biology," New York: Academic Press p 85.
Haldane JBS (1941). "New Paths in Genetics." New York: Harper.
Hamilton WD (1966). The moulding of senescence by natural selection. J Theor Biol 12:12.
Hayflick L, Moorhead PS (1961). The serial cultivation of human diploid cell strains. Exp Cell Res 25:585.
Linder E, Pasternack A, Edgington TS (1972). Pathology and immunology of age-associated disease of mice and evidence for an autologous immune complex pathogenesis of the associated renal disease. Clin Immunol Immunopathol 1:140.
Liu CS, Parsons CS, Hanawalt PC (1982). DNA repair response in human epidermal keratinocytes from donors of different ages. J Invest Dermatol 79:330.

Martin GM, Sprague CA, Norwood TH, Pendergrass WR (1974). Clonal selection, attenuation and differentiation in an _in vitro_ model of hyperplasia. Am J Pathol 74:137.

Medawar PB (1957). "The Uniqueness of the Individual." New York: Basic Books.

Merz GS, Ross JD (1973). Clone size variation in the human diploid cell strain WI-38. J Cell Physiol 82:75.

Robertson OH (1961). Prolongation of the life span of kokanee salmon (_Oncorhynchus nerka kneerlyi_) by castration before beginning of gonad development. Zoology 47:609.

Robertson OH, Hane S, Wexler BC, Rinfret AP (1962). The effect of hydrocortisone on miniature rainbow trout (_Salmo gardnerii_) Gen Comp Endocrinol 2:458.

Robertson OH, Wexler BC, Miller BF (1961). Degenerative changes in the cardiovascular system of the spawning Pacific salmon (_Oncorhynchus tshawytscha_). Circ Res 9:826.

Romquin N, Plouët J, Barritault D, Courtois Y. Human and bovine vascular endothelial cells: Comparative effect on cell growth and longevity of an eye derived growth factor (EDGF) and of extracellular matrix. Biol Cell (in press).

Sarber R, Hull B, Merrill C, Soranno T, Bell E (1981). Regulation of proliferation of fibroblasts of low and high population doubling levels grown in collagen lattices. Mech Ageing Dev 17:107.

Silberberg R (1972). Articular aging and osteoarthroses in dwarf mice. Pathol Microbiol 38:417.

Smith JR, Hayflick L (1974). Variation in the life-span of clones derived from human diploid cell strains. J Cell Biol 62:48.

Walford RL (1974). Immunologic theory of aging: Current status. Fed Proc 33:2020.

Weismann A (1891). "Essays on Heredity." Oxford: Clarendon Press.

Wexler BC (1976). Comparative aspects of hyperadrenocorticism and aging. In Everitt AV, Burgess JA (eds): "Hypothalamus, Pituitary and Aging," Springfield, IL: Charles C. Thomas, p 333.

Williams GC (1957). Pleiotropy, natural selection, and the evolution of senescence. Evolution 11:398.

Wodinsky J (1977). Hormonal inhibition of feeding and death in octopus: Control by optic gland secretion. Science 198:946.

DISCUSSION

DR. TEITELBAUM: You made a very important point regarding species specificity of this phenomenon, and I would like to call your attention to what happens if one oophorectomizes women instead of fish. They age faster, and develop cardiovascular disease and osteoporosis. As a matter of fact, women who go through menopause and are then treated with estrogens live longer than women who are not maintained on estrogens.

DR. BELL: It is very hard to compare one species with another; the constellation of defects that may exist in one species may be quite different in another. Your point is certainly well taken.

DR. TURTURRO: We agree with the point about keratinocytes. I made a point this morning to mention that we feel this exists because a subpopulation of cells has been studied that is continually replicating. This work was inspired by your reports on cell differentiation which clearly affects cell function.

If the complexity of functioning multicellular organisms results in their eventual death, then how would you explain that in certain cell lines, especially primate and mammalian lines, more progressively advanced organisms are the ones that survive the longest?

Further, you noted that in hypophysectomized animals all these changes occur, but it has to be made clear that hypophysectomy does not extend maximum achievable life expectancy.

DR. BELL: According to Everitt's data, there appears to be a 15 to 20% increase in life span if animals are hypophysectomized at 70 days of age.

DR. TURTURRO: In maximum achievable life span?

DR. BELL: In maximum life span in the rat. Coming to your point, if I understand you correctly, you say that proliferation is an important issue in studying DNA repair. I wonder how one knows that postmitotic cells don't repair their DNA? Is there good evidence for such a conclusion? In fact, there is considerable evidence to the contrary. I refer to the older work of Pelc and his associates, who for years reported unscheduled DNA snythesis in postmitotic cells in virtually every tissue of the organism using autoradiographic criteria, and I think the work is still sound.

When one looks at DNA repair in culture _in vitro_, is one looking only at cells that are replicating and not those that are out of cycle or the postmitotic? I think not. As we and others show, with fibroblasts a substantial proportion of the cell population _in vitro_ is out of cycle. How then can one say that the noncycling cells are not repairing DNA? I think it is a very difficult question to resolve, and it is still open. Criteria for identifying noncycling cells are needed to approach this problem.

DR. KING: I can confirm that. If one studies postmitotic myocardial cells _in vivo_ in rats after giving radioactive thymidine, one obtains incorporation of the isotope into DNA. Even though there is apparently no division as seen by a lack of mitotic figures, there is repair, or at least uptake which is indicative of repair. I like your concept of a "civil war" going on between all the interacting, homeostatic, cellular mechanisms. However, does the mouse, with three to four years maximum longevity, have so much more "civil war" than the human with a life span of 80-100 years, even though it is exposed to all the same environmental insults? My final comment is that even though you say you don't believe in the aging gene and I say I do; there is no evidence on either side. Remember that Huebner and Todern postulated an oncogene in the 1960's. Only in the last three or four years, work from your institution and others has led to acceptance that the oncogene does exist.

DR. BELL: It is very difficult to set aside the exceptions. For a long time the transformed cell _in vitro_ was an exception to the idea that cells are mortal and that they are clocked; that there is a ticket that they have punched every time they divide and are alloted a limited number of punches. It is exciting to see the emergence of new data which suggest that this phenomenon is characteristic not only of the transformed cell but also of karyotypically normal cell types as well. I think it is this kind of evidence that one has to point to as a basis for excluding the aging gene hypothesis. On the basis of data from transformed cells alone, there was doubt about ruling out an aging gene since transformation might involve a deletion of an aging locus which permits the cell to escape senescence. Now with the advance that normal cells can be cultivated indefinitely, it is much harder to argue for the aging gene hypothesis.

DR. TERRY: The cell wars must get terribly complicated in view of the finding that in a single organ of a single species such as the human brain, the cell number in the neocortex decreases markedly in the course of aging, while it does not decrease at all, apparently, in certain cranial nerve nuclei. I think that they must depend on the individual metabolic activity of that cell line to determine how serious the degenerative effect will be.

Now, given the interchangability in the early fetus from one cell area to another cell area within the nervous system, it is hard to believe that there is a gene which will control cell death; rather there must be some effect which comes on later, or else the repressor is also dependent upon the individual metabolic activity of that particular cell. It is almost beyond understanding.

DR. BELL: I appreciate your comment, and I agree with it. Dr. King should answer it, not I.

DR. KING: I am only saying the evidence for an aging gene is strictly speculative and hypothetical, and can be tested. There are excision enzymes which can take out portions of DNA, which, put in other cells, may produce structural and functional changes characteristic of aging cells.

DR. BELL: I don't think it is fair to compare the oncogene with a hypothetical aging gene. The oncogene may have to do with regulation of cell division and essentially little else. Either a cell remains in a particular state of differentiation out of the cell cycle, or a cell is catapulted into the cell cycle and remains there abnormally. A regulator of this process might explain the function of the oncogene, but the aging gene which you postulate would have to be much more complicated. You are asking that it control the proliferative potential of a cell by keeping track of the number of times the cell divides. This requires both a memory and the capacity to trigger a mechanism to self-destruct.

DR. KING: Working with idiotype memory is no problem.

DR. LANDFIELD: I think it might be helpful in considering this issue if we bear in mind that there are at least two separate issues under consideration here: the issue of whether some etiological aging factors are systemic and the issue of what initially triggers such systemic factors. With regard to the first issue, your data apparently argue against an aging gene within each cell line and therefore provide evidence that systemic factors are present. However, this does not necessarily indicate that there are no other genetically programmed changes in key regulatory systems. That is, although the physiological environment may be hostile to some cells and affect their survival, there might nevertheless be programmed changes in key regulatory systems (e.g., hormonal, immunological, etc.) that lead to this hostile cellular environment. I think the point that Dr. Turturro made earlier is also relevant to the question of whether complexity alone, in the absence of programmed changes, is sufficient to produce the hostile environment. If there is no critical regulatory change initially and if it is only the degree of multicellular complexity that generates "cell wars", why is it that the more complex animals do not age more rapidly? That is an interesting question that I didn't catch the answer to earlier.

DR. BELL: I didn't answer it. I think that it is arguable as to whether a large mammal or a mammal that appeared late in evolution is necessarily more complicated than a smaller one or one that appeared previously in evolution.

Comparative Pathobiology of Major Age-Related Diseases: Current Status and Research Frontiers, pages 89–108

ROLE OF THE NEUROENDOCRINE SYSTEM IN AGING PROCESSES

Joseph Meites, Ph.D.

Department of Physiology, Neuroendocrine Research Laboratory, Michigan State University, East Lansing, MI 48824

INTRODUCTION

The endocrine system and the central nervous system are the two great regulators of body functions, and there is growing evidence that they control many aging processes. Up to about 30 years ago it was widely believed that these two systems mostly operated independently of each other. As a result of the pioneer work of Geoffrey Harris in England, Ernst and Berta Scharrer in Germany, and Charles Sawyer and John Everett in the United States, it became clear that the endocrine system is largely regulated by the brain, particularly its hypothalamic portion, and the endocrine system, in turn, exerts a considerable influence on brain function. Inasmuch as the neuroendocrine system is known to control growth and function of many organs and tissues during the developmental and mature phases of life, it is logical to assume that it has an equally important role in regulating the decline in function of these organs and tissues during aging.

Early endocrine investigations focused mainly on the gonads, since the decline in gonadal function in old individuals appeared to be associated with many aging decrements. Brown-Séquard, often regarded as the "father of endocrinology," reported in 1889 that he had succeeded in rejuvenating himself at the age of 72 years by injecting himself with watery extracts of guinea pig and dog testes (Brown-Séquard 1889). The actual benefits from these gonadal extracts, so vividly described by Brown-Séquard, can be questioned, but his reports stimulated considerable interest in the relation of the endocrine system to aging phenomena, an interest that continues to the present day. We need only mention the widespread use of estrogens in postmenopausal women and of androgens in elderly men for treatment of various aging problems.

When the primacy of the pituitary as the "master gland" of the body was established in the 1930's and 1940's, it, rather than the gonads, was considered to exert the major endocrine influence on aging. However, the pituitary and its target glands (gonads, thyroid, adrenal cortex) were only considered to exert a secondary rather than a primary influence on aging processes. In a chapter on the relation of the pituitary to aging, Verzar (Verzar 1966), an internationally known gerontological investigator, concluded that "the pituitary, and especially the anterior pituitary, seems to have no primary role in the aging of the body." Today, as a result of the advances made in our knowledge of hypothalamic control of pituitary function, and the availability of radioimmunoassays (RIAs) for accurate measurement of pituitary and other hormones in the circulation, it is my belief that the hypothalamo-pituitary-target gland system may be the single most important regulator of aging changes in the body.

Our own studies on the laboratory rat show that the hypothalamo-pituitary unit is mainly responsible for cessation of estrous cycles in aging female rats, the decline in testosterone secretion in aging male rats, the occurrence of large numbers of spontaneous mammary and pituitary tumors in aging female rats and of pituitary tumors in aging male rats, and for the significant decline in growth hormone secretion with its many potential consequences. Furthermore, there is evidence that these aging processes in rats can be delayed, hastened, or reversed by appropriate neuroendocrine interventions. Some of the changes in neuroendocrine function that account for specific aging-related changes in body functions will be reviewed in the sections that follow.

GONADOTROPIC FUNCTION AND REPRODUCTION

Rats have a life span of about 2.5-3 years under favorable laboratory conditions, and as in man, females outlive males. Female rats come into puberty at 35-40 days of age and exhibit regular 4-5 day estrous cycles. At the age of about 8-15 months their cycles become <u>irregular</u> and lengthened; this is followed by a prolonged <u>constant estrous</u>

syndrome that may last for many months, and is characterized by ovaries with many follicles but no evidence of ovulation or corpora lutea (Figure 1); this is often followed by irregular and lengthy pseudopregnancies, characterized by ovaries with numerous corpora lutea that actively secrete progesterone (Figure 2). In the oldest rats, between 2-3 years of age, many of them exhibit an anestrous state, characterized by atrophic ovaries containing only small, undeveloped follicles, with little evidence of estrogen secretion as indicated by the infantile appearing uterus (Figure 3). It is of interest that the ovaries of all of these categories of rats, despite the reduction in ova and follicles, can be activated to normal or near normal function by appropriate stimulation with gonadotropic hormones or by transplanting them to younger cycling rats whose own ovaries have first been removed. This points to the hypothalamo-pituitary unit as primarily responsible for cessation of estrous cycles in aging female rats. This is in sharp contrast to the condition in aging women, whose ovaries begin to show dysfunction several years before the onset of menopause,

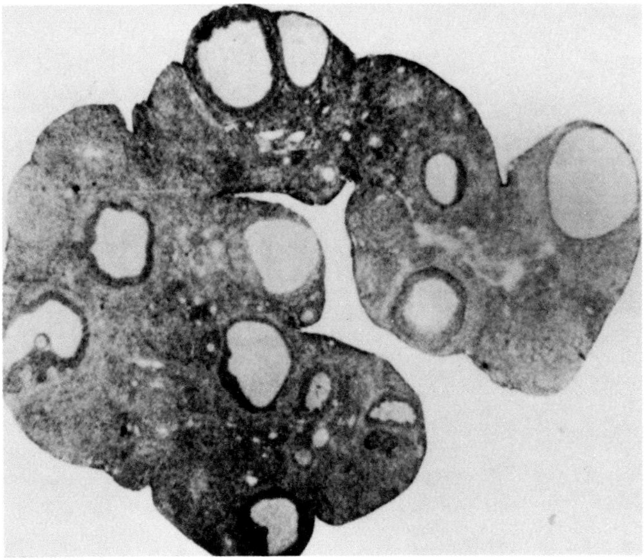

Fig. 1. Ovary from old constant estrous rat. Note well-developed follicles but no corpora lutea.

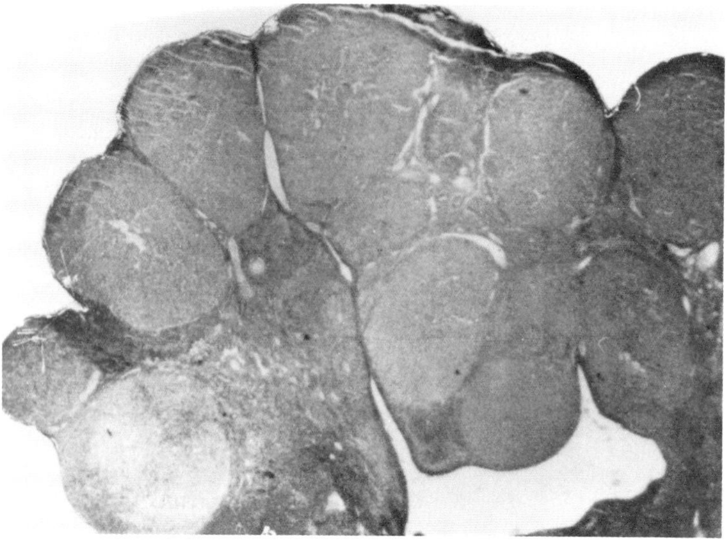

Fig. 2. Ovary from old pseudopregnant rat. Note numerous well-developed corpora lutea. These secrete progesterone due to high PRL secretion.

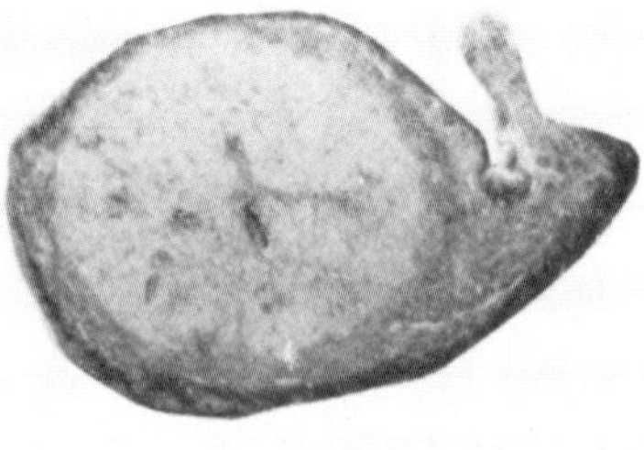

Fig. 3. Cross section of uterus from old anestrous rat. Note that lumen is closed, and general lack of estrogenic stimulation.

and in the postmenopausal state lose all follicles and ova, and become fibrotic, atrophic and unresponsive to gonadotropic hormone stimulation. Therefore loss of ovarian function is primarily responsible for cessation of menstrual cycles in aging women (Meites 1980, 1982).

There are many indications of subnormal hypothalamo-pituitary function in old non-cycling female rats. Thus there is no evidence of any cyclic surge of LH and FSH nor of a rise in estrogen secretion every 4-5 days, such as in normal cycling female rats. When old acycling female rats are ovariectomized, the increase in secretion of LH and FSH is markedly attenuated as compared to that in young ovariectomized rats. The old anestrous rats apparently show no rise at all in LH or FSH secretion after ovariectomy (Figure 4). The increase in LH secretion after ovariectomy in rats appears in the form of pulses, and it is of interest that the amplitude of these pulses is significantly lower in old than in young rats after castration.

The reduced capacity of old rats to secrete gonadotrophic hormones is due primarily to dysfunctions that develop in the hypothalamus. Sufficient LHRH has been shown to be present in the hypothalamus of old rats to induce LH and FSH release, but the hypothalamic neurotransmitters that normally regulate the release of LHRH into the pituitary portal vessels are altered during aging. The most important neurotransmitter that promotes LHRH and hence LH and FSH release is norepinephrine (NE), and its concentration and activity are significantly reduced in the hypothalamus of old rats (Figure 5). On the other hand, hypothalamic serotonin (5-HT), a neurotransmitter that under many conditions inhibits gonadotropin release, shows increased activity in old rats. We have also found that a major endogenous opiate, ß-endorphin, which inhibits LH secretion, is increased in the pituitary and circulation of old rats, and it, too, may serve to inhibit LH release (Simpkins et al 1977; Forman et al 1981).

In addition to the above changes in neurotransmitters, there also is evidence that the pituitary gland itself becomes less responsive to stimulation by LHRH in old rats. We have recently found that this is not due to loss of specific LHRH receptors in pituitary cells of old rats, but apparently is associated with internal changes within the gonadotropin secreting cells (WE Sonntag, V Hylka, J Meites, unpublished observations). There also is the possibility that the ovaries of old rats may be less responsive to gonadotrophic hormone stimulation.

Ovulation has been induced in old rats exhibiting the constant estrous syndrome by administration of LHRH or LH preparations, and resumption of estrous cycles was induced

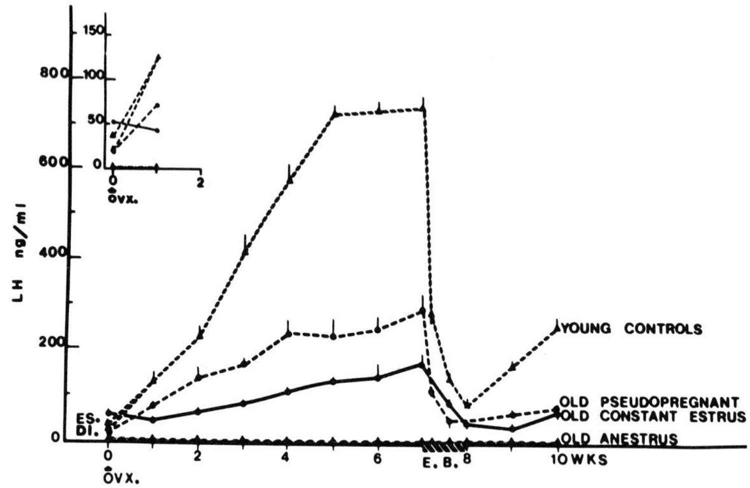

Fig. 4. Effect of ovariectomy (OVX) on LH rise in old versus young control rats. Note that the LH rise is greatest in young rats, and complete absence of LH rise in old anestrous rats. Administration of estradiol benzoate (EB) returned LH to pre-castration levels (Huang et al 1976).

by daily injection of L-dopa (Figure 6) or iproniazed, the latter a monoamine oxidase inhibitor that depresses metabolism of catecholamines (CAs) and hence increases CA activity. NE is of primary importance, since a definite role for DA in gonadotropin release is not established. Daily injection of progesterone or ACTH also are effective in reinitiating estrous cycles in old constant estrous rats, and also may act by increasing CA activity in the hypothalamus. An ergot drug, Pergolide, which is dopaminergic, has been reported to be effective in reinstating estrous cycles in old pseudopregnant rats, presumably by inhibiting prolactin secretion and thereby removing the major stimulus to progesterone secretion by the corpora lutea of these rats.

The reproductive decline in aging male rats, as in aging men, is more gradual than in female rats, and the capacity for producing offspring may remain to practically the end of life in healthy animals. Healthy elderly men in their 80's and 90's were reported to produce offspring from young wives (Harman 1983). However, both in male rats and

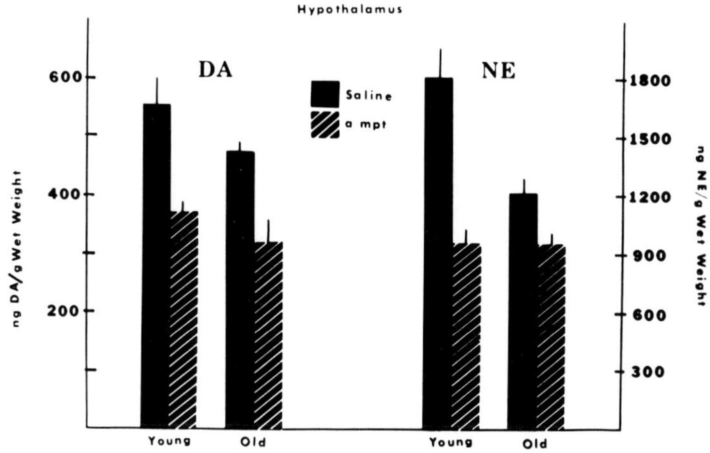

Fig. 5. Dopamine (DA) and norepinephrine (NE) concentrations and turnover in hypothalamus of old and young male rats. Female rats show similar changes with aging. Concentrations and turnover of DA and NE are lower in old rats, and are believed to mainly account for reduced LH and FSH and increased PRL secretion (Simpkins et al 1977, with permission).

men, most reports show there is a decline in testosterone secretion and sexual activity with aging, although the two are not necessarily closely associated. There is some evidence that selected healthy, middle-class, college-educated men may not show a decline in testosterone secretion with aging (Harman 1983), but these observations were based on single blood assays of testosterone. More recent work based on assays of blood testosterone throughout a 27-hour period showed there was less total testosterone in healthy old than in healthy young men (Bremner, unpublished observations).

The decline in testosterone secretion in old male rats is accompanied by a decrease in blood levels of LH and FSH (Simpkins et al 1977). As in old female rats, there is a decrease in hypothalamic NE and dopamine and an increase in serotonin activity in old male rats, as well as a diminished pituitary LH and FSH response to administration of LHRH. Thus, as in old female rats, the major cause for the reproductive decline in old male rats is due to dysfunction of the hypothalamo-pituitary unit. By contrast, in elderly

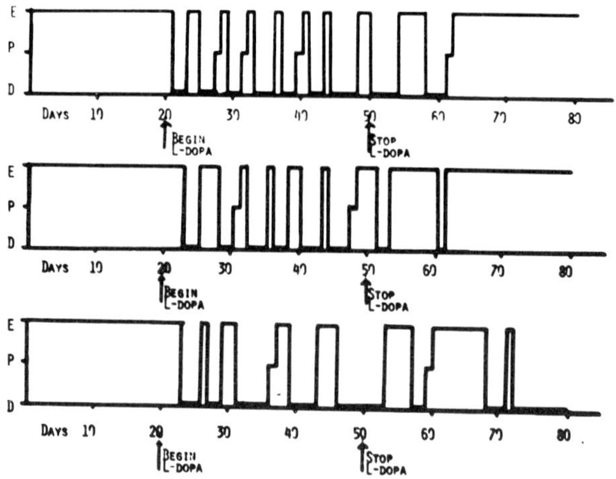

Fig. 6. Effect of twice-daily L-dopa injection in 3 individual old constant estrous rats. Note that estrous cycles returned within 48-72 hours after initiating L-dopa treatment, and that upper 2 rats returned to constant estrous state after L-dopa treatment was terminated.

human males, as in women, the reproductive decline is due mainly to faults that develop in gonadal function, resulting in decreased testosterone secretion and elevation of circulating LH and FSH levels that do not reach the even higher levels seen in postmenopausal women. There is some evidence that the pituitary LH and FSH response to gonadotrophic hormones is diminshed with age in men (Harman 1983).

PROLACTIN SECRETION AND DEVELOPMENT OF MAMMARY AND PITUITARY TUMORS

The decrease in capacity to secrete LH and FSH in old rats of both sexes is associated with a progressive increase in secretion of prolactin (PRL), which rises to greater heights in female than in male rats. The stimulus for the increase in PRL secretion comes mainly from the marked reduction in hypothalamic DA activity (Figure 5), and to a lesser extent from the increase in serotonin and perhaps also from greater opioid activity. DA is the major hypothalamic inhibitor of PRL secretion, and its decline results in elevated PRL secretion by the pituitary. We have recently observed that the major source of the DA that enters the pituitary portal vessels, namely the arcuate nucleus, shows extensive loss of dopaminergic neurons in old rats (Sarkar et al 1982, 1983). Serotonin and the endogenous opiates increase PRL secretion by indirect mechanisms, serotonin by enhancing release of PRL releasing factor (PRF) and the opiates by reducing DA and elevating serotonin activity. However, their role in the aging-related PRL increase is not clear at present. In postmenopausal women, there is a slight fall in PRL secretion, probably due to the decline in estrogen secretion, and in men there is no appreciable change in PRL secretion with age (Thorner 1977; Steger et al 1981).

The stimulus to increased PRL secretion in old female rats leads to a high incidence of spontaneous mammary and PRL-secreting pituitary tumors (prolactinomas). Prolactinomas also appear in old male rats. The mammary tumors are usually single benign fibroadenomas (Figures 7-8) that may reach an incidence of up to 80% in female Sprague-Dawley rats and up to 40% in Long-Evans rats. These mammary tumors are highly dependent on PRL secretion for their development and growth, although estrogen also is essential. We have shown that treatment of female rats that results in chronic elevation of PRL secretion, such as placing a lesion in the

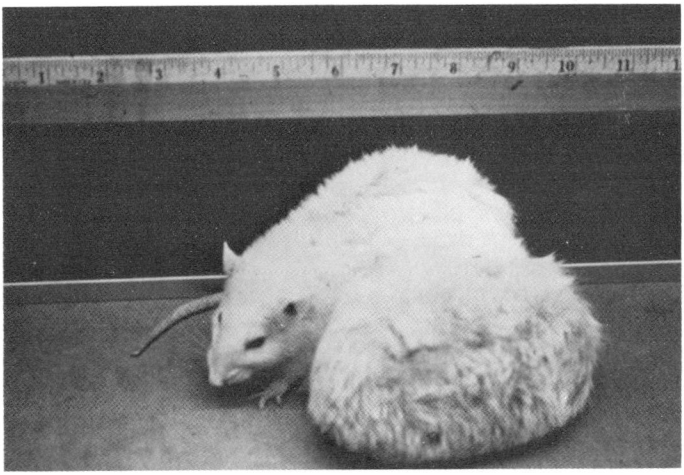

Fig. 7. Large spontaneous mammary tumor in old anestrous rat. These usually appear as a single tumor per rat.

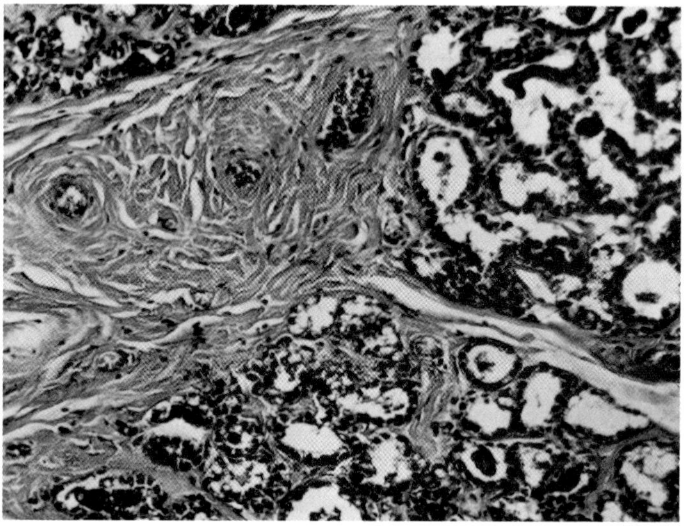

Fig. 8. Histological appearance of spontaneous mammary tumor in old female rat. Most of these tumors are benign fibroadenomas, as seen here.

median eminence to remove hypothalamic inhibition of PRL secretion, grafting of pituitaries underneath the kidney capsule, or prolonged administration of reserpine, hastens development of spontaneous mammary tumors in female rats (Welsch, Meites, 1978). On the other hand, chronic administration of L-dopa can inhibit development of mammary tumors, and induce regression of existing mammary tumors (K Quadri, J Meites, unpublished observations). In women, no definite association of PRL with development or growth of breast cancer has been demonstrated.

The incidence of pituitary tumors in old rats also is very high, particularly in rats between 2-3 years of age, and reaches 10-86% in females and a lesser percentage in males (Russfield 1966) (Figure 9). Most of these PRL-secreting tumors are stated to be chromophobic, but this is probably due to their rapid discharge of PRL granules. These prolactinomas release relatively enormous amounts of PRL, but only about 3% as much PRL is found per mg of pituitary tumor tissue as in normal rat pituitaries (Meites, Nicoll 1966). Regression of

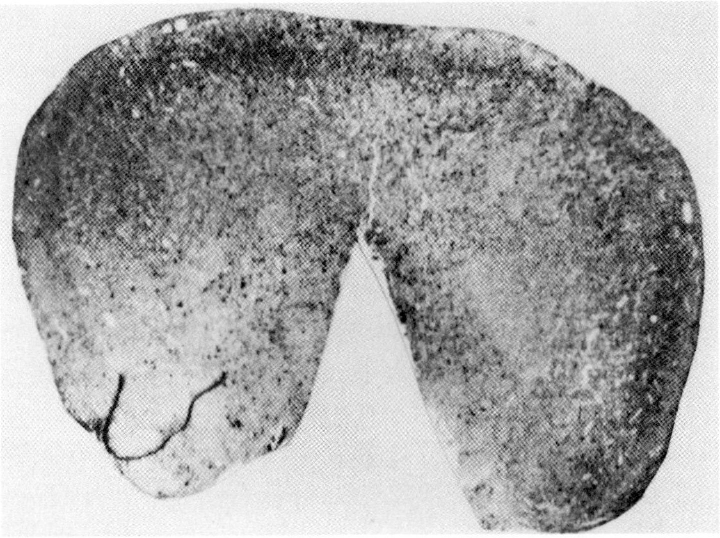

Fig. 9. Prolactinoma (anterior pituitary) in old anestrous rat.

prolactinomas and reductions in PRL release can readily be induced by administration of dopaminergic drugs (HH Huang, J Meites, unpublished observations). A transplantable rat pituitary tumor that secretes large amounts of PL and GH, the MtT.W15 tumor, was originally developed by the late Dr. Jacob Furth by prolonged estrogen treatment. This tumor was shown to regress and PRL secretion returned to normal levels after administration of a variety of ergot drugs (Quadri et al 1972). Subsequently, ergot drugs, particularly bromocryptine (Parlodel) were shown to be effective in reducing PRL secretion and inducing regression of PRL-secreting pituitary macro-adenomas in man (Post et al 1980).

Microadenomas of the pituitary, most of which are prolactinomas, were reported to show an incidence of 8-25% upon autopsy in human subjects, and these also exhibited some tendency to increase with age (Post et al 1980). There is no clear indication that prolactinomas in human subjects are associated with depressed hypothalamic DA activity, nor has it been proven that they result from prolonged exposure to estrogens, although estrogens can increase PRL secretion in man. In rats and mice, prolonged estrogen treatment can readily induce development of prolactinomas. Chronic estrogen treatment has been shown to damage dopaminergic neurons in the arcuate nucleus of rats (Brawer et al 1980). Some of the action of estrogen of DA activity may be exerted via its stimulation of PRL secretion, since chronic high circulating PRL also can damage dopaminergic neurons in the arcuate nucleus (Sarkar et al 1982).

GROWTH HORMONE AND PROTEIN SYNTHESIS

Growth hormone (GH) is the most important protein anabolic agent in the body, and is essential for protein synthesis throughout the life span of the individual. In addition to its important role in body and bone growth, it also promotes growth of the thymus and spleen, kidneys, liver, and other body tissues. It also promotes carbohydrate synthesis, and depresses fat formation. GH is believed to act by stimulating secretion of somatomedins which are produced in the liver, lungs, kidneys and other tissues. During aging in man and animals there is a decrease in protein synthesis in many body tissues (Richardson 1981; Florini, Roberts 1980), loss of bone, reduction in immunologic competency, and a decrease in kidney and liver function. In view of the recent evidence that GH secretion is reduced in aging rats and man, it is likely that this contributes importantly to the decrements in function of tissues and organs mentioned above. Before development of radioimmunoassays, we showed by bioassay that 3-5 times more GH was released by pituitary tissue from old (2 years) than from young (3-5 months) male rats when cultured _in vitro_ (Meites et al 1962).

In male rats, GH was shown to be secreted in a pulsatile manner, with about one large pulse released every 3-4 hours; each pulse rises from trough values of 25-50 ng/ml to peak values of 600 ng/ml or higher (Tannenbaum, Martin 1976). We have reported that the amplitude of GH pulses in old male rats is significantly lower than in young male rats, and that mean GH values in old rats only averaged 70.2 ± 7.6 ng/ml as against 175.3 ± 20.9 ng/ml in young rats (Sonntag et al 1980). There also is evidence that somatomedin levels in the circulation are reduced in old rats (Florini, Roberts, 1980). In elderly human subjects, there also is evidence for a decrease in GH secretion and attenuation of the nightly surge in GH release during sleep (Gregerman, Bierman 1974; Johanson, Blizzard 1981). There also is a reduction in plasma somatomedin C levels in elderly persons (Johanson, Blizzard 1981).

GH secretion is regulated by a hypothalamic growth hormone releasing factor (GRF) whose existence was first demonstrated in our laboratory (Deuben, Meites 1964) and whose structure was recently reported (Guillemin et al 1982; Thorner et al 1983), and by a GH release inhibiting factor (GIF or somatostatin) whose existence was first reported in 1968 (Krulich et al 1968) and whose structure was determined in 1973 (Brazeau et al 1973). We have reported indirect evidence indicating that more somatostatin is released by the hypothalamus of old than young rats (Sonntag et al 1981). In addition, several neurotransmitters, particularly NE and to a lesser degree, DA, promote GH release in rats and man, probably by stimulating release of GRF. Serotonin and acetylcholine also may increase GH secretion. In view of the decrease in both hypothalamic DA and NE previously demonstrated in old rats (Simpkins et al 1977), it seems likely that this constitutes the principal cause for the decrease in GH secretion in old male rats. Recently, we injected L-dopa, the precursor of DA and NE, twice daily into old male rats, and observed that this returned GH pulses to the same levels found in young male rats (Sonntag et al 1981). In elderly human subjects, there also is considerable evidence for a decrease in catecholamine concentration in the brain, including the hypothalamus (Robinson et al 1972), and this may contribute to the reduction in GH secretion. In addition we have recently found that human pancreatic GRF (1-44) has only about half as much ability to induce GH release *in vivo* in old as in young male rats, which would also contribute to reduced GH release in old rats (WE Sonntag, V Hylka, J Meites, unpublished observations).

The extent to which the decrease in GH secretion during aging is responsible for the age-related reduction in protein synthesis, loss of bone, decrease in immunologic, kidney or liver function, is unknown at present. We have recently compared protein synthesis in the diaphragm muscle of old and young male rats by measuring incorporation of ^{3}H-phenylalanine after correcting for pool size, and found it to be significantly lower in old male rats; injection of bovine GH into old male rats significantly increased incorporation of ^{3}H-phenylalanine in old male rats (WE Sonntag, V Hylka, J Meites, unpublished observations). We have also observed that daily injection of bovine GH into old rats significantly increased the weights of the kidneys, liver, spleen and heart of old male rats (LJ Forman, WE Sonntag, J Meites, unpublished observations). Probably part of this increase was in the form of protein.

CONCLUSIONS

Our studies clearly show that in aging female and male rats, there is a decrease in secretion of LH, FSH, estrogen, testosterone, and GH, and an increase in secretion of PRL. These changes in pituitary hormone secretion are due primarily to alterations in hypothalamo-pituitary function, of which the decrease in hypothalamic DA and NE concentrations and activities appear to be the most prominent features. These reductions in DA and NE may be due to loss of catecholaminergic neurons, a possible decrease in the enzymes that synthesize DA and NE, and a possible increase in the enzymes that metabolize these neurotransmitters. The decrease in NE is believed to result in reduced LHRH and GRF release from hypothalamus, leading in turn to lower LH, FSH and GH secretion, and the decrease in DA release leads directly to increased PRL secretion by the pituitary. Other neurotransmitters also may influence secretion of these pituitary hormones. There also is evidence for a lower pituitary responsiveness in old rats to LHRH and GRF. All of these changes in pituitary hormone secretion in old rats can be reversed by administration of L-dopa or other drugs that increase catecholamines in the brain generally and particularly in the hypothalamus.

Cessation of estrous cycles in old female rats, the decrease in testosterone secretion in old male rats, development of numerous mammary and pituitary tumors, and the decrease in GH secretion and its probably detrimental effects on protein synthesis and other body functions, are all consequences of the alterations in hypothalamic-pituitary activity during aging. It is clear that most of these aging changes in rats can be delayed or reversed by appropriate neuroendocrine intervention. What is not yet clear is the duration in time during which these changes can be prevented or reversed in aging rats. Chronic L-dopa treatment was reported to approximately double the life span of mice (Cotzias et al 1974, 1977), and chronic reduction in food intake was shown to approximately double the life span of rats (McCay et al 1943). All of these experimental studies in laboratory animals suggest possibilities for improving the quality of life during old age as well as extending life duration.

In the human species, much less is known about the function of the neuroendocrine system during aging and its relations to aging processes in the body than in rats and mice. This is not surprising since clinical studies on human subjects often follow leads generated by studies on animal models, and most of the information from animal studies on the neuroendocrinology of aging has been forthcoming only in the last 10-15 years. The reduced incidence of cardiovascular diseases and improved treatments for cancer in man should render the role of the neuroendocrine system in aging processes of even greater importance than in the past, and improve the possibilities for favorable neuroendocrine intervention. This should offer challenges as well as opportunities for research-oriented gerontologists.

ACKNOWLEDGEMENTS

The research from our laboratory was supported in part by NIH grant AG00416 from the National Institute on Aging. The work reported here was done in collaboration with HH Huang, J Simpkins, J Bruni, R Steger, W Sonntag, L Forman, D Sarkar, P Gottschall, V Hylka, K Quadri, J Lu, and JA Clemens.

REFERENCES

Brawer JR, Schipper H, Naftolin F (1980). Ovary-dependent degeneration in the hypothalamic arcuate nucleus. Endocrinology 107:274.

Brazeau P, Vale W, Burgus R, Ling N, Butcher M, Rivier J, Guillemin R (1973). Hypothalamic polypeptide that inhibits the secretion of immunoreactive pituitary growth hormone. Science 179:77.

Brown-Séquard CE (1889). Des effets produits chez l'homme par des injections sous-cutanées d'un liquide retiré des testicules frais de cobaye et de chien. CR Seances Soc Biol, Ser 9, 1:415.

Cotzias CC, Miller ST, Nicholson AR, Maston WM, Tong LC (1974). Prolongation of the lifespan in mice adapted to large amounts of L-dopa. Proc Natl Acad Sci USA 7:2466.

Cotzias CC, Miller ST, Tong LC, Papavisoliou PS, Wang YY

(1977). Levadopa, fertility and longevity. Science 196:549.

Deuben RR, Meites J (1964). Stimulation of pituitary growth hormone release by a hypothalamic extract _in vitro_. Endocrinology 74:408.

Florini JR, Roberts SB (1980). Effects of rat age on blood levels of somatomedin-like growth factors. J Gerontol 35:23.

Forman LJ, Sonntag WE, Van Vugt DA, Meites J (1981). Immunoreactive ß-endorphin in the plasma, pituitary and hypothalamus of young and old rats. Neurobiol Aging 2:281.

Gregerman RI, Bierman EL (1974). Aging and hormones. In Williams RH (ed): "Textbook of Endocrinology," 5th ed, Philadelphia: Saunders, p 1059.

Guillemin R, Brazeau P, Bohlen P, Esch F, Ling N, Wehrenberg W (1982). Growth hormone releasing factor from a human pancreatic tumor that caused acromegaly. Science 218:585.

Harman SM (1983). Relation of the neuroendocrine system to the reproductive decline in men. In Meites J (ed): "Neuroendocrinology of Aging," New York: Plenum, p 203.

Huang HH, Marshall S, Meites J (1976). Capacity of old versus young female rats to secrete LH, FSH and prolactin. Biol Reprod 14:538.

Johanson AJ, Blizzard RM (1981). Low somatomedin-C levels in older men rise in response to growth hormone administration. Johns Hopkins Med J 149:115.

Krulich K, Dhariwal APS, McCann SM (1968). Stimulatory and inhibitory effects of purified hypothalamic extracts on growth hormone release from rat pituitary _in vitro_. Endocrinology 83:783.

McCay CM, Sperling G, Barnes LL (1943). Growth, aging, chronic diseases, and life span in rats. Arch Biochem 2:481.

Meites J (1980). Decline in reproductive function with age in humans and rats. In Dietz AA (ed): "Aging--Its Chemistry," Washington, D.C.: Am Assoc Clin Chem, p 82.

Meites J (1982). Changes in neuroendocrine control of anterior pituitary function during aging. Neuroendocrinology 34:51.

Meites J, Hopkins TF, Deuben R (1962). Growth hormone production by rat pituitary _in vitro_. Fed Proc 21:96.

Meites, J, Nicoll CS (1966). Adenohypophysis: Prolactin. Annu Rev Physiol 28:57.

Post KD, Jackson KMD, Reichlin S (1980). "The Pituitary Adenoma." New York: Plenum.

Quadri SK, Lu KH, Meites J (1972). Ergot-induced inhibition of pituitary tumor growth in rats. Science 176:417.

Richardson A (1981). The relationship between aging and protein synthesis. In Florini JR (ed): "Handbook of

Biochemistry in Aging," Boca Raton, Florida: CRC Press, p 79.
Robinson DS, Nies A, Davis J, Bunney WE, Davis JM, Colburn RW, Bourne HR, Shaw DM, Coppen AJ (1972). Aging, monoamines and monoamine oxidase levels. Lancet I:290.
Russfield AB (1966). "Tumors of Endocrine Glands and Secondary Sex Organs." Washington, D.C.: US Government Printing Office, p 3.
Sarkar DK, Gottschall PE, Meites J (1982). Damage to hypothalamic dopaminergic neurons is associated with development of prolactin-secreting pituitary tumors. Science 218:684.
Sarkar DK, Gottschall PE, Meites J (1983). Relation of the neuroendocrine system to development of prolactin-secreting pituitary tumors. In Meites J (ed): "Neuroendocrinology of Aging," New York: Plenum, p 353.
Simpkins JW, Mueller GP, Huang HH, Meites J (1977). Evidence for depressed catecholamine and enhanced serotonin metabolism in aging male rats: Possible relation to gonadotropin secretion. Endocrinology 100:1672.
Sonntag WE, Forman, LJ, Miki N, Steger RW, Ramos T, Arimura A, Meites J (1981). Effects of CNS active drugs and somatostatin antiserum on growth hormone release in young and old male rats. Neuroendocrinology 33:73.
Sonntag WE, Steger RW, Forman LJ, Meites J (1980). Decreased pulsatile release of growth hormone in old male rats. Endocrinology 107:1875.
Steger RW, Huang HH, Meites J (1981). Reproduction. In Masaro EJ (ed): "Handbook of Physiology of Aging," Boca Raton, Florida: CRC Press, p 333.
Tannenbaum GS, Martin JB (1976). Evidence for an endogenous ultradian rhythm governing growth hormone secretion in the rat. Endocrinology 98:562.
Thorner MO (1977). Prolactin: Clinical physiology and the significance and management of hyperprolactinemia. In Martini L, Besser GM (eds): "Clinical Neuroendocrinology," New York: Academic Press, p 320.
Thorner MO, Spiess J, Vance MC, Rogol HD, Kaiser DL, Webster JD, Rivier J, Borges JL, Bloom SR, Cronin MJ, Evans WS, MacLeod RM, Vale W (1983). Human pancreatic growth-hormone-releasing factor selectively stimulates growth hormone secretion in man. Lancet I:24.
Verzar F (1966). Anterior pituitary function in age. In Harris GW, Donovan BT (eds): "The Pituitary Gland," Berkeley, California: University of California Press, p 444.
Welsch CW, Meites J (1978). Prolactin and mammary carcino-

genesis. In Sharma RK, Criss WE (eds): "Endocrine Control in Neoplasia," New York: Raven Press, p 71.

DISCUSSION

DR. RAISZ: I won't ask the question about the paradox that hypophysectomy and hypophysial stimulation both prolong life, but I will ask a different one. If beta-endorphin levels go up, isn't that another paradox in relation to ACTH response? Beta-endorphin is presumably cosecreted with ACTH. What happens to ACTH levels?

DR. MEITES: In our work we don't find any significant change in basal ACTH and corticosterone levels with age in the rat, but beta-endorphin levels are higher in old rats. Now, it is not necessarily true that both ACTH and beta-endorphin release have to go up or down together even though they are both produced by the pituitary gland. What I showed was the effect of corticotropin releasing factor (CRF) administration on pituitary release of ACTH and beta-endorphin in old and young male rats. We found that the pituitary of old rats is less responsive to CRF, and actually also is less responsive to growth hormone releasing factor (GRF), gonadotropin releasing hormone (GnRH), thyrotropin releasing hormone (TRH). So it is not only the hypothalamus that changes with aging but the pituitary response as well.

DR. TERRY: Where are the cell bodies which elaborate the enzymes which elaborate the dopamine and norepinephrine in the hypothalamus, and have these cells been counted?

DR. MEITES: The dopamine that inhibits prolactin secretion comes mainly from the arcuate nucleus, and norepinephrine from the lateral tegmental brain stem neurons and locus ceruleus. Dr. Peng has reported that in the preoptic area of old rats the cell count is reduced. This is the area in the rat, incidentally, that is very much involved with release of gonadotropins via LHRH. There also is evidence that neurons in the arcuate nucleus and locus ceruleus are lost with aging. What was your other question?

DR. TERRY: If these are intrinsic neurons within the hypothalamus, I know that in the Fischer rat they are significantly reduced, and so again, we find that it is not the secondary or tertiary product, as in this case the hormones, but rather cell numbers, cell death, which is producing the alteration.

DR. MEITES: There is also evidence that hormone receptors in the brain and in the hypothalamus of old rats are reduced. As far as the neurotransmitters are concerned, particularly the catecholamines, there is evidence that tyrosine hydroxylase, which is the rate-limiting enzyme for catecholamines, is reduced in the brains of both rats and human beings. Also the major enzyme that is concerned with the metabolism of catecholamines, monoamine oxidase, is reported to be increased. Thus there may be many causes for the changes in neurotransmitters with aging in the brain.

DR. LANDFIELD: As you know, we consistently find elevated corticosterone, and apparently ACTH, although that is less clear, in aged Fischer rats; and, of course, Wexler found similar results in Sprague-Dawley rats. Although you are working with the Long-Evans strain, and strain differences may be involved in the discrepant results, it also seems important to keep in mind how these hormonal responses are studied. For example, as you emphasized, your results on ACTH are limited to CRF stimulation conditions. If we anesthetize the animals we don't find an age-related rise in corticosterone. However, if we measure the response to stress in unanesthetized rats or under spontaneous resting levels, corticosterone is clearly elevated in aging rats. So the conditions under which these hormones are measured are of course very important.

The other point I want to make is that pituitary weight also needs to be taken into account. In the Fischer rat, pituitary weight is up with age which could account for quite a few of these hormonal changes during aging. Certainly, adrenal gland weight is up in the Fischer rat, and this is probably the basis for the elevated glucocorticoids in that strain. I also wanted to note that in humans the ACTH response to surgery or to metyrapone appears to be at least unchanged and possibly elevated with aging. Since the adrenal system appears potentially very important to age-related pathology, based on the Robertson and Wexler work in the Pacific salmon, and on other studies, it seems useful to clarify the sampling conditions and strain differences that may account for different results.

DR. MEITES: Yes. As far as weight of the pituitary is

concerned, in all the rat strains with which we have worked, namely the Sprague-Dawley, Long-Evans and Wistar strains, the pituitary weights are increased with aging.

Now, as far as ACTH and adrenocortical secretion in old rats and humans and many other species are concerned, I don't know any other hormones for which there are so many contradictory reports. You can find anything you want in the literature, evidence for increases in these hormones, decreases, no changes. We just have to work a little harder to try to clarify this situation.

DR. ROBINSON: Thank you, Dr. Meites, for an excellent presentation. I would like to bring to your attention some experiments I have done recently on some old male monkeys, in which we gave GnRH to stimulate the pituitary testicular axis. When we measured the testosterone in the old animals it was reduced, just like in the human population. We also measured the LH output by the pituitary using radioimmunoassay (RIA) and found it to be the same. But because we use a heterologous assay system for LH, we also decided to do bioassays for LH. What we found was that the LH molecule being secreted by the pituitary appeared to be somewhat different in these aged animals. The biological activity of the LH in the older animals was lower than that in the younger animals based on the rat interstitial bioassay system.

DR. MEITES: Thank you. I think these are very interesting results. Harman at the Gerontology Research Center in Baltimore recently reported that after administration of the LHRH peptide in several different age groups of men, the older men did show a decreased response with less LH and FSH released.

Comparative Pathobiology of Major Age-Related Diseases: Current Status and Research Frontiers, pages 109–125

AGE AND THE ENDOCRINE PANCREAS: EFFECT OF OBESITY

Eve P. Reaven, Ph.D., Donald L. Curry, M.D., and Gerald M. Reaven, M.D.

Geriatric Research, Education and Clinical Center Veterans Administration Medical Center, Palo Alto, CA 94304, and Department of Physiological Sciences, University of California, Davis, CA 95616

INTRODUCTION

Evidence from in vitro experiments involving either collagenase-isolated islets (Reaven et al 1979, 1983b; Kitahara, Adelman 1979; Reaven, Reaven 1981; Lipson et al 1981) or the intact perfused pancreas (Reaven et al 1983a) of rats of different ages suggests that there is a substantial decline in beta cell glucose-stimulated insulin release as rats age. The decrease in the beta cell response is progressive with age, decreasing with each 6-month interval examined (Reaven et al 1979). It has been observed in Sprague-Dawley rats at 6, 12, and 18 months of age (Reaven et al 1979) and in Fischer rats at 6 and 12 months of age (DL Curry, GM Reaven, EP Reaven, unpublished observations). It occurs in obese and in nonobese aging rats, alike (Reaven et al 1983a). Indeed, the seemingly ubiquitous nature of this finding has led us to suggest that the decline in beta cell function (in rats) may be an inevitable function of aging (Reaven et al 1983a).

Given this possibility (i.e., the irrevocable reduction of beta cell function with age), one must ask what impact such a state of affairs would have on the animal as a whole. The correct answer to this question will, no doubt, vary depending on the age of the animal and the environmental conditions under which he lives. For example, we have found that one variable, obesity, has an enormous impact on the rat, specifically as it influences the morphology of the endocrine pancreas when the animal enters middle age.

In this report we will summarize our findings on the endocrine pancreas of the aging obese rat, and will view the changes from the perspective of how structural changes in the encodrine pancreas contribute to the ability of the rats to secrete insulin. We will, at the end, make certain predictions as to the effect of further aging on such animals and discuss what relevance these findings may hold for human disease.

METHODS

In these studies, male, Sprague-Dawley rats were obtained from Charles River Breeding Laboratories at 40 days of age and were subsequently maintained in our facilities at 72-76°F until they were 12 months old. The rats were fed either pelleted standard laboratory chow (Ralston Purina, St. Louis, MO) *ad libitum*, or a calorie-restricted pelleted diet comprised of 1 part chow and 2 parts alpha cellulose (Teklad Industries, Madison, WI). The average body weight of the chow-fed rats at 12 months of age was ∿ 800 grams, whereas the calorie-restricted animals, of the same age, weighed approximately 300 grams less (Reaven et al 1983a).

When the rats reached 12 months of age, studies were carried out on the isolated pancreas of each animal to determine maximal glucose-stimulated insulin secretion (Reaven et al 1983a). At the conclusion of the secretory study, each pancreas was perfusion-fixed with 10% buffered formalin and processed for morphological studies (Reaven et al 1983a). For comparison, young male Sprague-Dawley rats weighing ∿ 250 g were directly obtained from the original breeder (Charles River Labs.) and studied in an identical fashion. Pancreas weights (Reaven et al 1983a) were obtained from additional rats of all three experimental groups.

The splenic region of each formalin-fixed pancreas was subsequently divided into horizontal slices, processed by standard techniques and embedded in paraffin for (1) hematoxylin-eosin or Masson's trichrome stains, or (2) immunocytochemical staining of insulin, glucagon and somatostatin. The latter was carried out with the use of immunostaining kits (Immulok, Carpenteria, CA).

For electron microscopy, pancreases of rats from the three experimental groups were perfused with glutaraldehyde (2% in 0.1 M cacodylate buffer) and prepared as previously described from this laboratory (Reaven et al 1979, 1983a). Observations were made on specimens taken only from the splenic region of the tissue.

All morphometric measurements were made using a point-counting grid method as previously described from this laboratory (Reaven et al 1983a). Measurements of islet content (per pancreas) were carried out at a magnification of 400x: estimations of islet composition, (e.g., percent connective tissue per islet, or percent insulin or glucagon-staining cells per islet) were carried out at a magnification of 800x on 50-80 islets from pancreas slices of each of four rats from each category.

RESULTS AND DISCUSSION

The pattern of pancreatic insulin secretion is qualitatively similar in all three groups of rats (Reaven et al 1983a), i.e., young rats and aging nonobese and aging obese rats show a sharp first phase insulin release and a more sustained second phase of release. Figure 1 indicates,

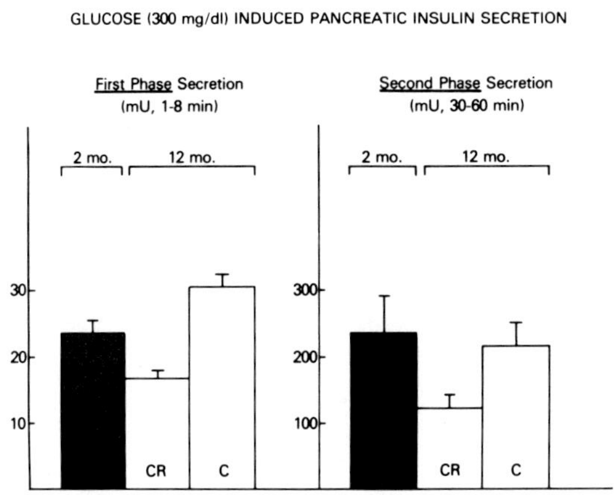

Fig. 1 First phase (1-8 min) and second phase (30-60 min) insulin release from perfused pancreases of 2-month-old (black bars) and 12-month-old nonobese, calorie-restricted (CR) and 12-month-old, obese, chow-fed (C) rats.

however, that quantitative differences exist between the groups. Thus, in both first and second phase release, aging obese rats secrete as much insulin as young animals--whereas aging, nonobese (calorie restricted) rats secrete less. However, in order to fully understand the effect of age on beta cell function, certain other considerations must be taken into account.

In the first place, there is quite a difference in the size and shape of the average islet from the two different groups of aging animals, as illustrated in the hematoxylin and eosin-stained sections of Figures 2 and 3. Islets of aging nonobese rats (Figure 2) generally resemble those of young rats, whereas many (approximately 50%) of the islets of aging obese rats appear to be enlarged, multilobulated and fibrotic (Figure 3). These observations on differences in size of the islets from the nonobese and obese animals have been quantified previously in collagenase-isolated islets (Reaven et al 1983b). The results show that the connective-tissue corrected volume of the average islet of an obese 12-month-old Sprague-Dawley rat is approximately double that of its calorically restricted, nonobese litter mate (and double the values of islets from young animals as well). Estimates of the connective tissue content of the various islets were obtained from sections of perfusion-

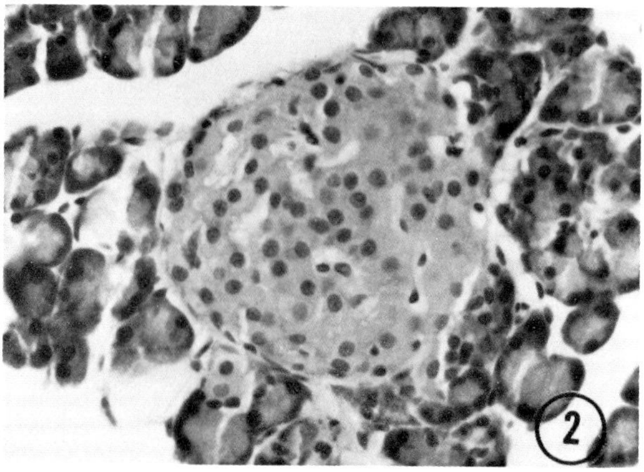

Fig. 2. Typical medium-sized islet from a nonobese, 12-month-old rat. H & E stain. X235.

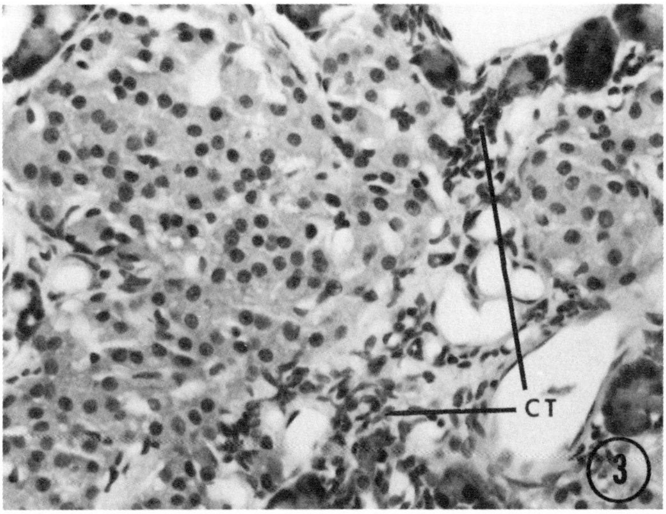

Fig. 3. Portion of enlarged, multilobulated, fibrotic islet typical of islets from obese, 12-month-old rats. Connective tissue (CT) infiltration of such islets is indicated. H & E stain. X235.

fixed pancreases of similar animals (Reaven et al 1983a), and suggest that the average islets from young rats have less than 5% of their volume composed of connective tissue (visualized by Masson's stain). In contrast, as much as 12% of the islets of nonobese 12-month-old rats and 25% of islets of obese rats may be composed of connective tissue. It is important to note, however, that even when corrected for these differences in islet connective tissue, the islets of the obese rat are still substantially larger than islets of the nonobese animal, and these differences are reflected in the fact that there is more endocrine tissue (per volume pancreas) in the aging obese animals than in the equally old nonobese animals (Reaven et al 1983a).

In addition to these changes in islet size and content within the pancreas, we have recently observed changes in the endocrine cell composition of the islets from obese rats. In Figure 4 we show a typical islet from a calorie-restricted, 12-month-old rat stained immunocytochemically for glucagon. The distribution of glucagon-producing cells (alpha cells) in

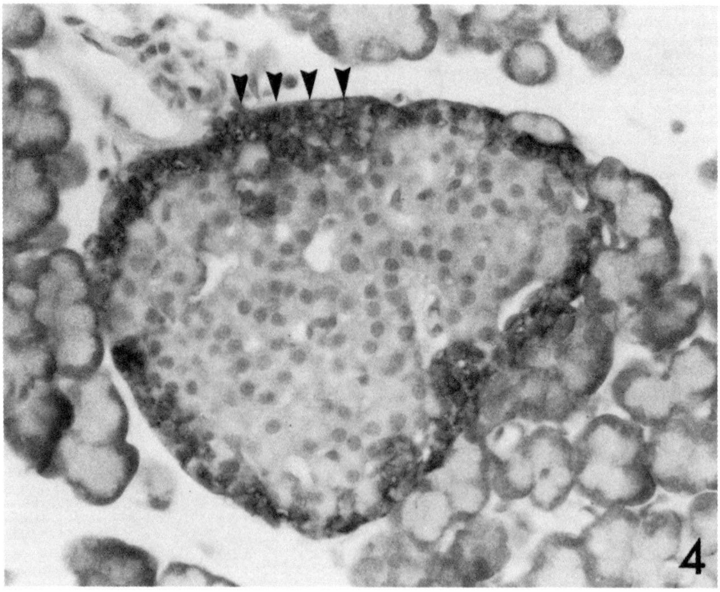

Fig. 4. Immunochemical stain typical for glucagon-producing cells (alpha cells) of islets of nonobese, 12-month-old rats. The pattern of staining (dark cells around rim of islet, see arrowheads) is identical to that found in islets of young rats (Orci, Unger 1975). X235.

these islets is similar to that found in young rats (Orci, Unger 1975); typically, as seen in Figure 4, alpha cells form a ring on the periphery of each islet. However, alpha cells in the enlarged, multilobulated islets of obese 12-month-old rats have a different distribution. Figure 5 illustrates the fact that very few alpha cells are found in such islets overall and, in general, one sees only an occasional cell in the periphery of most of these islets. However, in some enlarged islets, alpha cells seem to form cords radiating from the body of the islet (data not shown). Our preliminary estimates indicate that when all alpha cells are accounted for, they form 20-25 percent of the islets of the calorie-restricted animal and less than 10 percent (overall) of the islets of the obese rats. Somatostatin-producing cells appear to form only a minor (∿2%) proportion of the endocrine cells of the islet and their distribution appears similar in the islets of

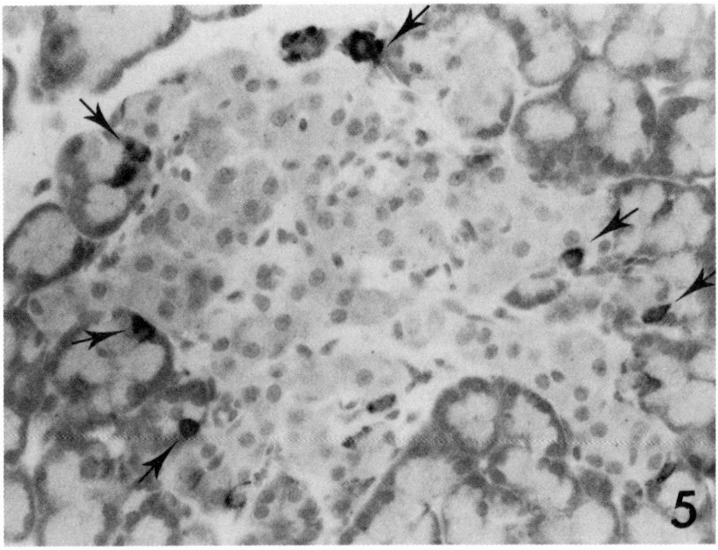

Fig. 5. Immunochemical stain typical for glucagon-producing cells (alpha cells) of the pleomorphic islets of 12-month-old, obese rats. Few alpha cells (arrows) are found in such islets and their location is erratic (see text). X235.

nonobese and obese animals. The impact of this reorganization of the islets is that the ratio of beta to alpha cells is increased in the islets of the obese animals and, as a result, the proportion of the pancreas volume (of the aging obese rat) occupied by beta cells, is even greater than previously estimated (Reaven et al 1983a).

In light of the above considerations, it is apparent that meaningful estimates of the effect of age on insulin secretory capacity depend upon accurate quantification of beta cell pool size. This was done for the pancreases of the rats used for the perfusion studies summarized in Figure 1, and these data are seen in Figure 6. The percent of the pancreas volume occupied by beta cell volume, for young rats, 12-month-old calorie-restricted nonobese rats, and 12-month-old chow fed, obese rats is presented in the left panel of Figure 6. When the figures in this column are multiplied by the total size of the average pancreas [expressed in the second panel as dry weight (Reaven et al 1983a)] for the rats of each

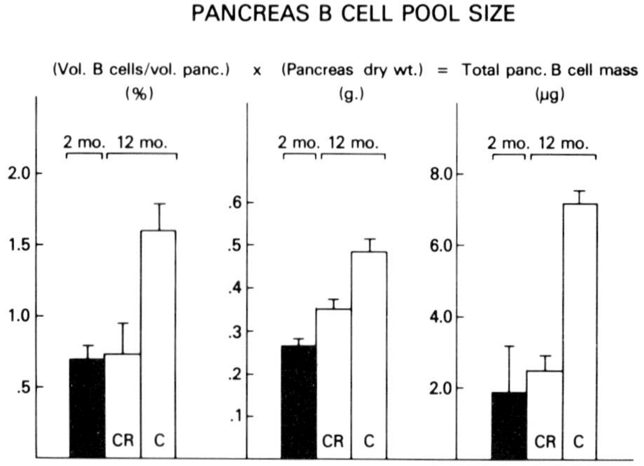

Fig. 6. Estimate of pancreas beta cell pool size for 2-month-old rats and 12-month-old nonobese and obese rats. (Percent beta cell volume per volume pancreas) x (pancreas mass) = beta cell mass per pancreas.

category, one obtains a figure for total beta cell mass per pancreas (right panel). This calculation suggests that the beta cell pool of the obese animal is ∿ 4 times that of young animals and more than 3 times that of its nonobese litter mate. As a result, when insulin secretion from the pancreas is expressed per beta cell per pancreas, it becomes clear that secretion per unit beta cell is equally (and severely) depressed in both obese and nonobese 12-month-old rats (Figure 7).

We have previously suggested that the obese animal (in contrast to the nonobese rat), is forced to compensate for the loss of beta cell insulin secretion by beta cell proliferation, since such an animal has lost peripheral tissue sensitivity to insulin (Reaven et al 1983b) and requires increased amounts of insulin to be secreted on a daily basis. Although the data shown here suggest that the obese animal successfully accomplishes this feat, it must be recognized that he does this at the expense of an abnormal-appearing endocrine pancreas.

It is of some interest to know whether this type of compensatory proliferation of beta cells can proceed indefi-

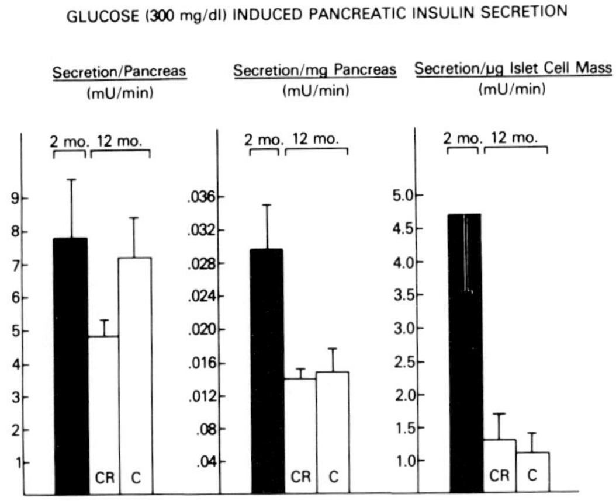

Fig. 7. Insulin release from the pancreas of 2-month-old rats (black bars) and 12-month-old nonobese (CR) and obese (C) rats expressed per pancreas, per pancreas weight, and per unit islet cell mass. Insulin secretion per pancreas (first panel) was based on steady-state (30-60 min) second phase values for insulin release (see Reaven et al 1983a; also Figure 1); insulin secretion per mg pancreas (second panel) represents the values from panel 1 divided by the averaged dry weight (see Reaven et al 1983a; also Figure 6) of pancreases from animals of each experimental category; insulin secretion per islet cell mass (panel 3) represents the values from panel 1 divided by estimated islet cell mass of pancreases from animals of each experimental category (see Reaven et al 1983a). Permission from John Libbey & Co.

nitely. Were this to be the case, then the loss of beta cell function with aging would be of academic interest only. On-going experiments in our laboratory on animals aging to 2 years, may ultimately provide some answers to this question. At the moment, however, we would predict that the capacity for the endocrine pancreas to compensate may have limits. Electron microscopic examination of the pleomorphic islets of the aging, obese animals shows that fragile, damaged and/or dead beta cells, such as seen in Figure 8B, occur in such islets with substantially greater frequency than in islets of the equally old, nonobese rats (Figure 8A). Although we have no way of demonstrating that the dual stress (of loss of beta cell function and loss of peripheral insulin sensitivity)

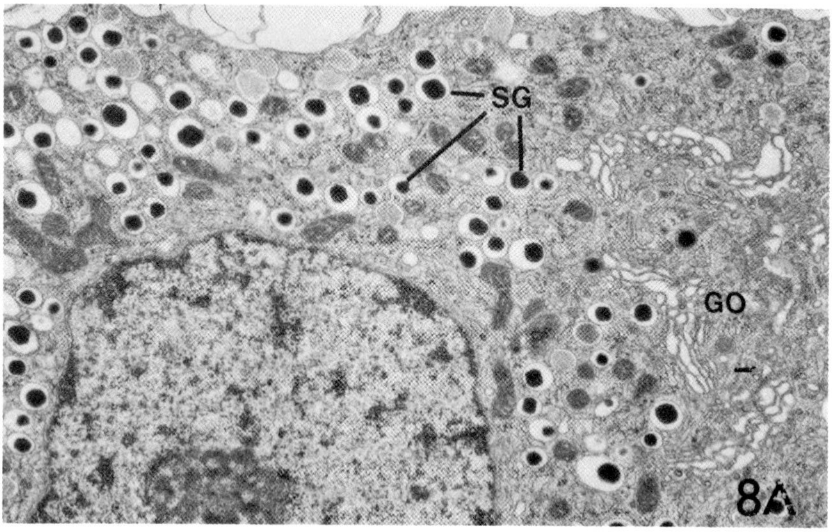

Fig. 8A. (See legend next page)

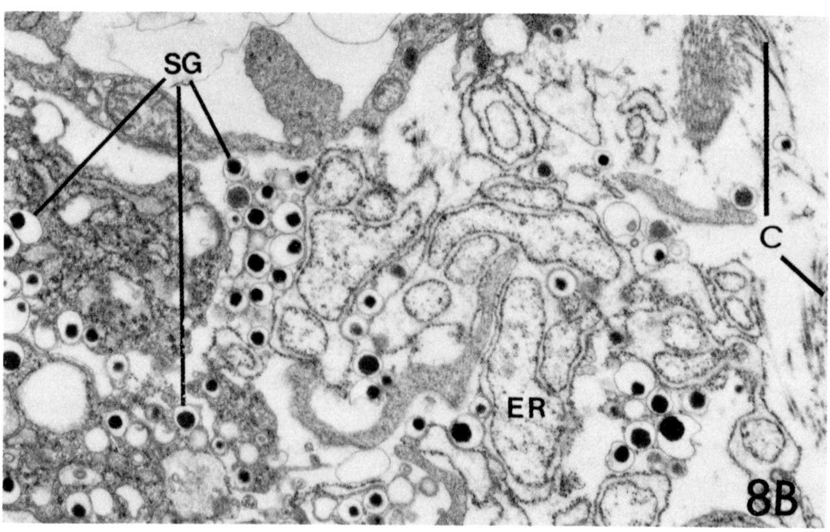

Fig. 8B. (See legend next page)

Fig. 8. Representative electron micrographs of portions of beta cells from 12-month-old nonobese rats (8A) and obese rats (8B). Qualitatively, beta cells from nonobese rats are similar to beta cells from islets of young rats: i.e., the relationships between intracellular organelles such as Golgi (GO) complexes, secretory granules (SG), etc., appear normal. In the enlarged, multilobulated, and fibrotic islets of obese rats, damaged beta cells, as in Figure 8B, are found with increased frequency. After perfusion-fixation, such cells appear to have lost their plasma membranes and show collagen fibrils (C) mixed with intracellular organelles such as secretory granules (SG), swollen endoplasmic reticulum (ER), etc. X12,000.

---

contributes to these changes and causes 'exhaustion,' and possibly death of beta cells, such a theory would be consistent with the findings and, at the same time, provide an explanation for the extensive fibrosis found in islets of the obese animals. One question which awaits additional information is whether the extent of such damage to the endocrine pancreas in the rat would ever be sufficient to produce overt hyperglycemia and diabetes mellitus.

Given these various knowns and unknowns, what can we say about the relevance of these events to human disease? Clearly we can only speculate on possibilities. There is evidence in man that insulin sensitivity (insulin-stimulated glucose uptake of peripheral tissues) declines with age (DeFronzo 1979; Rosenthal et al 1982). However, this insulin resistance is modest in magnitude when differences in degree of obesity are taken into account (Rosenthal et al 1982). We don't know whether beta cell function declines with age in man, nor do we know how successfully beta cells proliferate in humans. [It is of interest, in this regard, that beta cell proliferation appears to be a species-determined event, and that although it is active in rats, it does not occur in dogs and cats (see Gepts 1981).] Were both these problems to occur (i.e., loss of beta cell function and inability to replace beta cells with age), then one could imagine that the stage might be set for some individuals--who are insulin resistant, and who have for some reason sustained more loss of beta cell reserve than others--to become diabetic as they age.

CONCLUSION

These remarks can be summarized as in Figure 9. We believe that aging in rats has a profound effect on beta cell function. The impact of this on the endocrine pancreas depends to a large extent on whether or not peripheral tissues of the animal remain sensitive to the action of insulin. In the 12-month-old insulin-sensitive, nonobese animal with moderate insulin requirements, the impact of aging on the endocrine pancreas is minimal. In contrast, in the 12-month-old insulin-insensitive, obese rat with increased insulin requirements, there is extensive enlargement of the pancreatic beta cell pool, as a result of beta cell proliferation. The consequences of this event are pleomorphic, fibrotic islets with a substantial increase in fragile and/or damaged beta cells. Whether increased aging and continued high insulin demands will sufficiently exacerbate the situation, to lead to decompensation of the endocrine pancreas and development of diabetes mellitus in the obese rat, remains to be seen.

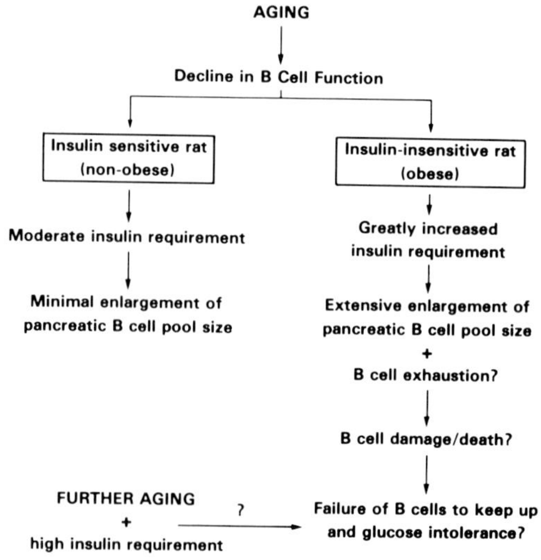

Fig. 9. Schematic representation of the effect of aging on the endocrine pancreas of the rat (B = beta cell).

REFERENCES

DeFronzo RA (1979). Glucose intolerance and aging. Evidence of tissue insensitivity to insulin. Diabetes 28:1095.

Gepts W (1981). Islet changes in human diabetes. In Cooperstein SJ, Watkins D (eds): "The Islets of Langerhans," New York: Academic Press, p 321.

Kitahara A, Adelman S (1979). Altered regulation of insulin secretion in isolated islets of different sizes in aging rats. Biochem Biophys Res Comm 87:1207

Lipson LG, Bobrycki VA, Bush MJ, Tietjan GE, Yoon A (1981). Insulin release in aging studies on adenylate cyclase, phosphodiesterase and protein kinase in isolated islets of Langerhans. Endocrinology 108:620.

Orci L, Unger RH (1975). Functional subdivision of islets of Langerhans and possible role of D cells. Lancet II:1243.

Reaven E, Curry D, Moore J, Reaven G (1983a). Effect of age and environmental factors on insulin release from the perfused pancreas of the rat. J Clin Invest 71:345.

Reaven EP, Gold G, Reaven GM (1979). Effect of age on glucose-stimulated insulin release by the ß-cell of the rat. J Clin Invest 64:591.

Reaven EP, Reaven GM (1981). Structure and function changes in the endocrine pancreas of aging rats with reference to the modulating effects of exercise and calorie restriction. J Clin Invest 68:75.

Reaven E, Wright D, Mondon CE, Solomon R, Ho H, Reaven GM (1983b). Effect of age and diet on insulin secretion and insulin action in the rat. Diabetes 32:175.

Rosenthal M, Doberne L, Greenfield M, Widstrom A, Reaven GM (1982). Effect of age on glucose tolerance, insulin secretion, and in vivo insulin action. J Am Geriatr Soc 30:562.

DISCUSSION

DR. SCARPELLI: Has anyone looked at the cytoskeleton in the beta cells of the older obese animals, since apparently the process of insulin secretion occurs by emiocytosis? Is it conceivable that there may be some defects in the cytoskeleton?

DR. REAVEN: What you may not know is that cytoskeletal research (microtubule research to be exact) is one of my main interests in life. So one of the first things I did on our initial tissues was to look at the cytoskeleton and, in fact, measure all kinds of possible organelle changes in beta cells from older animals. By the way, these were not the very obese animals I've just described. I found nothing of interest to report.

These, however, were collagenase-isolated islets. What we are going to do now, with the two-year-old rats that are coming due very soon, is to glutaraldehyde-perfuse their pancreases and look again for ultrastructural changes. My hunch is (based on the studies with collagenase-isolated islets) that we are not going to see much, i.e., we won't see many morphological changes in islets until they get to the fibrotic stage, despite the fact that the islets will show a decline in insulin secretion.

DR. SCARPELLI: From the initial response of islets of older obese animals to glucose one might suspect there are no differences in the entry of glucose into islet cells. Has that indeed been established by studying the entry of a nonmetabolizable compound such as 3-0-methylglucose?

DR. REAVEN: We have not used 3-0-methylglucose in our studies. However, our feeling is that glucose getting into the cell is not the problem, but that the decline in insulin secretion with aging has to do with glucose signalling once it is inside the cell. We are trying to get at this question now by studying various enzymatic changes in the islets of aging animals, and we have found some. But of course we don't know if these changes can account for the entire problem we see in the beta cells of aging animals.

DR. RAISZ: That was fascinating. Is it possible that the change in fibrosis is primary rather than beta cell exhaustion? Specifically, could there be a decrease in turnover of collagen or some change in glycosylation? For example, have you measured hemoglobin AIC in the obese animals?

DR. REAVEN: I don't think that the fibrosis comes first, but it is true we haven't looked at any of the circulating factors.

DR. BELL: Is it possible that the fibrosis which you indicate arises as a result of a change in biosynthetic activity of the beta cell might not be due to some other cell type in the islets; for example, to a fibroblastic cell? I am not convinced that the collagen fibrils which you showed are intracellular. It is very unusual to see formed collagen fibrils in the cytoplasm.

DR. REAVEN: I don't think they are inside the cell.

DR. BELL: I think there may be some doubt about the origin of the collagen fibrils. Do you suggest that the fibrils have been released from a lysed beta cell?

DR. REAVEN: Oh, no, I didn't mean to imply that. I am sorry. All I meant to say was that there are, in this islet, damaged and dead cells with damaged membranes and that as a result, one can see images where extracellular collagen fibrils seem to have mixed with the contents of broken cells. I didn't mean to imply that the collagen was inside a living beta cell.

DR. WILLIAMSON: I would like to congratulate you on those beautiful studies. I have a couple of questions and comments. I would agree with you that the presence of collagen in the islets does suggest injury and a response to injury. I would be curious to know what the cell type is that is producing collagen though.

I also have a question related to the granules that appear to be extracellular. You know, normally when the beta cell secretes insulin, the granules dissolve virtually instantly, as soon as they are extracellular. This makes me suspect that the extracellular granules you described may be artifacts reflecting damage to the islets after fixation. Maybe these islets are more fragile and are more easily ruptured during handling after fixation.

The second question I had was, do you have any information on just the blood glucose levels in the three groups of animals and changes in blood glucose levels after feeding them rat food rather than after an infusion of glucose?

DR. REAVEN: Yes. Actually, we published very similar pictures from isolated islets showing collagen mixed with granules. The pathologists to whom I showed the pictures did not find this to be very interesting because they felt it was probably a function of the collagenase that we had used to isolate the islets and that the islets from the old rats were more fragile, and perhaps more easily damaged, than islets of young rats. So when I began seeing these same kinds of images in islets fixed by perfusion, I began to take them more seriously.

But you are quite right. There is nothing that says that even with glutaraldehyde perfusion one couldn't damage certain cells more than others, by pressure, etc. I frankly find that to be unlikely, but it is a possibility.

DR. WILLIAMSON: What about the *ad libitum* fed animals? Are they actually compensated, that is, are their blood sugar levels really normal when they are eating rat chow in contrast to glucose load?

DR. REAVEN: This first slide shows insulin values. This was a somewhat earlier study; not the one I just reported on, but it shows age in months at the bottom. We studied *ad libitum*-fed animals at one and one-half, three, six and 12 months of age, and their insulin levels rise as early as three or four months of age and remain stable. This suggests to us that insulin resistance is not an age-dependent event but is, in fact, an obesity-dependent event. In animals which are exercising, or in calorie-restricted animals, the insulin levels remain quite normal. So, the animals maintain the euglycemia at the expense of their insulin levels.

DR. SCARPELLI: Have you looked at the peripheral content of insulin receptors in the obese as compared to diet-restricted animals?

DR. REAVEN: I haven't done that, but it is my impression from the literature that the number of insulin receptors decreases with obesity, not necessarily age.

DR. LANDFIELD: I would like to ask one quick question. What do you think of the possibility that the elevated corticosterone in these strains of rats is a factor in the peripheral resistance to insulin? Or have you looked at that?

DR. REAVEN: No, we haven't studied this.

DR. LORIA: Why did you use the term calorie-restricted rats? If I understood you correctly, in essence you are diluting your diet with "alphacel".

DR. REAVEN: Alpha cellulose.

DR. LORIA: Yes, alpha cellulose. In essence you are reducing both protein and lipids.

DR. REAVEN: Yes.

DR. LORIA: How do you know that these animals are specifically calorie-restricted and that they are not deficient in another nutrient, like protein?

DR. REAVEN: We reduce everything. The diet is actually vitamin and mineral enriched, as we add back vitamins and minerals. But the animals really aren't protein depleted because, you see, they eat double the amount of this diet. Indeed, when their consumption of protein was calculated, it was found to be well within normal limits.

II. THE MESENCHYME AND AGING

Comparative Pathobiology of Major Age-Related Diseases:
Current Status and Research Frontiers, pages 129–143

THE SYNOVIAL CELL

Endre A. Balazs, M.D. and
Janet L. Denlinger, Ph.D.

Matrix Biology Laboratory, Columbia University,
New York, NY 10032

The joint is one of the best examples of an organ where the normal aging process is altered by overuse, underuse or pathology. More correctly, early pathological changes, excessive wear and tear or too little use, when superimposed on the aging process result in new, age-related pathology. One cannot emphasize enough that in an organ like the joint normal aging is possible only when coupled with normal use. In exploring the parameters of normal aging one must determine, therefore, the bounds of normal function and usage of the joint.

Since the central theme of this paper is the synovial cell, we would like to describe briefly those parts of the joint which are under the direct influence of the function of these cells, that is, the synovial tissue, the synovial fluid and the surface layer of the articular cartilage.

SYNOVIAL TISSUE AND SYNOVIAL CELLS

Synovial tissue lines the inner surface of the diarthrodial joint capsule. This tissue is responsible for the metabolism of the synovial fluid, and as a loose, vascular connective tissue, acts as a potential "inflammation-mediating" structure. The synovial tissue consists of two parts: an inner lining layer adjacent to the joint space (the synovial intima, synovial lining or synovial membrane) and a supportive connective tissue layer, usually referred to as the subsynovial tissue. The microscopic and ultrastructural characteristics of synovial tissue have been reviewed in detail elsewhere

(Castor 1960; Barland et al 1962; Ghadially, Roy 1966, 1969; Roy, Ghadially 1967a; Schumacher 1975; Ghadially 1978; Hasselbacher 1981).

The term "synovial membrane" often used in the literature for the synovial intima is actually a misnomer, because it is not lined with endothelium, but is formed by connective tissue cells embedded in a loose matrix (Trueta 1968). There is no basal lamina separating the synovial intima from the synovial space or from the subsynovial tissue (Barland et al 1962; Coulter 1962; Ghadially, Roy 1966, 1969; Roy, Ghadially 1967a; Roy et al 1966). Key (1928) classified the subsynovial tissues as fibrous, adipose and areolar, but emphasized that these three types merge with each other continuously.

Two main cell types have been identified in the synovial intima (Barland et al 1962), but it may be that these are not actually two different types of cells, but the same cell exhibiting different morphology according to its various activities. The more frequently-occurring type A cell is characterized by large, numerous vacuoles, filopodia and mitochondria, intracellular fibrils, a prominent Golgi apparatus and evidence of pinocytosis and phagocytosis. This cell contains little rough endoplasmic reticulum. The less frequent B-type cell is characterized by abundant rough endoplasmic reticulum, few vacuoles, filopodia and micro-vesicles, and a less prominent Golgi apparatus. There are also intermediate-type cells which have both rough endo-plasmic reticulum and Golgi apparati. It is the presence of these intermediate cells which leads to the assumption that A and B cells are the same cell at different functional stages.

In terms of function, the A cells have been generally classified as phagocytic, macrophage-like cells, while B cells have been classed as secretory. However, it must be noted that it is only the resting macrophage which shows less endo-plasmic reticulum; stimulated macrophages show a hypertrophy of rough endoplasmic reticulum (Ghadially 1975). In patho-logical synovial tissue where there is increased phagocytic activity, there is an increase in intermediate and type B cells. This seems to be the result of the increase of endo-plasmic reticulum in the A cells, not a replacement of these cells by intermediate and B cells (Ghadially 1978). Both A and B cells may perform the functions of phagocytosis and secretion, but type A cells are the most active in phagocytosis (Mitnick et al 1978) and are also responsible for the synthesis of sodium hyaluronate (NaHA), which has been identified by autoradiography in the Golgi complexes and the large secretory vacuoles (Roy, Ghadially 1967b). The B cells, which are rich in rough endoplasmic reticulum, probably produce tissue-specific proteins. In conditions such as inflammation in which there is an increase in the protein concentration of the synovial fluid, there is also an increase in type B and intermediate cells (Roy, Ghadially 1967a).

The synovial intimal cells are embedded in a matrix of varying electron density, composed of collagen fibrils and electron-dense amorphous material (Ghadially, Roy 1966, 1969). The nature of this electron-dense material has not been determined, but is most likely composed of proteins and proteoglycans embedded in a molecular network of NaHA and precipitated during the fixation process. Between the collagen fibers of the matrix there is NaHA and proteoglycans of chondroitin sulfate and keratan sulfate. In the normal adult rabbit knee joint the chondroitin sulfate is present in the highest, and the keratan sulfate in the lowest, concentration (Table 1; Denlinger 1982).

Table 1

Glycosaminoglycans in the Synovial Tissue of Immobilized Rabbit Joints

	% Wet Tissue Weight		
	NaHA	KS	Ch-S
Normal	0.031 ± 0.008	0.012 ± 0.005	0.045 ± 0.011
7 Days Immobilized	0.067 ± 0.009	0.027 ± 0.011	0.065 ± 0.008
Significance	<0.01	<0.01	NS

Denlinger, 1982

The synovial tissue has a rich vascular and lymphatic supply. The capillary network extends to just beneath the synovial layer (Walmsley 1964) and most, but not all, of the capillaries of the synovial tissue are of the fenestrated type. These fenestrated capillaries are found in other tissues where rapid exchange of water and solutes occurs, such as renal glomeruli, ciliary body, and intestinal villi. A similar function for these capillaries in the superficial layers of the synovial tissue has been suggested (Sutter, Majno, 1964; Schumacher 1969; Mitnick et al 1978; Ghadially

1978; Hasselbacher 1981). Some capillaries, especially in the fibrous synovial tissue, have tight junctions and no fenestration.

The synovial lymphatics are less superficial and less numerous than the synovial capillaries (Davies 1946; Mitnick et al 1978). They drain into collecting vessels which anastomose with the lymphatic systems of the periosteum and the joint capsule. These lymphatic vessels are similar in structure to those in other areas of the body, having a thin endothelium closely associated with the surrounding matrix (Schumacher 1969, 1975; Rhodin, Sue 1979). These vessels probably serve to return water and solutes including NaHA to the circulation, but also may be important in clearing the joint of particles (Adkins, Davies 1940) and as a pathway for migratory cells.

SYNOVIAL FLUID

The synovial fluid is produced by the synovial tissue, and its most important component, NaHA, by the A cells. The synovial fluid owes its viscoelasticity to the large glycosaminoglycan molecule. This liquid compartment is not separated from the neighboring solid compartment by basal laminae. The main function of this fluid is to protect the internal surfaces (cartilage, synovial tissue) and to transport metabolites to and from the cartilage (for review, see Sundblad 1965; Balazs 1974; Swann 1978).

The synovial fluid also contains proteins, but at a much lower concentration than the serum in all species studied (Schubert, Hamerman 1968). The concentration of protein does not change with age in normal human knees and cattle joints (Table 2; Balazs 1968; Seppälä, Balazs 1969), but increases in all inflammatory and degenerative joint diseases. The concentration of NaHA varies from joint to joint and from species to species. In the human knee joint, after the age of 28 years, the concentration of NaHA drops significantly (Table 3). The molecular size of the NaHA, however, does not change with age, at least in the human knee joint (Balazs 1968, 1977; Table 3) and in bovine joints (Seppälä, Balazs 1969).

The elastoviscous nature of synovial fluids (human and bovine) was characterized by measurement of the dynamic shear moduli at various strain frequencies and various temperatures.

Table 2

Aging and Protein Concentration (mg/ml) of Human and Bovine Synovial Fluids

Age (years)	1.5-2.5	10-15	18-23	24-27	28-35	52-78
Human knee			21.0 ± 0.9	19.4 ± 1.3	18.5 ± 2.6	18.5 ± 1.6
Bovine hock	7.7 ± 2.0	9.4 ± 1.0				

Seppälä & Balazs, 1969

Table 3

The Molecular Weight and Concentration of NaHA in the Synovial Fluid of Knee Joints of Human Subjects of Various Ages.*

Age group (years)	Joints Analyzed	NaHA mg/ml	MW x 10^{-6}
18-20	36	3.8 ± 0.10	3.7 ± 0.07
21-23	30	3.8 ± 0.20	3.8 ± 0.07
24-27	31	3.4 ± 0.10	3.5 ± 0.10
28-35	18	2.5 ± 0.04	4.2 ± 0.22
52-78	34	2.5 ± 0.20	3.9 ± 0.14

*Data from the work of Balazs, Rydell, Seppälä, Duff, Merrill, Gibbs.

The three dynamic parameters determined by these methods are the rigidity modulus, the loss or viscous modulus and storage or elastic modulus. These moduli, when determined at a strain frequency (ω) range of 0.03 - 3.0 cycles sec^{-1} show considerable change. At low frequencies the viscous modulus is high and the elastic modulus is low, and at high frequencies the relationship is the reverse. The frequency at which the two moduli have the same numerical values (in dynes sec^{-2}) is called the crossover point. This frequency is characteristic for a given synovial fluid and describes the frequency of the energy which is approximately equally stored (elastic) and dissipated (viscous) in the fluid.

Table 4

Rheological Properties of Synovial Fluids Aspirated from the Knee Joints of Human Subjects of Various Ages*

Age (years)	Crossover point of two moduli (G'', G') cycles sec	Two moduli (G'', G') at crossover point dynes cm^{-2}
18-27	0.13 ± 0.020	332 ± 41
27-35	0.21 ± 0.004	59 ± 6
52-78	0.41 ± 0.012	61 ± 7

*Data from the work of Balazs, Rydell, Seppälä, Duff, Merrill, Gibbs.

The most striking rheological change in the human synovial fluid with age is the considerable decrease of its elastic properties. This change starts to occur during the third decade. The most dramatic difference in the elastic and viscous moduli was observed between the age groups of 18-27 and 27-39 years (Table 4). Later in life the elastic modulus further decreases and the viscous modulus increases. The rigidity modulus also decreases dramatically during the third decade of life. The crossover point of the viscous and elastic moduli moves with aging toward higher frequencies, and the numerical values of the two moduli also drop in the synovial fluids of individuals in the 27- to 78-year-old age group (Table 5). All these rheological changes of the synovial fluid around the end of the third decade of life indicate drastic aging changes. The decrease of elasticity and rigidity of the fluid and the shift of the crossover point to a higher frequency indicates that the NaHA in the fluid does not represent as effective mechanical protection as in the earlier part of life (Balazs 1968; EA Balazs, RW Rydell, PO Seppälä, IR Rydell, EW Merrill, DA Gibbs, unpublished observations).

Table 5

Rheological Properties of Synovial Fluid Aspirated from the Knee Joints of Human Subjects of Various Ages[1]

Age (years)	# of Samples	Elastic Modulus G'	Viscous Modulus G''	Rigidity Modulus G*
18-27	16	1170 ± 130	450 ± 82	1260 ± 88
27-39	18	226 ± 7	72 ± 8	233 ± 9
52-78	26	189 ± 33	101 ± 12	221 ± 39

Moduli in dynes cm^{-2} are measured at 2.5 cycles sec^{-1} and reduced to 37°C.

[1]Data from the work of Balazs, Rydell, Seppälä, Duff, Merrill, Gibbs.

One can better appreciate the real importance of these rheological changes if one considers that the targets for the main protective role of the synovial fluid are the cartilage surface and the synovial tissue. There is a free exchange and a steady state condition between the NaHA content of the fluid and the matrix of the synovial tissue and the cartilage surface.

It is of interest to compare the NaHA concentration in these matrix compartments. This comparison can be made only if one assumes a certain space available for these large molecules between the cells (synovial tissue) and between the collagen and proteoglycan molecules of the matrix (synovial tissue and cartilage surface). The only compartment where this real NaHA concentration can be measured directly is in the synovial fluid. In the rabbit knee joint such calculations were made (Denlinger 1982) and it was found that the lowest concentration of NaHA is in the synovial fluid

(3-4 mg/ml). In the synovial tissue the concentration is double (approximately 7 mg/ml) and in the cartilage surface layer it is even higher (approximately 15 mg/ml).

Since the NaHA is synthesized by the synovial cells and is transported to the two other tissues, the transport cannot be based only on diffusion. The fact that in the immobilized joint the NaHA content of both the synovial tissue and the fluid approximately doubles indicates that the movement of the joint also plays a role in pumping these molecules from the synovial tissue to the fluid (Table 1). The very high NaHA concentration in the cartilage surface can be explained only by movement from the synovial fluid through mechanical pressure. That is, the movement of the diarthrodal joint presses the synovial fluid and with it the NaHA into the loose collagen fibrillar network of the cartilage surface.

Rheological studies on the NaHA from the cartilage surface and from the synovial tissue are not reported, but it is reasonable to assume that molecular characteristics of NaHA in these tissues would be the same as those in the synovial fluid. We propose that the highly viscoelastic NaHA molecules are responsible for the structural integrity of the collagen network of the cartilage surface, and for that of the blood and lymphatic vascular system in the synovial tissue. The viscoelastic interfibrillar (collagen fibrils) fluid protects the lumen of the vessels from constriction during flexion and extension of the joint. The function of the NaHA in protecting blood vessels from constriction is very similar to that in the umbilical cord, where the blood vessels are also embedded in a viscoelastic NaHA matrix. In both cases the extreme movement (flexion-extension) of the tissues exposes the vessel system to mechanical dislocation, to potential damage to the vascular intima and consequent decrease of blood flow.

CARTILAGE SURFACE LAYER

The lamina splendens (MacConaill 1951) is the thin (1-3 μm) surface layer of the articular cartilage which is made up of highly-ordered thin fibrils (4-12 nm thick; Silberberg et al 1961; Weiss et al 1968). This cell-free layer exhibits straining characteristics very distinct from those of the deeper layers of the articular cartilage (Balazs, Gibbs 1970). It was shown that this layer is imbibed with synovial fluid, and therefore the NaHA content of it is considerably higher than that of the deeper layers of the cartilage (Balazs et al 1966; Balazs 1968). With hyaluronic acid-specific enzymes most of this layer can be removed from the surface. It was also shown that in young and adult bovine cartilage this layer, unlike the rest of the cartilage, contains fibronectin, which somehow interacts with the NaHA (Denlinger 1982).

Scanning electron microscopic studies (Gardner, Woodward 1969; Clarke 1971a,b; Walker et al 1969) of dried surfaces of lamina splendens showed a variety of "pits", "ridges" and "humps" which were generally regarded as artifacts due to the dehydration process and the accumulation of dried synovial fluid. It was also pointed out that some of these surface structures are different in the young, mature and aged cartilage (Longmore, Gardner 1975; Ghadially et al 1978). The proteoglycan and NaHA content of the lamina splendens also changes with aging (Stockwell, Scott 1965; Balazs et al 1966; Stockwell 1970). The erosion or fibrillation of the joint surface in pathological conditions is regarded as the initiation of more serious joint pathology. The importance of the lamina splendens in the protection of the cells and matrix of the cartilage has been well recognized both in terms of lubrication and shock absorption. Nevertheless its role in the normal aging processes and its pathology is not understood.

THE SPECIAL FUNCTION OF THE SYNOVIAL CELLS AND AGING

We would like to suggest that the synovial cells (A and B cells) be called hyalocytes, because they are very similar in morphology to the histiocytes of the vitreous (Szirmai, Balazs 1958; Bloom, Balazs 1965; Freeman, et al 1968, 1979). They also show the same two major functions: production of NaHA and phagocytosis. This means that they provide the cellular function responsible for the maintenance of both tissue compartments. The molecular structural similarity of these two predominantly extracellular matrix-containing compartments has been pointed out previously (Balazs, Denlinger 1979).

How the aging process in the joint is related to the function of the synovial cells is not known. One can speculate that the dramatic decrease of the NaHA concentration in the joint of normal young adults (over 30 years of age) is due to the decrease of the synthetic activity of these cells. But it is also possible that the lower concentration is the result of the increased rate of outflow of these molecules through the lymphatic system of the synovial tissue. A marked increase in the vascularization of the synovial tissue after infancy was reported (Barnett et al 1961). How the other important function of these cells--the phagocytic activity--changes during aging is not known.

One must assume that the hyalocytes of the joint, just as the hyalocytes of the vitreous, are constantly removed and replaced by blood monocytes. If this is the case, then the mobility of the joint must play an important role in this exchange, because of its effect on the blood and lymph capillary systems. The integrity of these two capillary systems is essential for the metabolic supply of the cartilage and the turnover of the NaHA in the entire matrix system of the joint. Thus the key to the normal and pathological aging of the joint must be found in the normal or abnormal movement pattern of the joint, that is, its normal and abnormal use (underuse and overuse).

There is ample evidence that the extreme form of underuse, the immobilization of the joint, causes such drastic changes that complete joint destruction follows (Finsterbush, Friedman 1973; Wigren, Wik 1974; Akeson et al 1968). The concomitant rapid increase of NaHA and protein content of the synovial tissue, fluid and cartilage surface was reported (Table 6, Denlinger 1982). This is probably the earliest (seven days) and most dramatic occurrence in the joints after immobilization which clearly emphasizes the importance of NaHA and the normal

Table 6

Proteins and NaHA in the Synovial Fluid of Immobilized Rabbit Joints

	Exudate ml	Proteins mg	NaHA mg
Normal	none	5.1 ± 0.6	0.58 ± 0.07
7 days Immobilized	0.2 - 1.5	32.6 ± 7.0	1.26 ± 0.19

Denlinger 1982

movement pattern for joint function. Since in aging and in joint pathology the NaHA decreases, one cannot parallel the occurrences during immobilization with those of aging.

The overuse of the joint can be described in race horses. It is well established that injuries to the cartilage surface are the most common intra-articular damage in extreme use of the joint (Adams 1966; Nilsson 1973). It was reported that the protein concentration in the synovial fluid of normal horses in training is significantly greater than that of those at rest. The intrinsic viscosity of the NaHA in the synovial fluid of horses in training is significantly lower than in those at rest, but the concentration of NaHA is not changed (Persson 1971). While our knowledge of the effect of overuse of the normal joint is very incomplete, the few data available suggest that overuse has a profound effect on the composition of the matrix of the synovial tissue, fluid and cartilage surface. Thus the movement (folding and unfolding) and lack of movement of the synovial tissue provides the controlling factor for the NaHA content of the joint. This can be for two reasons: one is that the massaging action or the lack of it in the lymph vessels causes a change in the rate of "pumping out" of the fluid and its NaHA. In addition, the movements can cause changes in the rate of blood supply to the hyalocytes and thereby alter the rate of synthesis of NaHA. The combination of these two conditions would suggest that in the underuse of the joint the lymph vessels carry away less synovial fluid and the dilated leaky capillaries produce a greater than normal volume of synovial fluid and stimulate NaHA synthesis (Table 1). During overuse the lymph system carries away more synovial fluid and the mechanically constricted capillaries cause a decrease of the volume of synovial fluid and NaHA synthesis. It is obvious that in this scenario the normal aging process is protected only by the absence of the extreme conditions of overuse and underuse.

Further experimentation is needed not only to understand the aging process in joint structures, but also to focus on the activity of the synovial cells under normal and pathological conditions. By investigating the abnormal occurrences which affect joint function and usage, one can determine the factors which contribute to age-related and pathology-related changes in joint structure and function. The reactions of synovial cells, fluid and tissues to aging and pathology, as well as their relationship to the cartilage surface layer, are interrelated, and in turn cannot be separated from the environment in which they occur.

REFERENCES

Adams OR (1966). "Lameness in Horses." Philadelphia: Lea & Febiger.
Adkins EW, Davies DV (1940). Absorption from the joint cavity Q J Exp Physiol 30:147.
Akeson WH, Amiel D, LaViolette D, Secrist D (1968). The connective tissue response to immobility: An accelerated aging response? Exp Gerontol 3:289.
Balazs EA (1968). Viscoelastic properties of hyaluronic acid and biological lubrication. Univ Mich Med Ctr J Suppl:255.
Balazs EA (1974). The physical properties of synovial fluid and the special role of hyaluronic acid. In Helfet AJ (ed): "Disorders of the Knee," Philadelphia: J. B. Lippincott, p 63.
Balazs EA (1977). Intercellular matrix of connective tissue. In Hayflick L, Finch CE (eds): "Handbook of the Biology of Aging," New York: Van Nostrand Reinhold, p 222.
Balazs EA, Bloom GD, Swann DA (1966). Fine structure and cartilage. Fed Proc 25:1813.
Balazs EA, Denlinger JL (1979). Vitreous and joint: Comparative morphology and biochemistry. Atti Fond Giorgio Ronchi XXXIV (6):637.
Balazs EA, Gibbs, DA (1970). The rheological properties and biological function of hyaluronic acid. In Balazs E (ed): "Chemistry and Molecular Biology of the Intercellular Matrix," New York: Academic Press, p 1241.
Barland P, Novikoff AB, Hamerman D (1962). Electron microscopy of the human synovial membrane. J Cell Biol 14:207.
Barnett CH, Davies DV, MacConaill MA (1961). "Synovial Joints--Their Structure and Mechanics." London: Longmans Green and Co., Ltd.
Bloom GD, Balazs EA (1965). An electron microscopic study of hyalocytes. Exp Eye Res 4:249.
Castor WC (1960). The microscopic structure of normal human synovial tissue. Arthritis Rheum 3:140.
Clarke IC (1971a). Surface characteristics of human articular cartilage--a scanning electron microscope study. J Anat 108:23.
Clarke IC (1971b). Articular cartilage: A review and scanning electron microscope study. J Bone Joint Surg 53-B:732.
Coulter WH (1962). The characteristics of human synovial

tissue as seen with the electron microscope. Arthritis Rheum 5:70.
Davies DV (1946). The lymphatics of the synovial membrane. J Anat 80:21.
Denlinger JL (1982). Metabolisme de l'hyaluronate de sodium au niveau des tissus articulaires et oculaires. Thèse presentee a l'Universite de Lille 1 pour obtenir le titre de Docteur d'Universite en Sciences Naturelles.
Finsterbush A, Friedman B (1973). Early changes in immobilized rabbits knee joints: A light and electron microscopic study. Clin Orthop Rel Res 92:305.
Freeman MI, Jacobson B, Balazs EA (1979). The chemical composition of vitreous hyalocyte granules. Exp Eye Res 29:479.
Freeman MI, Jacobson B, Toth LZ, Balazs EA (1968). Lysosomal enzymes associated with vitreous hyalocyte granules. I. Intracellular distribution patterns of enzymes. Exp Eye Res 7:113.
Gardner DL, Woodward D (1969). Scanning electron microscopy and replica studies of articular surface of guinea-pig synovial joints. Ann Rheum Dis 28:379.
Ghadially FN (1975). "Ultrastructural Pathology of the Cell." London: Butterworths.
Ghadially FN (1978). Fine structure of joints. In Sokoloff L (ed): "The Joints and Synovial Fluid," Vol 1, New York: Academic Press, p 105.
Ghadially FN, Moshurchak EM, Ghadially JA (1978). A maturation change in the surface of cat articular cartilage detected by the scanning electron microscope. J Anat 125:349.
Ghadially FN, Roy S (1966). Ultrastructure of rabbit synovial membrane. Ann Rheum Dis 25:318.
Ghadially FN, Roy S (1969). "Ultrastructure of Synovial Joints in Health and Disease." London: Butterworths Ltd, p 98.
Hasselbacher P (1981). Structure of the synovial membrane. Clin Rheum Dis 7:57.
Key JA (1928). The synovial membrane of joints and bursae. In Cowdry EV (ed): "Special Cytology," New York: P. B. Hoeber, p 735.
Longmore RB, Gardner DL (1975). Development with age of human articular cartilage surface structure. Ann Rheum Dis 34:26.
MacConaill MA (1951). The movements of bones and joints. IV. The mechanical structure of articulating cartilage. J Bone Joint Surg 33-B:251.
Mitnick H, Hoffstein S, Weissmann G (1978). Fate of antigen

after intravenous and intra-articular injection into rabbits. Arthritis Rheum 21:918.
Nilsson G (1973). Lameness and pathologic changes in the distal joints and the phalanges of the Standardbred horse. Acta Vet Scand [Suppl] 14:83.
Persson L (1971). On the synovia in horses. Acta Vet Scand [Suppl] 33:29.
Rhodin JAG, Sue SL (1979). Combined intravital microscopy and electron microscopy of the blind beginnings of the mesenteric lymphatic capillaries of the rat mesentery. Acta Physiol Scand [Suppl] 463:51.
Roy S, Ghadially FN (1967a). Ultrastructure of normal ray synovial membrane. Ann Rheum Dis 26:26.
Roy S, Ghadially FN (1967b). Ultrastructure of synovial membrane in human hemarthrosis. J Bone Joint Surg 49-A:1636.
Roy S, Ghadially FN, Crane WAJ (1966). Synovial membrane in traumatic effusion. Ultrastructure and autoradiography with tritiated leucine. Ann Rheum Dis 25:259.
Schubert M, Hamerman DA (1968). "A Primer on Connective Tissue Biochemistry." Philadelphia: Lea & Febiger.
Schumacher HR (1969). The microvasculature of the synovial membrane of the monkey: Ultrastructural studies. Arthritis Rheum 12:387.
Schumacher HR (1975). Ultrastructure of the synovial membrane. Ann Clin Lab Sci 5:489.
Seppälä P, Balazs EA (1969). Hyaluronic acid in synovial fluid. III. Effect of maturation and aging on the chemical properties of bovine synovial fluid of different joints. J Gerontol 24:309.
Silberberg R, Silberberg M, Vogel A, Wettstein W (1961). Ultrastructure of articular cartilage of mice of various ages. Am J Anat 109:251.
Stockwell RA (1970). Changes in the acid glycosaminoglycan content of the matrix of aging human articular cartilage. Ann Rheum Dis 29:509.
Stockwell RA, Scott JE (1965). Observations on the acid glycosaminoglycan (mucopolysaccharide) content of the matrix of aging cartilage. Ann Rheum Dis 24:341.
Sundblad L (1965). Glycosaminoglycans and glycoproteins in synovial fluid. In Balazs EA, Jeanloz RW (eds): "The Amino Sugars: The Chemistry and Biology of Compounds Containing Amino Sugars," Vol IIA, New York: Academic Press, p 229.
Sutter ER, Majno G (1964). Ultrastructure of the joint capsule in the rat: Presence of two kinds of capillaries. Nature 202:920.
Swann D (1978). Macromolecules of synovial fluid. In

Sokoloff L (ed): "The Joints and Synovial Fluid," Vol I, New York: Academic Press, p 407.

Szirmai J, Balazs EA (1958). Studies on the structure of the vitreous body. III. Cells in the cortical layer. Arch Ophthalmol 59:34.

Trueta J (1968). "Studies of the Development and Decay of the Human Frame." London: Pitman, p 170.

Walker PS, Sikorski J, Dowson D, Longfield MD, Wright V, Buckley T (1969). Behaviour of synovial fluid on surfaces of articular cartilage. A scanning electron microscope study. Ann Rheum Dis 28:1.

Walmsley R (1964). Syndesmology or arthrology. In Romanes GJ (ed): "Cummingham's Textbook of Anatomy," 10th edition, London: Oxford University Press, p 213.

Weiss C, Rosenberg L, Helfet AJ (1968). An ultrastructural study of normal young adult human articular cartilage. J Bone Joint Surg 50-A:663.

Wigren A, Wik O (1974). The influence of hyaluronic acid on immobilized knees: An experimental study on adult rabbits. Ups J Med Sci [Suppl] 16:1.

Comparative Pathobiology of Major Age-Related Diseases: Current Status and Research Frontiers, pages 145–158

HORMONAL REGULATION OF MESENCHYME; WITH SPECIAL REFERENCE TO THE REGULATION OF BONE FORMATION AND RESORPTION

Lawrence G. Raisz, M.D.

University of Connecticut Health Center, Farmington, CT 06032

Disorders of bone and connective tissue are an important part of the pathobiology of aging (Raisz 1982a). The skeleton is unique among mesenchymal tissues in serving simultaneously for structure and as a storehouse for minerals, so that it is frequently called upon to perform functions which are mutually incompatible. This system is regulated by a number of different local and systemic hormones which can be grouped into 1) calcium regulating hormones which are largely responsible for the metabolic functions of the skeleton such as parathyroid hormone (PTH), 1,25 dihydroxyvitamin D (1,25-$(OH)_2D_3$ or calcitriol) and calcitonin (CT), 2) growth hormones which are responsible for regulating overall gain or loss of skeletal mass including insulin, insulin-like growth factors (IGF) and glucocorticoids, and 3) local hormones which are important in maintaining the mechanical functions of the skeleton and the ability to respond to local stress. These include prostaglandins (PG), osteoclast activating factor (OAF) and bone-derived growth factors (Raisz, Kream 1981).

Among the connective tissues, bone turns over more rapidly than subcutaneous tissue, tendon, fascia and cartilage. Moreover, the process of bone turnover is anatomically definable in terms of specific sites of osteoclastic bone resorption and osteoblastic bone formation. In the adult human skeleton, these processes are coupled; that is to say, the most common sites of bone formation are those at which prior resorption has taken place, both in Haversian remodeling of osteons and in surface remodeling of trabecular and endosteal bones. In contrast to other connective tissues in which the fibroblasts which produce the extracellular matrix also appear to be important in its degradation, bone resorption and formation are carried out by different cell lines. The bone forming cell or osteoblast is a highly differentiated collagen synthesizing mesenchymal cell, probably derived from a predetermined osteoprogenitor cell (Owen 1978), while the bone resorbing cell or osteoclast is of hematogenous origin, perhaps of the same family as the macrophage, but showing important structural and functional differences. In addition, macrophages serve a scavenger function in the degradation of connective tissues and may be particularly important in pathologic destruction.

Connective tissue turnover is dependent not only on the function of the differentiated cells, but on the rate at which these cells can be renewed. This is particularly true for bone, in which remodeling depends on cell replication since both the osteoclast and the osteoblast have finite life spans and limited functional capacity. Thus hormones may not only regulate the function of these cells directly, but might also alter the rates of renewal and differentiation of the respective precursor pools. Aging is often accompanied by impairment of cell renewal. This may be intrinsic, but could also be related to decreased secretion of hormones.

Different connective tissue components do not change in a uniform manner with aging. The mass of bone and muscle decreases substantially with age, while the relative proportion of fat increases. Aging-related changes may vary greatly at specific sites. There is marked loss of trabecular bone mass with age, with slower loss of cortical bone mass in the appendicular skeleton (Riggs et al 1981) and no loss of bone mass in the cranial vault. Finally, periosteal bone may increase, both by symmetric increases in periosteal diameter of long bones and in the form of osteophytes in patients with osteoarthritis. Although there is a general loss of cartilage and synovial tissue with age, the rates differ greatly in different areas, being greatest in those which are under the greatest stress. Against this background, I will summarize the major actions of several hormones on connective tissue, particularly bone, and indicate what is known about age-related changes in their secretion or tissue effects.

PTH may produce both catabolic and anabolic effects on bone *in vivo* (Parsons 1976). Its major physiologic function is to maintain serum calcium concentration. This is brought about largely by stimulation of osteoclastic bone resorption. However, it has not been possible to show PTH receptors on osteoclasts or to isolate a precursor population of these cells which is stimulated by PTH directly. This has led to the alternative theory that PTH acts on osteoblasts and that its action on osteoclasts is indirect. Osteoblast-like cells isolated from bone, as well as osteosarcoma cells which have an osteoblastic phenotype, show PTH receptors and can respond to PTH with an increase in cyclic AMP, activation of protein kinase and subsequently a decrease in alkaline phosphatase and in collagen systhesis (Kream et al 1980). Accompanying these effects there may be an increase in cell replication. It is not known whether the cells which replicate are precursors of osteoblasts or osteoclasts. An increase in cell replication is not necessary for either the inhibitory effect of PTH on osteoblasts or the stimulatory effect on osteoclasts. Despite these catabolic actions, animals given intermittent injections of relatively low doses of PTH can show an increase of trabecular bone mass and perhaps also cortical bone mass. Baylink and his associates have suggested that this effect is secondary to the release of a skeletal growth factor from the matrix by increased bone resorption (Howard et al 1981). PTH might stimulate bone formation by increasing the production of some systemic hormone, such as $1,25\text{-}(OH)_2D_3$. PTH may also increase bone mass by stimulating cell replication and matrix synthesis in cartilage cell.

In patients, hyperparathyroidism is generally associated with a decrease in bone mass and hypoparathyroidism with an increase in mass (Seeman et al 1982). The effect of age on parathyroid hormone secretion is not completely established. Most data suggest that PTH concentrations and biological effects are increased in elderly individuals. This may be due to the cumulative effect of calcium deficiency in the elderly and could result in enhanced bone resorption and impaired bone formation. PTH levels are relatively high in some patients with osteoporosis, although not sufficiently high to produce the hypercalcemia associated with primary hyperparathyroidism. One reason for elevated PTH might be impaired intestinal calcium absorption. This in turn could be due to impaired $1,25\text{-}(OH)_2D_3$ synthesis.

The direct effects of $1,25\text{-}(OH)_2D_3$ on bone are remarkably similar to those of PTH (Raisz 1980a). Resorption is stimulated and formation is inhibited. The major difference is that $1,25\text{-}(OH)_2D_3$ does not act through cyclic AMP and that it does not appear to stimulate cell replication in bone to the same extent as PTH. These catabolic effects of 1,25-$(OH)_2D_3$ on bone are difficult to reconcile with the requirement of vitamin D for skeletal growth. They may only come into play at high concentrations of the hormone which are produced during periods of calcium and phosphate deficiency. Under such conditions, net bone growth is impossible and stimulation of resorption and inhibition of formation would provide extra calcium and phosphate for soft tissue needs, as well as for mineralization of matrix that has already been formed and for fracture repair. Like PTH, 1,25-$(OH)_2D_3$ has been reported to stimulate cartilage growth, but in some experiments it appears that 24,25-$(OH)_2D_3$ is more potent. The importance of this metabolite in skeletal growth and development is much debated. Recent studies suggest that 24,25-$(OH)_2D_3$ is not necessary for skeletal development in chicks and rats and that 1,25-$(OH)_2D_3$ is the essential hormone in the vitamin D system. Low concentrations of vitamin D can increase trabecular bone mass, but high concentrations produce hypercalcemia and impairment of growth, often associated with renal damage.

The synthesis of 1,25-$(OH)_2D_3$ is generally decreased in older individuals. This may be related to the fact that renal mass decreases with age. Beyond this, there appears to be an impaired response of the kidney to PTH suggesting that the 1-α hydroxylase system which synthesizes 1,25-$(OH)_2D_3$ is selectively impaired. There have been some reports that the ability to synthesize 1,25-$(OH)_2D_3$ is particularly impaired in patients with osteoporosis, but this difference is not seen in all studies and is not large.

The role of calcitonin in connective tissue physiology has not yet been fully defined. CT is known to inhibit bone resorption, and osteoclasts appear to have receptors for this hormone. In contrast, there is no evidence for receptors or for important direct effects on osteoblasts. The most likely physiologic role of CT in mammals is to inhibit bone resorption after oral calcium loads and thus prevent excessive hypercalcemia and hypercalcuria. Calcitonin secretion, particularly in response to calcium, appears to decrease with age and this decrease is much more prominent in women than in men. There are data suggesting that the impairment of calcitonin secretion plays a role in osteoporosis (Stevenson et al 1982). This could be due to the fact that with aging there is decreased calcium absorption in the gut and so repeated oral calcium loads produce less hypercalcemia, less stimulus to the C-cells and progressive atrophy of these cells. The response to parenteral as well as oral calcium is eventually impaired.

Other systemic hormones which influence the mesenchyme are not as selective for bone as the calcium regulating hormones. Among these, the most important are insulin, insulin-like growth factor (IGF) or somatomedin, thyroid hormone and glucocorticoids (Raisz, Kream 1981). Although growth hormone has powerful effects on mesenchymal growth, it probably acts only indirectly through stimulation of IGF secretion. Insulin and IGF appear to be partners in stimulating mesenchymal growth. Both hormones can bind to the other's receptor. In bone, the insulin receptor appears to be most important in regulating osteoblast collagen synthesis, while the IGF receptor appears to be more important in stimulating the replication and differentiation of osteoblast precursor cells. With the two hormones together at low concentrations or either hormone alone at high concentrations there is a pleiotypic growth response involving both cell replication and increased matrix formation. The effects of IGF on cartilage are similar. Receptors for both hormones have been found, although the effects of insulin appear not to be as selective for matrix synthesis as in bone. Thyroid hormones are essential for mesenchymal growth and development *in vivo*, but their specific role has not been well-defined. In cartilage, thyroid hormones can act synergistically as co-factors in the response to IGF.

These hormones may play a role in the atrophy of mesenchymal tissues with aging. Insulin secretion is not generally decreased with age, although the rapid insulin response to glucose may be blunted. On the other hand, there is evidence for insulin resistance in older connective tissues. IGF secretion probably decreases with age. It is not clear to what extent this is due to decreased growth hormone secretion or to decreased hepatic response to growth hormone. Growth hormone and IGF are still effective in stimulating growth of older tissues and hence might be useful in the reversal of aging-related mesenchymal tissue atrophy.

Of the hormones which influence the mesenchyme, glucocorticoids probably have the most dramatic effects (Raisz 1980b). Glucocorticoid excess can produce a marked loss of bone, muscle and subcutaneous tissue and growth arrest in children. The only tissue which increases in mass is adipose tissue, although the increase is often localized in the trunk with a loss of subcutaneous fat in the extremities. The mechanism of glucocorticoid effects has been extensively studied, but no single hypothesis covers all the observations. A decrease in cell replication has been observed in many tissues, including cartilage and bone, and this may be the primary mechanism for loss of mass. Glucocorticoids do not have a direct inhibitory effect on osteoblastic collagen synthesis in bone. On the contrary, in fetal bone cultures collagen synthesis and alkaline phosphatase levels are increased acutely, although in long-term cultures there is a decrease related to a decrease in cell replication (Dietrich et al 1979). The stimulatory effect of glucocorticoids is not dose-related, but appears to be a permissive, all-or-none effect. Glucocorticoids are probably essential for the full differentiated function of mesenchymal cells. Similar glucocorticoid requirements have been described in other tissues, for example, the ability of the lung to develop surfactant. In bone organ cultures treated with glucocorticoids for several days, the progressive decrease in collagen synthesis can be attributed to an effect on a periosteal cell. Even early in the glucocorticoid response, periosteal DNA and protein synthesis are impaired.

In vivo, one of the most important effects of glucocorticoid excess is to produce osteopenia. While this may in part result from the inhibitory effects on bone cell replication, it is also associated with an increase in bone resorption. In vitro glucocorticoids do not stimulate bone resorption, but rather inhibit it. However, there could be an indirect stimulatory effect, due to the ability of glucocorticoids to inhibit calcium absorption in the intestine and produce secondary hyperparathyroidism.

There is great interest in the role of local regulatory hormones in the control of mesenchymal tissues. Endogenous prostaglandin production has been demonstrated in these tissues and evidence that the endogenous PG's are important in their function and development is accumulating rapidly (Raisz 1982b). The fact that glucocorticoids inhibit prostaglandin production has been instrumental in demonstrating the importance of PG's in many developmental processes. For example, the formation of cleft palate after the administration of glucocorticoids during fetal life appears to be related to an inhibition of prostaglandin production and can be reversed by the administration of the precursor, arachidonic acid. This and other evidence indicates that glucocorticoid effects are on arachidonic acid release rather than on the conversion of the precursor to prostaglandins. In bone, the inhibition of growth by glucocorticoids can be reversed by treatment with prostaglandin E_2 at 10^{-8} to 10^{-7} M. PGE_2 is the only potent stimulator of bone resorption thus far identified which can also increase bone formation. This increase appears to be related to stimulation of precursor cell replication or differentiation and not to a direct enhancement of collagen synthesis by mature osteoblasts. High concentrations of PGE_2 (10^{-6} and 10^{-5} M) can inhibit collagen synthesis. This biphasic effect may also occur in cartilage, where evidence for both stimulation and inhibition of growth have been obtained with PG's. The ability of PG's to affect bone *in vivo* has now been demonstrated in a clinical experiment in which PGE_1 was infused in infants to maintain patency of the ductus arteriosus and stimulated periosteal new bone formation. Prostaglandins can stimulate cell replication in other connective tissues, particularly skin, and have been implicated in the pathogenesis of certain dermatologic lesions.

There are many other possible mesenchymal growth regulating factors whose function and importance have not yet been fully elucidated (Canalis 1983). These include epidermal growth factor, which can stimulate bone resorption both directly and by increasing prostaglandin synthesis, and can stimulate cell replication but inhibit collagen synthesis in organ cultures of fetal rat calvaria. Similar effects have been observed with fibroblast growth factor and platelet-derived growth factor. Bone itself can produce several factors which can enhance cell replication, and similar factors are produced by cartilage (Canalis et al 1980; Kato et al 1981). Bone and cartilage cells as well as fetal fibroblasts have been shown to produce a factor which is biologically and immunochemically similar to IGF. However, in adult animals IGF is produced largely by the liver.

No summary of hormone effects on mesenchyme could be complete without a discussion of sex hormones. Estrogen withdrawal at the menopause is associated with thinning of subcutaneous tissue and loss of bone mass. However, it has not been possible to demonstrate any direct effects of estrogen on bone and hence an indirect mechanism has been postulated, such as an effect of estrogen on the calcium regulating hormones. Estrogen administration has been shown to increase 1,25-$(OH)_2D_3$ production and calcitonin secretion (Gallagher et al 1980). Circulating IGF levels are decreased by estrogen, but whether or not local production is altered in the same direction has not been determined. Androgens have anabolic effects on bone *in vivo*, but these may be indirect through effects on muscle. Age-related loss of androgen secretion or sensitivity may be important in connective tissue atrophy. The most important conclusion that one can make about sex hormones and mesenchyme is that we do not know the precise mechanisms for their effects on target tissues other than the classical ones such as breast, uterus and gonads. There are sex hormone receptors in the hypothalamus and it is possible that some of their effects *in vivo* are mediated indirectly through effects on the secretion of hypothalamic hormones which regulate pituitary function. In conclusion, aging-related changes in mesenchymal tissues, particularly bone, are probably the result of changes in both the production of and response to systemic hormones and local factors which regulate the formation and degradation of connective tissue.

REFERENCES

Canalis E (1983). Effect of hormones and growth factors on alkaline phosphatase activity and collagen synthesis in cultured rat calvariae. Metabolism 32:14.

Canalis E, Peck WA, Raisz LG (1980). Stimulation of DNA and collagen synthesis by autologous growth factor in cultured fetal rat calvaria. Science 210:1021.

Dietrich JW, Canalis EM, Maina DM, Raisz LG (1979). Effects of glucocorticoids on fetal rat bone collagen synthesis *in vitro*. Endocrinology 104:715.

Gallagher JC, Riggs BL, DeLuca HF (1980). Effect of estrogen on calcium absorption and serum vitamin D metabolites in postmenopausal osteoporosis. J Clin Endocrinol Metab 51:1359.

Howard GA, Bottemiller BL, Turner RT, Rader JI, Baylink DJ (1981). Parathyroid hormone stimulates bone formation and resorption in organ culture: Evidence for a coupling mechanism. Proc Natl Acad Sci USA 78:3204.

Kato Y, Nomura Y, Tsuji M, Ohmae H, Kinoshita M, Hamamoto S, Suzuki F (1981). Cartilage-derived factor (CDF). II. Somatomedin-like action on cultured chondrocytes. Exp Cell Res 132:339.

Kream BE, Rowe DW, Gworek SC, Raisz LG (1980). Parathyroid hormone alters collagen synthesis and procollagen mRNA levels in fetal rat calvaria. Proc Natl Acad Sci USA 77:5654.

Owen M (1978). Histogenesis of bone cells. Calcif Tissue Res 25:205.

Parsons JA (1976). Parathyroid physiology and the skeleton. In Bourne GH (ed): "The Biochemistry and Physiology of Bone," Vol IV, New York: Academic Press, p 159.

Raisz LG (1980a). Direct effects of vitamin D and its metabolites on skeletal tissue. Clin Endocrinol Metab 9:27.

Raisz LG (1980b). Effect of corticosteroids on calcium metabolism. Prog Biochem Pharmacol 17:212.

Raisz LG (1982a). Osteoporosis. J Am Geriatr Soc 30:127.

Raisz LG (1982b). Prostaglandins and skeletal metabolism. In Lee JB (ed): "Prostaglandins," New York: Elsevier, p 351.

Raisz LG, Kream BE (1981). Hormonal control of skeletal growth. Annu Rev Physiol 43:225.

Riggs BL, Wahner HW, Dunn WL, Mazess RB, Offord KP, Melton LJ III (1981). Differential changes in bone mineral density of the appendicular and axial skeleton with aging. Relationship to spinal osteoporosis. J Clin Invest 67:328.

Seeman E, Wahner HW, Offard KP, Kumar R, Johnson WJ, Riggs BL (1982). Differential effects of endocrine dysfunction on the axial and the appendicular skeleton. J Clin Invest 69:1302.

Stevenson JC, White MC, Joplin GF, MacIntyre I (1982). Osteoporosis and calcitonin deficiency. Br Med J 285:1010.

DISCUSSION

DR. SCARPELLI: When I saw the cross section of bone following the infusion of PGE_1 it resembled what one sees in cases of pulmonary osteoarthropathy. Is there evidence that the PGE_1 effect is involved in the pathogenesis of this condition?

DR. RAISZ: I don't know of any, but it fits beautifully because of the relation to lung lesions. The lung is a great producer of PGE_2 and since it doesn't have to pass through the lung it will remain biologically active in the arterial circulation and, therefore, could affect bone.

We have done infusion experiments using PGE_2 locally and can produce a change in the rat calvaria which looks very much like hypertrophic pulmonary osteoarthropathy.

DR. SCARPELLI: So it is PGE_2 that does it?

DR. RAISZ: We used PGE_2. Most people use PGE_1 because it is easier to get, but there is no biological difference between PGE_2 and PGE_1. In the bone those are the only two potent agents. Everything else is quite weak.

DR. WILLIAMSON: I have a question about the experiments in which you showed a decrease in proline incorporation into collagenase-digestable protein induced by calcitriol. Did you do any parallel experiments to look at release of prelabelled collagen by calcitriol?

DR. RAISZ: Yes. The rate of collagen degradation is accelerated in a bone-resorbing system. I mentioned earlier that those studies were done in two different tissues. To study bone resorption we used long bones from 19-day-old fetal rats. Those are poised to resorb, and so we have a lot of osteoclastic bone resorption.

To study bone formation we used 21-day-old fetal rat calvaria. There are relatively few osteoclasts present, and we don't see as much degradation.

With $1,25\text{-}(OH)_2D_3$ we don't see any effect on degradation of the newly synthesized collagen. Finally, the most recent data we have is that a cDNA probe for type I procollagen that Dr. Rowe has developed at the University of Connecticut does recognize fewer mRNA molecules in tissue that has been treated with $1,25\text{-}(OH)_2D_3$.

DR. POTTENGER: Certainly there are a lot of people on indomethacin chronically. Has anybody noted that this may cause osteoporosis?

DR. RAISZ: I didn't go into our problems with indomethacin but we cannot replicate the effects of glucocorticoids with it. Whether this is because there is something else about the drug or we are getting incomplete local inhibition of PGE_2, I don't know. There aren't many people on enough indomethacin to block all local prostaglandin synthesis, and it has been very disappointing in the hypercalcemia of malignancy, even when prostaglandin production is increased.

There are some animal studies suggesting that indomethacin treatment at high doses decreases bone turnover. However, there is also impairment of renal function in the whole animal, and also slow wound healing. It is going to be difficult to use inhibitors unless we have a really clean drug, if there is such a thing.

DR. TURTURRO: Are all the bones of the body equally susceptible to this PGE_2 and this glucocorticoid stimulation, and do you find differences in development in different parts of the bone?

DR. RAISZ: We haven't looked at many different bones. We certainly find that glucocorticoids inhibit bone growth universally. Trabecular bone and rapidly growing fetal bone are clearly more susceptible than adult cortical bone, but that could simply be the result of the fact that the adult cortical bone is turning over less rapidly.

There is endosteal resorption with prostaglandins and periosteal apposition. This is also the pattern of bone growth normally. So, there are differences between periosteum and endosteum in the response to this hormone. There is not as much periosteal change elsewhere in the skeleton as there is in the weight-bearing long bones of the dog. There is some change in the vertebrae.

DR. REAVEN: Have you anything to say about the effects of exercise, fitness and aging in regard to bones?

DR. RAISZ: There is no question that exercise increases bone mass. This group is probably at the right age to remind you that Rod Laver's left radius and ulna were 25 percent bigger than his right, and for those of you who are too young, he was the John McEnroe of my generation.

Bone mass increases have been clearly demonstrated with exercise programs. Could there be humoral mediators of exercise? If there is an analogy between exercise and direct mechanical stress, the latter has been shown to increase prostaglandin production by bone cells.

DR. REAVEN: How about ballerinas?

DR. RAISZ: There is another problem. There is something called "athletic amenorrhea" syndrome. Women athletes who exercise or lose enough body fat (as in anorexia nervosa) stop having periods and they lose sex hormone secretion. It isn't a simple correlation but amenorrhea does reverse the beneficial effects of exercise. There are astounding data from California which show a 20% decrease in trabecular bone mass in women who run and are amenorrheic. These women run 50 miles or more a week, and that is a special case.

DR. REAVEN: Have you studied aging individuals who are fit?

DR. RAISZ: We have looked only at activity in the aging. There is a rough correlation between bone mass and activity, but there are so many other things that go with activity in terms of diet and health concern that I don't think that correlation is good enough. There are a couple of clinical trials which show that an exercise program in postmenopausal women with fractures will increase bone mass.

DR. ZOOK: Do you have a hormonal explanation for electrical stimulation of bone fracture repair?

DR. RAISZ: No one has yet put together electrical stimulation with a humoral factor. Electrical stimulation will increase the replication of bone cells, and Dr. Gideon Rodan has shown direct effect on DNA synthesis from electrical stimulation and magnetic fields, but whether there is a humoral mediator, we don't know.

DR. VAN SICKLE: Is there an effect of prostaglandins on adipose bone marrow?

DR. RAISZ: I don't know the answer to that question. I have never seen any data on that.

DR. VAN SICKLE: The reason I ask the question is that there is a naturally occurring disease in some families of German Shepherd Dogs called panosteitis. The disease results in a medullary formation of bone with endosteal resorption and periosteal addition which looks very similar to what you are showing as resulting from prostaglandin administration.

DR. RAISZ: That would be very interesting to investigate.

DR. VAN SICKLE: We have looked at the cortisol levels. However, we couldn't find any correlation between stage of disease and hormone level.

The other interesting item is that the one common etiological factor that we could find in looking at both males and females was stress.

DR. MEITES: You mentioned that very little is known about how estrogen acts on bone. I think there are data going back quite a long time showing that estrogen increases growth hormone secretion. For example, Andrew Frantz at Columbia has reported that in normal men and women estrogens increase growth hormone in the circulation, and there is also some evidence, I believe, that estrogen increases parathyroid hormone in the circulation as well.

DR. RAISZ: Well, with respect to the first, the problem is that estrogens decrease somatomedin levels. That has been shown in younger individuals and, more recently, Ernest Schwartz has shown that even in older individuals estrogen administration decreases somatomedin.

If we accept that growth hormone acts on bone largely through somatomedins, and the somatomedin levels go down, then it is hard to explain any trophic effect on bones from estrogen via growth hormone, but it is not a settled issue.

As far as the effect of estrogen on parathyroid hormone levels are concerned, there aren't any major effects. The major effect *in vivo* in a postmenopausal woman with hyperparathyroidism is decreased bone resorption and serum calcium levels without any drop in PTH levels. So, there is an opposition to the action of parathyroid hormone.

The problem is that you cannot show estrogen receptors in bone or any direct action of estrogen at physiologic or even reasonable pharmacologic concentrations to inhibit bone resorption.

DR. WISSLER: The cardiology community is excited these days about a group of drugs called calcium channel blockers that seem to be almost miraculous in terms of their effects on mesenchyme. They appear to do a lot relative to smooth muscle, to cardiac muscle and probably cardiovascular conduction processes. Do they have any special effect on bone metabolism?

DR. RAISZ: At the high concentrations at which they probably become nonspecific membrane stabilizers they act very much like other membrane stabilizers, like lidocaine or diphenylhydantoin. At the low concentrations which are effective for cardiac muscle we don't see much effect. This may be related to the fact that we do not have the specific kind of calcium channel in bone cells that are present in muscle cells.

Comparative Pathobiology of Major Age-Related Diseases: Current Status and Research Frontiers, pages 159–174

PATHOBIOLOGY OF OSTEOARTHRITIS

Lawrence A. Pottenger, M.D., Ph.D.

Assistant Professor of Orthopaedic Surgery,
The University of Chicago, Chicago, IL 60637

Osteoarthritis (OA) is a gradually progressive, destructive disease of joints characterized by four classical X-ray findings: joint space narrowing indicative of cartilage loss, sclerosis and remodeling of subchondral bone, juxta-articular bone cysts, and peripheral bony outgrowths or osteophytes. Clinical symptoms such as pain and loss of function usually appear after X-ray changes have become advanced. Joint changes are generally irreversible and there is little evidence that current drug therapy is beneficial beyond symptomatic relief.

OA has been arbitrarily divided into two subgroups, "primary" where there is no obvious antecedent cause and "secondary" where an etiologic factor can be identified. Common causes of secondary osteoarthritis include: a) inflammatory joint disease, such as septic arthritis, rheumatoid arthritis and gout, b) mechanical abnormalities which alter the normal weight distribution across a joint so as to produce abnormally high focal loads, such as incongruent healing of an intra-articular fracture, genu varum and Perthes' disease and c) destruction of cartilage with chondrocyte death. Secondary OA has also been noted to result from occupations in which specific joints are heavily used (Lee et al 1974).

The chronic nature of osteoarthritis and late appearance of symptoms probably masks many causes of cartilage damage. Indeed, the concept of "primary" osteoarthritis may disappear as we increase our understanding of etiologic mechanisms.

CARTILAGE STRUCTURE

Human articular cartilage can be structurally divided into four zones (Weiss 1979). The most superficial zone or tangential zone consists of densely interwoven collagen fibers running parallel to the surface. Immediately below is a transitional zone where tangential fibers turn in to connect with fibers of the radial zone which are oriented perpendicular to the underlying bone. Fibers in the radial zone are continuous with the bottom layer or zone of calcified cartilage. Chondrocytes are sparsely but uniformly distributed throughout the tissue. In adult life, under normal circumstances, chondrocytes very rarely divide (Mankin 1982). Most articular cartilage contains no nerves or vessels. Chondrocytes are nourished and waste metabolites are eliminated by diffusional exchange with synovial fluid (McKibbin, Maroudas 1979).

The extracellular matrix of cartilage contains 3 groups of macromolecules: collagen, proteoglycans, and matrix proteins. Collagen accounts for more than 50% of the dry weight of cartilage. The vast majority is type II collagen in the form of a fine mesh with average fibril diameter of approximately 10-20 nm (Linsenmayer 1982).

Proteoglycans can be extracted from cartilage with chaotropic agents such as 4 molar guanidine HCl. Individual proteoglycan molecules have a molecular weight of approximately 2 million daltons (Hascall 1981). They consist of a "core protein" of approximately 200,000 daltons to which 80-100 chondroitin sulfate chains and 10-15 keratan sulfate chains are attached. One end of the core protein molecule contains a region, devoid of carbohydrate chains, which can form a strong non-covalent bond with hyaluronic acid. Immediately adjacent, there is a region which contains mainly keratan sulfate chains while the chondroitin sulfate chains are dispersed throughout the remaining part of the molecule.

Thirty to 50 individual proteoglycans bind to long hyaluronic acid chains forming aggregates as large as 100 million daltons (Muir 1981). Binding of proteoglycans is strengthened by "link" proteins (MW 44,000 or 48,000) which simultaneously bind to both hyaluronic acid and core protein (Hardingham 1979). Proteoglycan aggregates are so large that they are physically trapped within the collagen mesh

(Pottenger et al 1982).

Even with the same cartilage, the molecular weight of proteoglycans varies greatly (Heinegard 1977). This heterogeneity is thought to be in both the glycosaminoglycan side chains and the core protein. As much as 30% of the proteoglycans within cartilage cannot bind hyaluronic acid (Pottenger et al 1983). Some of these non-binding proteoglycans may be early degradation products which are still too large to diffuse from the collagen mesh (Sandy et al 1978). However, novel low molecular weight proteoglycans have recently been found which do not appear to be chemically related to aggregating proteoglycans (Heinegard et al 1981).

Physical interaction between proteoglycans and collagen is responsible for many of the biomechanical characteristics of cartilage. The large number of fixed negative charges on proteoglycans attract high concentrations of mobile cations thus raising the osmotic pressure and creating a tendency for proteoglycans to expand. Osmotic pressures as high as 3 atmospheres are maintained within cartilage because the expansion is resisted by the tensile strength of collagen (Urban et al 1979). When an external force is applied, water is extruded, proteoglycans are compressed, and the osmotic pressure is locally increased. The extruded water acts as a lubricant for joint motion (Swanson 1979). Upon removal of the force, the cartilage expands to its original size.

CHANGES WITH AGE

Many investigators have noted changes in the composition of articular cartilage proteoglycans at the time of skeletal maturation. In humans (Roughley, White 1980), pig (Simunek, Muir 1972), steer (Sweet et al 1979) and dog (Inerot et al 1978) the percentage of chondroitin sulfate within proteoglycans decreases while that of keratan sulfate and protein increases. The size of the proteoglycan monomers decreases slightly, but there is no change in the ability of proteoglycans to form aggregates with hyaluronic acid. In steers and dogs, average chondroitin sulfate chain length is slightly decreased while in pigs and humans the chains remain the same length but are reduced in number. With maturation, chondroitin-6-SO_4 becomes the predominant isomer synthesized whereas prior to that time chondroitin-4-SO_4 is predominant. Thus far, the studies have not been thorough enough to demonstrate significant changes in proteoglycan composition later in life when OA becomes predominant.

Water content, cell density and collagen density do not appear to vary with age after maturity (Muir 1979). However, recent reports suggest that cartilage tensile stiffness and fatigue resistance gradually decrease with age (Kempson 1979) while collagen fibril diameter increases (Weiss 1979).

CARTILAGE CHANGES IN OSTEOARTHRITIS

Animal models have been extremely important for the study of early OA because it is impossible to determine if a mild human lesion seen at autopsy would have progressed to typical OA. Spontaneous OA is seen in horses (O'Brien et al 1977), cattle, swine, dogs, mice, hamsters and guinea pigs (Moskowitz 1972). In addition, many forms of mechanical and chemical cartilage damage in animals will go on to produce histologic changes similar to OA in humans. Mechanical methods are generally used because they are biochemically less ambiguous than chemical methods. In rabbits, OA has been produced by compressing immobilized knee joints (Langenskiold et al 1979), and by partial meniscectomy alone (Moskowitz et al 1979) or in conjunction with removal of the cruciate ligaments (Telhag, Lindberg 1972). It has been produced in dogs by section of the the anterior cruciate ligament (McDevitt, Muir 1976).

In most mechanically induced models of OA, and in human OA, the sequence of histologic changes is quite similar (Moskowitz 1972). One first sees irregularity and fissuring of superficial layers of the tangential zone. As the abrasion continues chondrocytes disappear from the tangential and transitional zones and large fissures develop in the radial zone extending down to the layer of calcified cartilage. Cells nearest the fissures die; cells slightly farther away proliferate forming clusters of actively synthesizing cells (Rothwell, Bentley 1973). As the fissures become confluent, the radial zone becomes filled with hair-like projections of fragmented cartilage known as fibrillations. Eventually, the "hairs" are abraded away leaving exposed subchondral bone.

Proteoglycans can be stained in tissue with Safranin O (Weiss 1979). The stain normally appears homogenously spread throughout the cartilage with mild increases in pericellular areas. With fibrillation, there is a dramatic loss of intercellular staining and a "halo-like" accentuation of staining around chondrocyte clusters, suggesting that proteoglycans are being synthesized but are not staying in the tissue. Degenerated cells do not have proteoglycan halos.

BIOCHEMICAL CHANGES IN OSTEOARTHRITIS

Chemical characterization of OA cartilage is difficult because of the great local variation in the condition of cartilage. The central area of an OA joint may be totally denuded of cartilage. It is usually surrounded by a rim of fibrillated tissue which increases in height toward the periphery. Often a portion of cartilage at the edge remains structurally intact. When sampling for biochemical studies, it is very important to document the condition of the cartilage. Mankin et al (1971) have suggested a system for grading the severity of osteoarthritic cartilage which has found general acceptance.

Environmental factors may also affect joints in ways which are difficult to predict. If the joint is painful, the person or animal may refrain from using it. Immobilized joints often show atrophy of cartilage with loss of Safranin O staining. In dogs, the loss of staining appears to be due to a reversible proteoglycan aggregation defect which allows proteoglycans to escape from the cartilage (Palmoski et al 1979).

As one would expect from histological studies, biochemical changes in both human OA and animal models include increased DNA synthesis which eventually decreases as the disease becomes severe and decreased concentrations of proteoglycans in proportion to the severity of the disease (Mankin et al 1971). The concentration of collagen remains unchanged except in areas where cartilage is completely missing (Mankin, Lippiello 1970).

In human tissue, the loss of proteoglycans (measured as uronic acid or hexosamine) closely parallels variations in the histologic severity of the disease even within the same joint (Maroudas et al 1973; Mankin et al 1971). Non-fibrillated areas of OA joints contained normal concentrations of proteoglycans (Maroudas et al 1973). Proteoglycan concentrations are increased close to viable chondrocytes but greatly decreased away from chondrocytes (Mitchell et al 1981). Rabbit (Moskowitz et al 1979) and dog (McDevitt, Muir 1976) models of OA show similar reductions of proteoglycans.

The size of individual proteoglycan monomers has been reported to decrease slightly in human OA (Vasan 1980), but remains unchanged in naturally occurring bovine OA (Axelsson, Bjelle 1979) and dog models (Inerot et al 1978). Similarly, chondroitin sulfate chain length was noted to decrease in human but not bovine disease. In human disease as well as dog models, the ratio of chondroitin sulfate to keratan sulfate is much higher than age matched controls. This is thought to represent a change to synthesis of proteoglycans characteristic of immature animals, perhaps in response to accelerated synthesis.

Most proteoglycans from both human (Santer at al 1981) and dog (Inerot et al 1978) OA cartilage are capable of forming aggregates with hyaluronic acid; however, an abnormally high percentage of proteoglycans are incapable of forming aggregates (McDevitt, Muir 1981) and the size of aggregates tends to be smaller than normal (Vasan 1980).

The decreased concentration of proteoglycans in OA cartilage is due either to increased degradation or loss of proteoglycans from the articular surface. Much higher percentages of proteoglycans can be extracted from OA cartilage with low ionic strength solutions (Sweet et al 1977). This is probably in large part due to the inability of collagen from fibrillated cartilage to physically retain proteoglycans. Microfragmentation of normal articular cartilage allows increased extractability with low ionic strength solutions (Hecht et al 1983). It may also be due to partial degradation of proteoglycans by proteoglycanases (Barrett 1981).

Chondrocytes in OA cartilage increase their synthesis of proteoglycans, presumably in response to decreased tissue concentrations (Mankin et al 1971). Explants of human tissue show increased incorporation of $^{35}SO_4$ into proteoglycans in all but the most severely diseased tissue. This has also been demonstrated in isolated osteoarthritic chondrocytes (Teshima et al 1983).

Similarly, incorporation of radioactive precursors into collagen increases from 3- to 5-fold in experimental OA (Floman et al 1979). The specific activity of collagen increases much more than other cartilage proteins, suggesting that the increase is not merely due to a generalized increase in metabolic activity. Since the concentration of collagen in fibrillated cartilage remains unchanged, (Mankin et al 1971) both synthesis and degradation of collagen must be increased.

The chemical composition of OA collagen remains relatively unchanged in spite of its gross physical disruption. Chondrocytes continue to synthesize type II collagen (Goldwasser et al 1982). Small amounts of type V and type I collagen have also been identified by immunohistochemical staining in areas of degenerating chondrocytes (Gay, Rhodes 1981).

It is very difficult to derive information about the structural integrity of OA collagen fibrils through mechanical testing because fibrillated cartilage is grossly disrupted. However, intact OA cartilage near areas of fibrillation has been shown to have less tensile stiffness than age matched controls (Kempson 1979). OA cartilage is also much more susceptible to thermal shrinkage than normal, which suggests that the integrity of individual collagen fibrils has been altered (Herbage et al 1972).

Increased cartilage water content is one of the earliest and most consistent changes noted in OA. Human osteoarthritic cartilage contains approximately 9% more water than controls (Mankin, Thrasher 1975). Experimental canine OA tissue contains 3 to 4% more water than normal (Inerot et al 1978). A single mechanical impact to dog knees has been shown to increase water content without causing fibrillation or proteoglycan loss (Donohue et al 1983).

Increased water content likely results from swelling of damaged cartilage which can no longer completely restrain the swelling pressure of proteoglycans. It may, in part, be due to water molecules occupying space previously occupied by proteoglycans which have disappeared.

CARTILAGE REPAIR

Most of the characteristic microscopic and biochemical changes of OA cartilage can be attributed to a normal reparative process in reaction to loss of cartilage continuity (Mankin 1982). Cartilage does not have a blood supply and therefore cannot manifest a typical inflammatory response followed by scar formation unless the subchondral bone is penetrated. Superficial abrasions show characteristic changes; there is death of chondrocytes near newly created cartilage surfaces. Slightly deeper, chondrocytes proliferate and accelerate their synthesis of proteoglycans and other matrix proteins.

Presumably, if the edges of a defect were held in close apposition, formation of new collagen fibers would cross the defect and thus heal the lesion. In reality, this rarely occurs because of constant joint motion. Cartilage lacerations remain unchanged for years (Mankin 1982). Abrasion of cartilage alone, however, does not produce OA in experimental animals (Thompson 1975), whereas models which produce widespread chondrocyte death or persistent mechanical trauma rapidly lead to typical OA. It appears likely that chondrocytes in fibrillated tissue can synthesize a sufficient amount of matrix components to prevent further destruction as long as the mechanical demands upon them are not excessive. The inability of cartilage to effectively repair itself produces a situation in which repetitive minor trauma can lead to progressive deterioration.

ROLE OF MECHANICAL STRESS

There is a general consensus among most investigators that OA begins with cartilage damage. Examination of animal models suggests that to produce progressive OA there must be either continuing abnormal mechanical stresses, or the original cartilage damage must be great enough that even normal stresses cause propagation of cartilage damage throughout the joint. The spread of damage may be very slow, but it is relentless because of its mobility to heal.

Freeman (1975) hypothesized that mechanical fatigue of cartilage is the major etiologic factor in primary OA and is responsible for propagation of cartilage damage in secondary OA. He pointed to the studies of Kempson and Weightman

(Kempson 1979), showing decreased collagen tensile stiffness and fatigue resistance with age, as evidence that cartilage becomes more susceptible to mechanical disruption with advancing age. Proteoglycans are thought to be lost from cartilage through leakage into synovial fluid rather than through degradation by proteoglycanases. Local loss of proteoglycans leads to focal decompression of the cartilage with transfer of load bearing to remaining intact cartilage.

Radin et al (1982) suggested that mechanical disruption of cartilage might increase as the subchondral bone becomes sclerotic and thus loses its shock absorbing ability. They reported that *in vitro* cartilage wear using impulsive loading was much greater if the subchondral bone was stiffened with methyl methacrylate.

In the same study, it was reported that glutaraldehyde treatment of the cartilage substantially decreased the rate of articular wear. Schwartz et al (1980) have reported that OA can be prevented in a guinea pig model by feeding large doses of ascorbic acid. Both of these studies suggest that progression of the disease may be reduced by strengthening collagen cross-links.

ROLE OF INFLAMMATION

Though OA is not considered to be an "inflammatory" arthritis there is much evidence that a low grade inflammation exists in most OA joints. Joint fluid cell counts are usually mildly elevated. Patients have symptoms unrelated to activity which often respond to anti-inflammatory drugs. Many patients have obvious synovitis by physical examination and at time of total joint replacement. The frequent association of mild inflammation with OA prompted Ehrlich (1978) to postulate that OA is primarily a low grade inflammatory arthritis.

The most likely stimulus to inflammation in mechanically induced OA is cartilage debris. Inflammatory arthritis has been produced in rabbits by injection of proteoglycans (Friedlaender et al 1980) and type II collagen (Trentham et al 1977). Cartilage wear particles stimulate cultured synovial cells and macrophages to secrete proteases and collagenase (Evans 1981).

Leukocytes in synovial fluid also release several enzymes capable of degrading cartilage matrix (Barrett 1981). The most important of these enzymes is probably elastase which can degrade both proteoglycans and collagen cross-linkages, thus completely solubilizing cartilage.

Cartilage concentrations of proteoglycan degrading enzymes including metal dependent neutral proteoglycanase, serine protease (Walton et al 1981), and cathepsin D (Howell 1975) are all increased in OA. Collagenase levels are also increased in human disease (Woessner et al 1981) and experimental canine OA (Pelletier et al 1981). Enzymatic degradation of cartilage, however, is controlled by a complex combination of enzyme activators and inhibitors. Finding an elevation of a particular enzyme does not necessarily indicate that increased degradation is occurring. OA cartilage has also been shown to contain trypsin activators not present in age matched controls (Walton et al 1981).

To determine whether the propagation of OA is primarily mechanical or inflammatory, one would have to analyze proteoglycans and collagen coming from the joint surface. If it were mechanical, the molecules would not be degraded; if it were inflammatory, they would be partially degraded. It is likely that both mechanical disruption and inflammation are important and that their relative significance varies from joint to joint.

THERAPEUTIC INTERVENTION

Perhaps the greatest detriment to establishing meaningful therapeutic intervention in patients with osteoarthritis is that they are relatively asymptomatic until joint destruction becomes severe. Presently, it is not possible to separate the person with mild OA that will eventually become severe from the vast numbers of people with mild OA whose disease either progresses very slowly or not at all. Options for meaningful therapeutic intervention become very limited in severe disease because of the gross bony changes and extensive loss of cartilage.

From considerations of the pathobiology of OA there appear to be four possible therapeutic approaches to the maintenance of joint function: removal of adverse mechanical influences, elimination of inflammation, fortification of remaining cartilage and replacement of destroyed cartilage with either fresh cartilage or synthetic low friction material. Several of these approaches are presently being used with limited success. Certain types of OA in weight bearing joints improve after osteotomy of the bone to redirect mechanical forces. Non-steroidal anti-inflammatory drugs often give dramatic temporary relief of symptoms. Permanent relief appears impossible in joints with gross bony deformity because of the mechanical aspects of the disease.

Studies of cartilage transplantation are still in their infancy (Lane et al 1977). Application of these procedures to OA will be particularly complicated because of deformities in the bone. Recently, rib perichondrium has been used in place of cartilage; it forms hyaline cartilage on joint surfaces (Coutts et al 1983).

As with most chronic diseases our goal should ultimately be aimed at prevention and treatment of early disease. Presently, the definitive treatment for most cases is to replace the joint when the disease becomes severe.

REFERENCES

Axelsson I, Bjelle A (1979). Proteoglycan structure of bovine articular cartilage. Scand J Rheumatol 8:217.

Barrett AJ (1981). Which proteinases degrade cartilage matrix? Semin Arthritis Rheum 11:52.

Coutts RD, Amiel D, Woo SLY, Woo YK, Akeson WH (1983). Establishment of an appropriate model for the growth of perichondrium in a rabbit joint milieu. Trans Orthop Res Soc 8:196.

Donohue JM, Oegema TR, Thompson RC, Buss D (1983). Morphological and biochemical changes in adult articular cartilage following indirect blunt trauma. Trans Orthop Res Soc 8:243.

Ehrlich GE (1978). Osteoarthritis. Arch Intern Med 138:688.

Evans CH (1981). Cellular mechanisms of hydrolytic enzyme release in osteoarthritis. Semin Arthritis Rheum 11:93.

Floman T, Eyre DR, Glimcher MJ (1979). Focal biochemical changes in rabbit articular cartilage in late experimental osteoarthrosis. Trans Orthop Res Soc 4:132.

Freeman MAR (1975). The fatigue of cartilage in the pathogenesis of osteoarthrosis. Acta Orthop Scand 46:323.

Friedlaender GE, Landenbauer-Bellis IM, Chrisman OD (1980). Cartilage matrix components as antigenic agents in an osteoarthritis model. Trans Orthop Res Soc 5:170.

Gay S, Rhodes RK (1981). Immunohistologic demonstration of distinct collagens in normal and osteoarthritic joints. Semin Arthritis Rheum 11:43.

Goldwasser M, Astley T, van der Rest M, Glorieux FH (1982). Analysis of the type of collagen present in osteoarthritic human cartilage. Clin Orthop Res 167:296.

Hardingham TE (1979). The role of link protein in the structure of cartilage proteoglycan aggregates. Biochem J 177:237.

Hascall VC (1981). Biology of carbohydrates. In Ginsburg V, Robbins P (eds): "Proteoglycans: Structure and Function," Vol 1, New York: John Wiley & Sons, p 1.

Hecht JD, Pottenger LA, Lyon NB, Webb JE (1983). The effect of cartilage fragment size on sequential associative-dissociative extraction of normal human cartilage proteoglycans. Trans Orthop Res Soc 8:200.

Heinegard D (1977). Polydispersity of cartilage proteoglycans: Structural variations with size and buoyant density of the molecules. J Biol Chem 252:1980.

Heinegard D, Paulsson M, Inerot S, Carlstrom C (1981). A novel low molecular-weight chondroitin sulfate proteoglycan isolated from cartilage. Biochem J 197:355.

Herbage D, Huc A, Chabrand D, Chapuy MC (1972). Physicochemical study of articular cartilage from healthy and osteoarthritic human hips. Biochim Biophys Acta 271:339.

Howell DS (1975). Degradative enzymes in osteoarthritic human articular cartilage. Arthritis Rheum 18:167.

Inerot S, Heinegard D, Audell L, Olsson S-E (1978). Articular-cartilage proteoglycans in aging and osteoarthritis. Biochem J 169:143.

Kempson BE (1979). Adult articular cartilage. In Freeman MAR (ed): "Mechanical Properties of Articular Cartilage," London: Pitman Medical, p 333.

Lane JM, Brighton CT, Ottens HR, Lipton M (1977). Joint resurfacing in the rabbit using an autologous osteochondral graft. J Bone Joint Surg 59-A:218.

Langenskiold A, Michelsson J-E, Videman T (1979). Osteoarthritis of the knee in the rabbit produced by immobilization. Acta Orthop Scand 50:1.

Lee P, Rooney PJ, Sturroch RD, Kennedy AC, Dick CW (1974). The etiology and pathogenesis of osteoarthritis: A review. Semin Arthritis Rheum 3:189.

Linsenmayer TF (1982). Cell biology of extracellular matrix.

In Day ED (ed): "Collagen," New York: Plenum Press, p 5.

Mankin HJ (1982). Current concepts review: The response of articular cartilage to mechanical injury. J Bone Joint Surg 64-A:460.

Mankin HJ, Dorfman H, Lippiello L, Zarins A (1971). Biochemical and metabolic abnormalities in articular cartilage from osteo-arthritic human hips. J Bone Joint Surg 53-A:523.

Mankin HJ, Lippiello L (1970). Biochemical and metabolic abnormalities in articular cartilage from osteo-arthritic human hips. J Bone Joint Surg 52-A:424.

Mankin HJ, Thrasher AZ (1975). Water content and binding in normal and osteo-arthritic human cartilage. J Bone Joint Surg 57-A:76.

Maroudas A, Evans H, Almeida L (1973). Cartilage of the hip joint. Topographical variation of glycosaminoglycan content in normal and fibrillated tissue. Ann Rheum Dis 32:1.

McDevitt CA, Muir H (1976). Biochemical changes in the cartilage of the knee in experimental and natural osteoarthritis in the dog. J Bone Joint Surg 58-B:94.

McDevitt CA, Muir H (1981). Proteoglycan aggregation in early experimental osteoarthrosis. Ann Rheum Dis (Suppl 4):37.

McKibbin B, Maroudas A (1979). Adult articular cartilage. In Freeman MAR (ed): "Nutrition and Metabolism," London: Pitman Medical, p 461.

Mitchell N, Harrod J, Shepard N (1981). Pericellular proteoglycan concentrations in early degenerative arthritis. Trans Orthop Res Soc 6:154.

Moskowitz RW (1972). Experimental models of degenerative joint disease. Semin Arthritis Rheum 1:95.

Moskowitz RW, Howell DS, Goldberg VM, Muniz O, Pita JC (1979). Cartilage proteoglycan alterations in an experimentally induced model of rabbit osteoarthritis. Arthritis Rheum 22:155.

Muir H (1979). Adult articular cartilage. In Freeman MAR (ed): "Biochemistry," London: Pitman Medical, p 145.

Muir H (1981). Proteoglycans: State of the art. Semin Arthritis Rheum 11 (Suppl 1):7.

O'Brien T, Lippiello L, Mankin HJ (1977). Osteoarthritis in the race horse: An experimental model. Trans Orthop Res Soc 3:274.

Palmoski M, Perricone E, Brandt KD (1979). Development and reversal of a proteoglycan aggregation defect in normal canine knee cartilage after immobilization. Arthritis

Rheum 22:508.
Pelletier JP, Altman RD, Pelletier JM, Woessner JF, Pardo V, Howell DS (1981). Collagenolytic enzymes in osteoarthritic dog cartilage. Trans Orthop Res Soc 6:332.
Pottenger LA, Lyon NB, Hecht JD, Neustadt PM, Robinson RA (1982). Influence of cartilage particle size and proteoglycan aggregation on immobilization of proteoglycans. J Biol Chem 257:11479.
Pottenger LA, Lyon NB, Webb JE (1983). Proteoglycan extraction of sized cartilage particles. Arch Biochem Biophys (in press).
Radin EL, Swann DA, Paul IL, McGrath PJ (1982). Factors influencing articular cartilage wear _in vitro_. Arthritis Rheum 25:974.
Rothwell AG, Bentley G (1973). Chondrocyte multiplication in osteoarthritic articular cartilage. J Bone Joint Surg 55-B:588.
Roughley PJ, White RJ (1980). Age-related changes in the structure of the proteoglycan subunits from human articular cartilage. J Biol Chem 255:217.
Sandy JD, Brown HLG, Lowther DA (1978). Degradation of proteoglycan in articular cartilage. Biochim Biophys Acta 543:536.
Santer V, White RJ, Roughley PJ (1981). Proteoglycans from normal and degenerate cartilage of the adult human tibial plateau. Arthritis Rheum 24:691.
Schwartz ER, Oh W, Leveille CR (1980). Osteoarthritis in guinea pigs: Effects of vitamin C. Trans Orthop Res Soc 5:214.
Simunek Z, Muir H (1972). Changes in the protein-polysaccharides of pig articular cartilage during prenatal life, development and old age. Biochem J 126:515.
Swanson SAV (1979). Adult articular cartilage. In Freeman MAR (ed): "Friction, Wear and Lubrication," 2nd edition. London: Pitman Medical, p 415.
Sweet MBE, Thonar EJ-MA, Immelman AR, Solomon L (1977). Biochemical changes in progressive osteoarthrosis. Ann Rheum Dis 36:387.
Sweet MBE, Thonar EJ-MA, Marsh J (1979). Age-related changes in proteoglycan structure. Arch Biochem Biophys 198:439.
Telhag H, Lindberg L (1972). A method for inducing osteoarthritic changes in rabbits' knees. Clin Orthop Res 86:214.
Teshima R, Treadwell BV, Mankin HJ (1983). Proteoglycan synthesis and size in cell suspensions of human normal and osteoarthritic chondrocytes. Trans Orthop Res Soc 8:169.

Thompson RC (1975). An experimental study of surface injury to articular cartilage and enzyme responses within the joint. Clin Orthop Res 107:239.

Trentham DE, Townes AS, Kang AH (1977). The arthritogenicity of type II collagen: A new animal model. Arthritis Rheum 20:138.

Urban JPG, Maroudas A, Bayliss MT, Dillon J (1979). Swelling pressures of proteoglycans at the concentrations found in cartilaginous tissues. Biorheology 16:447.

Vasan N (1980). Proteoglycans in normal and severely osteoarthritic human cartilage. Biochem J 187:781.

Walton EA, Upfold LI, Stephens RW, Ghosh P, Taylor TKF (1981). The role of serine protease inhibitors in normal and osteoarthritic human articular cartilage. Semin Arthritis Rheum 11:73.

Weiss C (1979). Normal and osteoarthritic articular cartilage. Orthop Clin N Am 10:175.

Woessner JF, Pelletier J-P, Pelletier JM, Enis J, Howell DS (1981). Direct measurement of cartilage collagenolytic activity in human osteoarthritis. Semin Arthritis Rheum 11:58.

DISCUSSION

DR. BERENSON: You mentioned that in repair, cartilage only shows type II collagen. Would synovial tissue produce type I, and could there be an admixture in certain areas of healing near the surface that might be a mixture of types I and II?

DR. POTTENGER: Cartilage trauma which involves penetration of the subchondral bone leads to a proliferation of the capillaries from the marrow space. They will migrate up and form typical granulation tissue which then is converted to hyaline cartilage. While it is granulation tissue it has type I collagen. When it becomes hyaline cartilage it develops type II collagen. The orientation of these new collagen fibers is such that they cannot mechanically sustain the loads, and so the new cartilage rapidly degenerates into fibrocartilage. The collagen then becomes type I again.

The synovium really does not play a part in cartilage repair that I am aware of, but the situation of capillaries growing through the subchondral bone is not present in osteoarthritis until there is abrasion all the way down to bone.

DR. WILLIAMSON: In view of all the proteases that you indicated are present in the damaged cartilage, I wondered if you did the leakage experiments in the presence of protease inhibitors?

DR. POTTENGER: Yes. All of them were done with inhibitors. One last comment. What I am saying is that osteoarthritis is not closely related to age except in the area of tensile strength, and the thought that it is invariably a part of aging is not correct. Secondly, the problem is not in the cells but in the extracellular matrix because the cells cannot repair the cartilage and therefore cannot respond effectively to the changes. So, it is really a matrix form of aging.

Comparative Pathobiology of Major Age-Related Diseases: Current Status and Research Frontiers, pages 175–188

EXPERIMENTAL MODELS OF OSTEOARTHRITIS

D. C. Van Sickle, D.V.M., Ph.D.

Professor and Head, Anatomy Department,
School of Veterinary Medicine, Purdue University,
W. Lafayette, IN 47907

INTRODUCTION

A little over a decade ago osteoarthritis (degenerative joint disease), a disease which affects the weight-bearing joints in 90% of the human population over 40 years of age (Moskowitz 1972), was considered to be an inevitable accompaniment of aging. Then scientific investigators began to discover that chondrocytes were not somnolent but could divide and increase proteoglycan synthesis, especially during the early stages of disease (Mankin 1976). These findings resulted in a more positive scientific attitude towards combating osteoarthritis. Perhaps the appearance of the disease, possibly by adequate exercise or by judicious pharmaceutical usage, could be delayed or, at best, be prevented. To realize these possibilities, the early biochemical, cellular and tissue changes which accompany osteoarthritis needed to be elucidated. This appeared to be an almost impossible task since the etiology of the early pathogenesis of the disease is still unknown and the disease initially is not painful enough to cause affected people to seek medical treatment. Therefore, the animal models of osteoarthritis were developed to study the early stages of the disease.

At first some of the models were used only to study cartilage metabolism; others mimicked rheumatoid arthritis; while others mimicked only certain aspects of osteoarthritis.

To aid in the differentiation of the various arthritides, a set of definitions and experimental conditions needed to be established. Osteoarthritis, osteoarthrosis (deformans) or degenerative joint disease (DJD) is an age-related alteration of a synovial joint in which there is a central focal degeneration of adult articular cartilage (the character of the lesion is dependent upon the load history of the cartilage) with secondary periarticular osteophytosis, thickening of the joint capsule, possible subchondral cyst formation, and sclerosing of the subchondral bone which results in eburnation. Osteoarthritis is a disease of adult articular cartilage--that aneural, avascular hyaline cartilage which covers the articular surface of synovial joints and which consists of a non-mineralized portion, separated from a calcified portion by a thin dynamic calcification front called the tidemark. This point must be kept firmly in mind, especially when evaluating research in which abattoir specimens of domestic animals have been utilized. Most of these animals are immature (e.g., the pig is not skeletally mature until 3 years of age, yet the market age of most pigs is 4-5 months). Their articular cartilage is not a prototype of adult articular cartilage. Rather it is a composite of two layers of hyaline cartilage--that avascular portion adjacent to the synovial cavity which will never ossify and will develop into the adult articular cartilage, and that portion between the presumptive articular cartilage and the secondary center of ossification which pre- and postnatally contains cartilage canals and will participate in endochondral ossification, resulting in radial enlargement of the secondary center of ossification. The chondrocytes of these two areas appear to be different and *in vitro* differences are beginning to become apparent (Sachs et al 1982). Since the researcher is already plagued with a number of variables in osteoarthritis research, it seems unwise to add another by working with juvenile models.

It is also helpful to separate those experimental models which deal with osteoarthritis (OA) from those dealing with rheumatoid arthritis (RA) since there are many facets of these diseases which are different, yet which the public press indiscriminately refers to as "arthritis". The reader is referred to a current review entitled "Animal Models of Degenerative Joint Disease" for OA models (Adams, Billingham 1982) and another entitled "Experimental Models of Arthritis" (Heymer et al 1982) which deals principally with rheumatoid arthritis models, to learn the existing level of knowledge in each field.

The objective of this paper is to present: a) the pathology of the natural degenerative joint disease of the canine shoulder; b) an experimental model of spondylosis in a subhuman primate and c) a filipin induced DJD model in the equine carpus. Most of this research was done in the author's laboratory in cooperation with Drs. Harvey, Kincaid, Wilsman, Pijanowski, McIlwraith, Hillberry, Kinzel, and Scheer. It was due to their innate intelligence, enthusiasm, hard work, and desire to answer vexing biological questions that the following projects were accomplished.

A NATURAL MODEL OF DEGENERATIVE JOINT DISEASE IN THE CANINE SHOULDER

In several reviews of animal models of degenerative joint disease (Adams, Billingham 1982; Sokoloff 1969), there is no statement that a naturally occurring model of canine degenerative joint disease exists, followed by a description of the osteoarthritis which occurs secondarily to hip dysplasia in the young German Shepherd Dog. A degenerative joint disease of the canine shoulder has been reported in the USA (Van Sickle 1980) and in Sweden (Ljunggren, Olsson 1975). It occurs not in the hip as in man but in the quadruped's shoulder which is the largest joint of the principal weight bearing forelimb (60-70% of the total weight) (Thompson 1961).

Investigation in the USA involved two canine populations (a) 100 German Shepherd Dogs which had been used as USAF sentry dogs and were 3-13 years of age and (b) 47 privately owned dogs from 3-18 years of age which ranged in size from Toy Manchester to Great Danes. The German Shepherd Dogs were used as a quasi control since they had to be of a minimum standard (age known, clinical history, weight) to be selected for the program, were trained in similar manner, performed similar work, and received adequate nutrition and veterinary care. The shoulder, elbow, and hip joints of all the dogs were examined grossly and the lesion quantified as to size and location. The mid-sagittal section of each humeral head was selected, fixed in 10% formalin, decalcified in a 50-50 mixture of formic acid and sodium citrate, processed under vacuum for histopathology, sectioned on a sliding microtome, evaluated quantitatively and qualitatively, and recorded.

Up to 4.5 years of age, the articular cartilage, joint capsule, and transitional zone of the joint margins appeared normal while at 5-6.5 years of age, one of two different lesions began to appear in the articular cartilage of the central-caudal region of the articular surface of the humeral head. In almost half the cases there was a small central-caudal focal loss of articular cartilage (5-10 mm in diameter 20 mm from the caudal margin); in the rest of the cases there was a central-caudal blister with radiating lines in the same location. On histopathology, no blister was found--only a condensation of chondrocytes and matrix. This was attributed to the dehydration of the histological processing. The articular cartilage on the dorsal plateau had undergone superficial fraying. In 5% of the cases there was an initiation of osteophytosis formation at the transitional zone of the lateral amd medial joint margins. By 7.5-8 years of age, 25% of the humeral heads had very evident articular marginal osteophytosis and an encompassing osteophyte was forming in the intertubercular groove. Deep fibrillations, some extending to the tideline with the majority extending into the middle parts of the middle zone, were observed principally in the central-caudal region. In 10% of this age group, the entire transverse expanse of the articular cartilage of the central-caudal region of the humeral head was undergoing some degree of degeneration. Macrophages were observed to be attached to the acellular glycosaminoglycan-poor tips of the fibrillated cartilage. In the synovial membrane, collagenous fibers were becoming more evident in the subintimal tissue and there was a round cell infiltration of this region which consisted of lymphocytes and plasmacytes. By 9-10 years of age, the central-caudal focal loss of articular cartilage had increased in diameter 10-15 mm) and in depth (superficial and middle layers were absent and the deep layer either absent of fibrillated). The lateral and medial osteophytosis at the joint margin was becoming more evident and appeared to extend more caudally. The intimal cells of the synovial membrane were arranged in layers and the subintimal deposition of collagen was very evident. At 10.5-13 years of age, a 20 mm diameter of articular cartilage of the central-caudal region of the humeral head was replaced by eburnated bone. There was a completely encircling marginal osteophyte, and the joint capsule was 3 mm thick (5-6 times thicker than at 6 years of age).

Several factors of the described pathogenesis require further emphasis. The osteophytosis and reaction of the joint capsule occurred secondarily to the articular cartilage degeneration. The point as to whether synovitis occurs first and then the articular cartilage degeneration or vice versa is a classical argument among rheumatologists. The 9-13.5

year old USAF sentry dogs were reported to have lost physical stamina and were losing the ability to work effectively for 8-hour shifts. It was also reported that they were losing muscle mass which is important to maintain muscle forces across the joint providing for a stable joint as well as providing proper compressive forces which assist in maintaining healthy cartilage.

The lesion was found in a similar articular location in the privately owned dogs, but depending upon the breed, amount of exercise and other variables, it did not develop as uniformly and the final lesion usually took longer to develop.

The articular cartilage degeneration was so chronologically similar that German Shepherd Dogs could be aged to within six months of their known age. This is also the same lesion area of canine osteochondrosis which occurs much earlier (3-9 months of age); the subsequent secondary osteoarthritis reaches the same degree of severity by 6 years of age. This is approximately the same chronology for the pathology of canine osteoarthritis (6-12 years of age).

A major question asked was: what is so special about the central-caudal region of the humeral head? Using an interdisciplinary approach a team of veterinarians and mechanical engineers designed a spatial linkage and developed computer programs as well as methods to attach the rig solidly to the foreleg (Kinzel et al 1972, 1976; Scherrer et al 1979). By reviewing the sequential computer plots, the amount of time and area of articular surface of the humeral head utilized during locomotion could be visualized. It was found that the central-caudal region of the humeral head was rarely used in normal locomotion but when it was, it appeared to be under shear stress. From the initial study of OA, it was learned that the dorsal plateau where lesions were not found was thinner while the central-caudal area was thicker (Van Sickle, Harvey 1970). This finding was substantiated and the dorsal plateau was found to stain (using Alcian blue in 0.9M $MgCl_2$) as if it contained more chondroitin sulfate and less keratan sulfate than the thicker caudal area (Kincaid, Van Sickle 1981).

These biomechanical histochemical studies have been responsible for the generation of new research protocols in which exercised cartilage and its role in DJD will be investigated.

AN EXPERIMENTAL MODEL OF SUBHUMAN PRIMATE SPONDYLOSIS

In an attempt to determine the effect of subcritical (i.e., no direct injury producing) $+G_z$ impact on the baboon spine, the following research was accomplished and reported (Van Sickle, Kazarian 1982).

Twelve male baboons (Papio anubis) were acquired, conditioned, and radiographed in anterior-posterior (AP) and lateral positions to determine spinal normalcy. During June 1974, at time of impact, eight animals weighing 20 kg were tranquilized with ketamine hydrochloride (6 mg/kg IM). They were placed in a seat in a sitting position, restrained with a torso harness, a lap belt and leg belts, with the head nestled between the arms which were acutely flexed at the elbows. The wrists were fastened to the top of the chair. The chair was raised to a predetermined height and dropped once. The calibration signal and deceleration-time history were photographed. The impact time histories were recorded, using a piezoelectric accelerometer located beneath the seat pan and the impact vehicle base. The deceleration-time history resulted in an average plateau of 40 G's with a time duration of 10-13 msec. Following impact, each baboon was radiographed in the AP and lateral positions and both views were accomplished at 15, 30, 45 and 60 days post-impact and then every six months until euthanasia (Figure 1). The four controls were handled in an identical manner except for not being impacted. In 1979 five of the impacted baboons were euthanatized and necropsied and in 1980 the remaining animals were euthanatized, necropsied, and hard and soft tissue histopathology accomplished.

Clinically, the baboons had no apparent post-impact discomfort. Radiographically there was no apparent spinal damage; however, 50% of the subjects appeared to have a minor subluxaton in the thoracolumbar transregion when compared with the pre-impact radiographs. By 12 months post-impact, 75% of the baboons which had a slight T-L subluxation had an increased density within the anterior portion of the annulus fibrosus. In two of the baboons, the anterior borders of the lumbar vertebrae were becoming indistinct and, in many of the animals, decreased height of the intervertebral disc (IVD) spaces was evident. Within 36 months post-impact, there was very evident osteophytosis on the caudal-inferior aspect of L_3-L_5 while L_2 had an increased density of the centrum. In one baboon, the T_{12}-T_{13} disc space

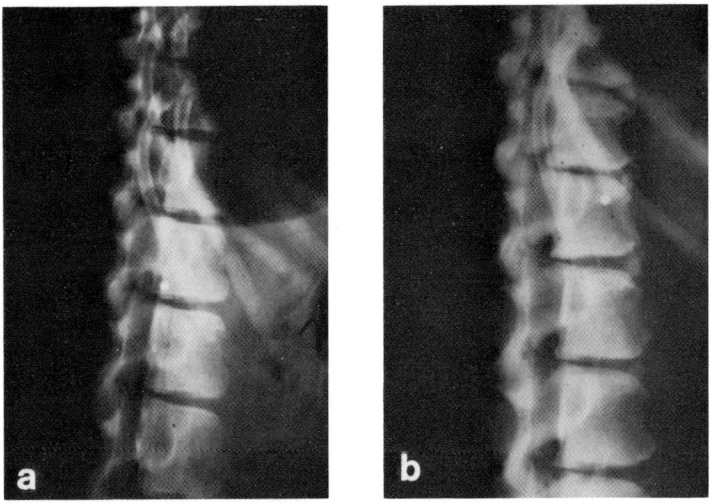

Fig. 1. Radiographs of the lateral aspect of the thoracolumbar region of the spine of E18: (a) immediately post-impact and (b) 27 months post-impact. On the (b) radiograph, anterior radiodensities are apparent at T_{12}-T_{13}, T_{13}-L_1 and L_1-L_2 IVD.

was obliterated and increased densities were evident on the anterior portion of the annulus fibrosus from T_{10}-L_5. In fact, L_1-L_2, L_1-T_{13} and T_{12}-T_{13} IVD spaces were bridged by osteophytosis. Within the same time frame, the articular facets were enlarging (as much as 3 times larger than controls) especially those of T_{11}, T_{12}, and T_{13}. By time of euthanasia the spinal columns of all the impacted animals had varying degrees of pathology. This variation may have been due to the amount of natural trauma to which the baboon is subjected prior to becoming an experimental subject.

At necropsy, the spines from the thoracolumbar area to the sacrum had large osseous bulbous enclosed IVD spaces. This reaction appeared to be greater in the lumbar region; however, by comparing the degree of osteophytosis with the size of centrum, the greatest degree of bony reaction was at the thoracolumbar region where there is normally a sharp morphological difference between facets of each region. Schmorl's nodes were observed in the medullary cavity of L_1 of several baboons. The muscle mass of the dorsum of the subjects did not appear atrophied when compared with the controls.

The histopathology verified the radiographic and gross findings. In addition, a burst cortical fracture was found associated with one of the Schmorl's nodes. The osteophytes were composed of lamellar cancellous bone surrounded by hemopoietic marrow. In general, the large initial osteophyte appeared to develop inferiorly to the superior edge of the involved vertebrae. The articular cartilage of the facets had an uneven articular surface and the superficial layer was missing in some areas or was acellular in others. There were areas of multiple tidemarks indicating the progressive remodelling of osteoarthritis (Johnson 1959).

The baboons, following one impact, had developed a time dependent spondylosis characterized by decreased IVD spaces, followed by osteophytosis, hyperostosis of the centrum with decreased height and articular facet osteoarthrosis. This correlates well with a recent hypothesis that the IVD and two facet joints are a tripoidal joint where failure in one segment will have secondary effects on the other two. Also a number of animal experiments have been described where spondylosis has developed following a single trauma; however, these experiments required invasive techniques which clouded the results of the experiment (Schmorl, Junghanns 1971).

In light of the serial radiographic, gross pathologic, and histopathologic results indicating a decreased IVD space at the thoracolumbar region, the secondary margination of anteriolateral osteophytosis, the secondary osteoarthrosis of the articular facets and the presence of Schmorl's nodes in the lumbar region, this model has been classified as spondylosis deformans traumatica. Research is continuing to identify the initial stages of this important disease of the elderly.

EXPERIMENTAL MODEL OF EQUINE DEGENERATIVE JOINT DISEASE

This model of osteoarthritis was developed to mimic the equine clinical condition and is interesting because it is an adaptation from a rabbit model (Weissman et al 1967). Following a pilot study, a more definitive study on the effect of filipin injection into the equine intercarpal joint was done. Four hundred μg of filipin, a polyene antibiotic, dissolved in 1 ml of DMSO were injected intra-articularly (IA) weekly for eight weeks and euthanasia was performed at twelve weeks. An acute synovitis occurred in the induction phase with regression of inflammation and the development of chronic joint capsular changes in the subsequent stabilization period. Utilizing arthroscopic examination, synovial fluid analysis, synovial membrane biopsies, serial radiography and necropsy results, it was determined that the model correlated well with what is believed to occur in the early stages of equine DJD of the carpus (McIlwraith et al 1979).

In another study, the experimental animals were given 12 consecutive weekly IA carpal injections of 600 µg of filipin in 1 ml of DMSO and were euthanatized 4 weeks after the last injection. The ponies were exercised for 1 hour/day throughout the experiment. Articular cartilage from 4 sites in each intracarpal joint was examined histologically and histochemically (McIlwraith, Van Sickle 1981), and synovial membrane was studied ultrastructurally (McIlwraith 1979). Clincal changes were similar to the earlier study, but the radiographic changes were more pronounced with exostosis on the dorsal surface of the carpal bone as well as a marginal osteophytosis. Superficial fibrillation of the articular cartilage with chondrocytic necrosis was found in the areas where there was a decrease of matrical staining, presumably from loss of glycosaminoglycans. This decreased staining was theorized to be evidence of "a decreased synthetic activity by the chondrocytes and destruction of the proteoglycan integrity by lysosomal enzyme." (McIlwraith, 1979) This was accompanied by hypertrophy of the remaining chondrocytes and chondrone formation (chondrocytic clusters).

The synovial membrane had a broad spectrum of pathological changes from intimal hyperplasia to frank ulceration in the more severely affected joints. This damage was more severe than seen in clinical cases. The ultrastructural changes paralleled those of the histopathology. No primary pathology of the intimal vessels was evident.

This model was chosen because it was postulated that the filipin caused disruption of the lysosomal membrane, and when the enzymes were released, caused depolymerization of the proteoglycan and loss of glycosaminoglycans (Weissman et al 1969) a pathogenesis which has been postulated for the initial stages of osteoarthritis (Bollet 1969; Howell 1976; Ali 1979). However, it was impossible to determine if the filipin acted on the chondrocytic lysosomes, the synovialcytic lysosomes, or both. The 400 μg level of filipin produced a model of experimental osteoarthritis which, using a number of parameters, simulated the clinical condition. Unfortunately, filipin is no longer available and other polyene antibiotics (e.g., amphotericin) do not seem to be as adaptable to IA use as filipin. While these investigations may be only historical, one of the valuable spinoffs was to allow for the histochemical characterizations of equine articular cartilage (McIlwraith, Van Sickle 1981). This biological data will serve as a foundation for future studies of equine arthritides.

CONCLUDING REMARKS

A naturally occurring model of canine degenerative joint disease has been presented along with two experimental models, utilizing diverse species of varying size. The etiologies simulated in the two experimental models have been traumatic and chemical. In the natural pathogenesis of degenerative joint disease, it is postulated that the accumulated microtrauma or microtrauma due to a change in locomotion may be enough to trigger the release of cellular proteases which cause depolymerization of the proteoglycan releasing the denatured glycosaminoglycans. It is apparent, as one follows the pathogenesis of an arthritic lesion, that when the lesion is seen grossly, it was present earlier histologically and earlier still at the ultrastructural and biochemical levels. This then is the goal of the utilization of experimental animal models of osteoarthrosis--the detection of the first molecular or biochemical change due to the initiation of osteoarthrosis so that ameliorating therapy--physical and/or chemical--can be immediately employed to delay or suppress the progression of osteoarthrosis.

REFERENCES

Adams ME, Billingham M (1982). Experimental models of degenerative joint disease. In Berry CL (ed): "Bone and Joint Disease," New York: Springer-Verlag, p 265.

Ali SY (1979). New knowledge of osteoarthrosis. J Clin Pathol [31 Suppl] 12:191.

Bollet AJ (1969). An essay on the biology of osteoarthritis. Arthritis Rheum 12:152.

Heymer B, Spaniel R, Haferkamp O (1982). Experimental models of arthritis. In Berry CL (ed): "Bone and Joint Disease," New York: Springer-Verlag, p 123.
Howell, DS (1976). Osteoarthritis - etiology and pathogenesis. In AAOS: "Symposium on Osteoarthritis," St. Louis: C. V. Mosby, p 44.
Johnson LC (1959). Kinetics of osteoarthritis. Lab Invest 8:1223.
Kincaid SA, Van Sickle DC (1981). Regional histochemical and thickness variations of adult canine articular cartilage. Am J Vet Res 42:428.
Kinzel GL, Hillberry BM, Hall AS, Van Sickle DC, Harvey WM (1972). Measurement of the total motion between two body segments. II. Description of application. J Biomech 5:283.
Kinzel GL, Van Sickle DC, Hillberry BM, Hall AS (1976). Preliminary study of the in vivo motion in the canine shoulder. Am J Vet Res 37:1505.
Ljunggren F, Olsson SE (1975). Osteoarthrosis of the shoulder and elbow joint in dogs: A pathologic and radiographic study of necropsy material. Am Vet Rad Soc J 16:33.
Mankin HJ (1976). Biochemical changes in articular cartilage in osteoarthritis. In AAOS: "Symposium on Osteoarthritis," St. Louis: C. V. Mosby, p 1.
McIlwraith CW (1979). Ultrastructural and Histochemical Studies of Filipin Induced Equine Arthritis. Ph.D. Thesis, Purdue University, W. Lafayette, IN.
McIlwraith CW, Fessler JF, Blevins WE, Page EH, Rebar AH, Van Sickle DC, Coppoc GL (1979). Experimentally induced arthritis of the equine carpus: Clinical determinations. Am J Vet Res 40:11.
McIlwraith CW, Van Sickle DC (1981). Experimentally induced arthritis of the equine carpus: Histochemical changes in the articular cartilage. Am J Vet Res 42:209.
Moskowitz R (1972). Experimental models of degenerative joint disease. Semin Arthritis Rheum 1:95.
Sachs BL, Goldberg VM, Moskowitz RW, Malemud CJ (1982). Response of articular chondrocytes to pituitary fibroblast growth factor (FGF). J Cell Physiol 112:51.
Scherrer PK, Hillberry BM, Van Sickle DC (1979). Determining the in vivo areas of contact in the canine shoulder. J Biomech Eng 101:271.
Schmorl G, Junghanns H (1971). "The Human Spine in Health and Disease." New York: Grune & Stratton, p 305.
Sokoloff L (1969). "The Biology of Degenerative Joint Disease." Chicago: University of Chicago Press, p 19.

Thompson D (1961). "On Growth and Form." Cambridge: University Press, p 246.
Van Sickle DC (1980). Primary osteoarthritis of the canine shoulder. Kal Kan Symp 4:53.
Van Sickle DC, Harvey WM (1970). A study of the gross characteristics of degenerative joint disease of the canine shoulder. Report to Seeing Eye, Inc, Morristown, New Jersey.
Van Sickle DC, Kazarian LE (1982). Chronic effects of $^{+}G_{Z}$ impact on the baboon spine. In AGARD Conference: "Impact Injury Caused by Linear Acceleration Mechanisms, Prevention and Cost." Neuilly Sur Seine, France: AGARD CP 322, p 1-1.
Weissman G, Pras M, Rosenberg L (1967). Arthritis induced by filipin in rabbits. Arthritis Rheum 10:325.
Weissman G, Spilberg I, Krakauer K (1969). Arthritis induced in rabbits by lysates of granulocytic lysosomes. Arthritis Rheum 12:103.

DISCUSSION

DR. POTTENGER: Were your horses still walking on that leg?

DR. VAN SICKLE: Yes. We routinely exercised them an hour a day on a circular mechanical carousel; one-half hour clockwise and one-half hour counterclockwise.

DR. POTTENGER: The loss of proteoglycans around the cells suggests that the metabolism or some hormonal factor is causing the chondrocytes to digest their own matrix rather than a mechanical loss.

DR. VAN SICKLE: Right. Filipin provides an initial articular inflammatory disease which subsides into a chronic one.

DR. POTTENGER: Loss of proteoglycans around cells is usually seen with inflammatory diseases and often in situations where animals refuse to bear weight because of pain.

DR. VAN SICKLE: Yes. The animals were hesitant at first, but they eventually walked normally on the carousel. The remainder of the time, we left them free in a paddock.

DR. HOWARD: I don't know exactly which species of baboon you were working with, but 20 kg is not necessarily fully mature. We see arthritis occasionally in aged rhesus monkeys. You didn't show young and aged baboon controls. I am wondering if you followed controls or if you would have found aged baboons with the compression pathology that you showed but who had not undergone the experimental compression? I hate to think that one three-foot fall brought on all of that spinal pathology.

DR. VAN SICKLE: Presently, we are working with the Southwest Research Institute which is providing us with spines from known aged baboons. We don't know the ages of our experimental subjects. You are right, they had the ring apophysis on the vertebrae at time of impact, so they were youngsters. However, this was the weight of animals which were available to us. The prior traumatic history of our subjects was unknown, and that is the reason I argue against using just a pre- and post-radiographic study, allowing the individual to be his or her own control. There is the possibility that some of these baboons might have developed idiopathic spondylosis, and this may account for the range of pathological reactions we observed in the spines of different individuals.

DR. LEVY: Did you section any of the blisters that you described in the dog?

DR. VAN SICKLE: Yes.

DR. LEVY: I think it is important to know what that early lesion is. It may give us a lead as to its pathogenesis.

DR. VAN SICKLE: Yes. We tried to, and initially we thought we had missed the blisters because we only observed a condensation in the articular cartilage in the region of the blister which we attributed to the histological processing We plan to study them by frozen section prepared in a cryostat to minimize the distortion of conventional dehydration and paraffin embedding.

It is presently a well accepted fact that one of the first consequences of initial osteoarthritis is an imbibition by the articular cartilage of water resulting in swelling. Therefore, I am wondering if this is what we may be observing.

DR. SIMMONS: Obviously there are implications in your baboon model for the type of trauma suffered by Army helicopter pilots.

DR. VAN SICKLE: Yes. This is actually why the baboon model was initiated. The Army asked us to look at the biodynamic effects of physical forces encountered by helicopter pilots while flying.

DR. SIMMONS: Now that we have had 15 or so years' experience with helicopters, do you know if there is any evidence that we are seeing increased back problems?

DR. VAN SICKLE: It may be, because there have been changes in helicopter seats. Hydraulic absorbers have been installed on the seats and other design changes have been made to the seat. In 1974 it was just a bucket seat, as you well may know.

As far as epidemiology is concerned, a large percentage of USAF pilots who have medical waivers are those who develop back problems. We are starting to follow these individuals very closely and are also quite interested in those who have experienced ejection.

DR. SAUNDERS: Why is the condition you described in the German Shepherd Dog restricted to a single joint? I don't think you told us that.

DR. VAN SICKLE: The reason why the canine shoulder is involved rather than the hips is that if one takes a 100-pound Great Dane and places his front legs on a scale there will be approximately 60 pounds of weight transmitted through those forelegs and only 40 pounds transmitted to the hindlegs. Consequently, if any damage occurs at the hips, the center of gravity moves forward over the shoulder and increased weight is added to the front legs.

D'Arcy Thompson reported some years ago that the four-legged animal supports a large share of its weight on the forelimbs and uses its hindlegs principally for propulsion.

DR. SAUNDERS: Could there be more damage to the joints below the shoulder joint?

DR. VAN SICKLE: I wonder about this also but I couldn't find any damage there.

Comparative Pathobiology of Major Age-Related Diseases: Current Status and Research Frontiers, pages 189–205

OSTEOPENIA, OSTEOCLASTS AND MACROPHAGES

Steven L. Teitelbaum, M.D. and
Arnold J. Kahn, Ph.D.

Washington University Medical Center,
St. Louis, MO 63110

INTRODUCTION

Osteopenia is a generic term which includes the family of diseases characterized by insufficient skeletal mass. In fact, most generalized disorders of bone are osteopenic, whether they occur in children (e.g., osteogenesis imperfecta) or adults (e.g., post-menopausal osteopenia).

Because of the clinical heterogeneity of osteopenic diseases, they undoubtedly reflect a potpourri of pathogenetic mechanisms. Regardless of pathogenesis, however, each form of osteopenia is characterized by a net increase in bone resorption, relative to formation. Hence, the activity of the principal, and perhaps exclusive bone resorbing cell, the osteoclast, is pivotal to development of all forms of skeletal demineralization.

Ultrastructural studies of osteoclasts have yielded many clues regarding the mechanisms of bone resorption. It is known, for example, that these cells attach to bone surfaces via an actin-rich, organelle-free zone (Holtrop, King 1977). This _clear zone_ surrounds and isolates the region of osteoclast membrane involved in bone degradation, thereby probably providing a "resorptive microenvironment". The resorption portion of the membrane is also the most distinctive component of the osteoclast. It consists of complex finger-like infoldings and is hence known as the "ruffled membrane" (Figure 1). This structure, which is the _sine qua non_ of the resorbing osteoclast, is generated by a variety of agents which promote bone matrix degradation, such as parathyroid hormone (King et al 1978), 1,25-dihydroxyvitamin D_3 ($1,25(OH)_2D_3$) (Holtrop et al 1981) and prostaglandin E_2 (Schelling et al 1980). Alternatively, calcitonin which inhibits bone resorption, leads to rapid disappearance of membrane ruffling (Kallio et al 1972).

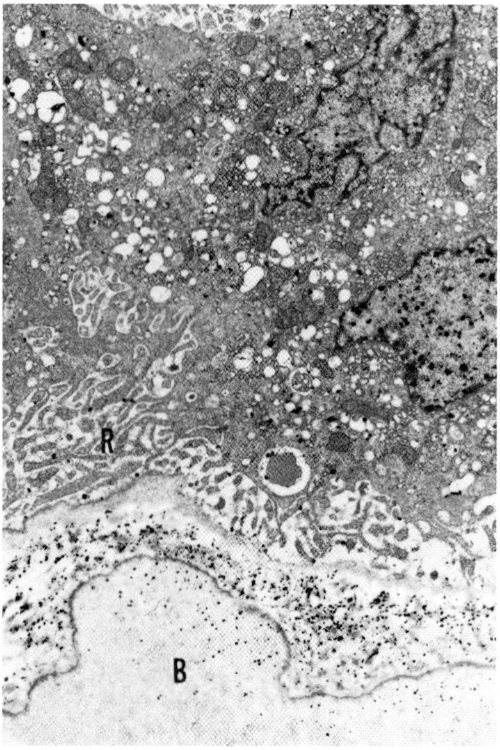

Fig. 1. Osteoclast resorbing bone (B). The complex cytoplasmic infoldings (R) represent the ruffled membrane. The black material on the bone is acid phosphatase reaction product representing lysosomal enzyme secretion by the osteoclast (Electron micrograph, X2000).

These morphological changes which accompany alterations of osteoclast activity are dramatic, yet little is known about how they occur, or in fact, precisely how osteoclasts degrade bone. We believe most of the confusion surrounding the cellular mechanisms of bone resorption, reflects the traditional models used to study the process. Bone resorption experiments have almost always been performed in whole animals (Heath et al 1972) or on organ culture of fetal bone rudiments (Brand, Raisz 1972). These systems are of great cellular complexity and hence, it is difficult, if not impossible, to distinguish the activities of osteoclasts from those of other resident cells. A case in point is lysosomal enzyme secretion. Osteoclasts are rich in these hydrolases (Holtrop, King 1977), and enzymatic activity in tissue culture medium often parallels enhanced resorption (Vaes 1968) (Figure 1). On the other hand, it has yet to be proven that these secreted lysosomal enzymes play a role in bone matrix degradation (Lerner 1980).

A more problematic issue relates to the mechanisms by which "bone-seeking" hormones effect osteoclasts. We noted above that a variety of these agents induce rapid and profound change in osteoclast morphology, yet it is unclear if this multinucleated cell is the primary target of all or any of these hormones. It is possible, for example, that parathyroid hormone exerts its effects on osteoclasts via intermediary (modulating) cells, and a recent and widely considered hypothesis proposes this to be the case (Rodan, Martin 1981). In any event, the issue remains unresolved.

Clearly, the most effective means by which physiology of osteoclasts could be studied would be on pure populations of these cells. Unfortunately, however, techniques are not currently extant whereby osteoclasts may be isolated and maintained in sufficient purity and numbers to perform meaningful experiments. On the other hand, our laboratory has in the past few years focused on developing bone resorption assays based upon the use of mononuclear and multinuclear phagocytes as surrogate osteoclasts (vida infra).

OSTEOCLAST ONTOGENY

Our focus on macrophages as experimental models of bone resorbing cells was prompted by the abundant data indicating that these cells are developmentally related to osteoclasts. To us, persuasive evidence that this ontogenetic relationship exists is provided by the following observations; 1) the appearance of labeled osteoclasts at bone fracture sites in rats receiving injections of thorotrast-labeled macrophages (Göthlin, Ericsson 1976), 2) the appearance of labeled nuclei in osteoclasts of vitamin D-treated mice injected with monocytes labeled with ^{3}H-thymidine (Tinkler et al 1981), 3) the formation of osteoclasts, *in vitro*, in cultures containing a) adherent bone marrow cells (largely macrophages) and fetal (osteoclast-free) calvaria (Ko, Bernard 1981), and b) bone marrow macrophages and embryonic, non-vascularized, cartilaginous (osteoclast-free) bone rudiments (Burger et al 1982). Also consistent with a common lineage of monocytes and osteoclasts, is the observation that both cell types are defective in human (Coccia et al 1980) and murine (Minkin 1981; Chambers, Loutit 1979) osteopetrosis. Based on these findings, it would appear that the pivotal issue in osteoclast lineage is no longer whether the precursor is hematopoietic or not, or whether it belongs to the monocyte family, but rather, at which stage in monocyte differentiation the cells acquire the capacity to give rise to osteoclasts.

MACROPHAGE-MEDIATED BONE RESORPTION

While the above discussion documents the ontogenetic relationship of osteoclasts and macrophages, it does not establish the latter as appropriate models of bone resorbing cells. We addressed this issue a few years ago by determining if monocytes or macrophages (and more recently, macrophage-like cell lines) resorb bone, *in vitro*, in an "osteoclast-like" manner. The essential limitation to resolving this problem is, of course, the fact that the precise means by which osteoclasts degrade bone are poorly understood. In any event, we found that like osteoclasts, mononuclear phagocytes extracellularly degrade the organic and inorganic matrices of bone, and do so in a manner which requires contact between the cell and matrix (Kahn et al 1978; Teitelbaum et al 1979). Similar to osteoclasts, macrophages secrete lysosomal enzymes onto the resorptive surface of bone and attach to the matrix via an actin-rich clear zone (Kahn et al 1978). The physiological significance of these findings is underscored by the recent report of Tran Van et al (1982), indicating that mononuclear phagocytes resorb bone *in vivo*.

These accumulated observations suggest that macrophages are the most appropriate, available models of bone resorbing cells which can be isolated and maintained in culture. This conclusion led to the development of a series of *in vitro* resorption assays using pure populations of mononuclear and multinuclear macrophages and bone (Figures 2,3,4). In the subsequent section we briefly review how the sequence of cellular events which culminate in bone matrix degradation has been analyzed using macrophage-based systems. In reviewing the following material, it is important to realize that 1) these assays involve the separate addition of cells and bone (or its components) to the culture vessel and 2) the bone is devitalized so as to obviate any influence of endogenous cells.

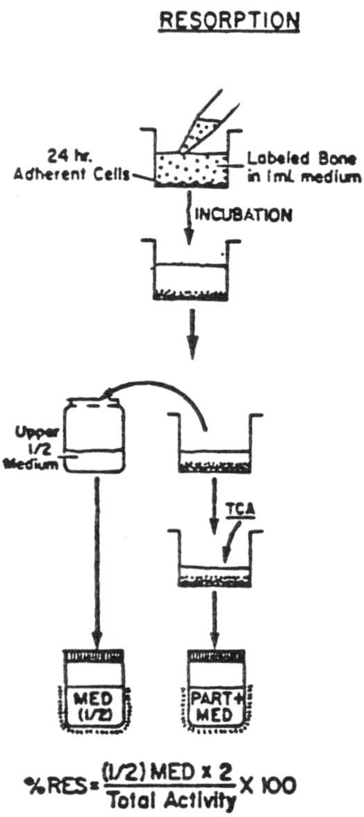

Fig. 2 (legend on next page)

Fig. 2. Macrophage-based resorption assay. Macrophages are purified by their adherence to tissue culture plastic. Radio-labeled, devitalized bone particles are then added to the culture dishes which are then incubated for up to 96 hours after which, the upper half of the medium is gently aspirated and its radioactivity determined. The residual (non-resorbed) bone is dissolved in concentrated trichloro-acetic acid (TCA) and its radioactivity also determined. The magnitude of resorption is expressed in terms of the radioactivity released into the medium. This value is corrected to express cell-mediated (net) isotope release by subtracting the percentage of isotope mobilized from bone in the absence of cells.

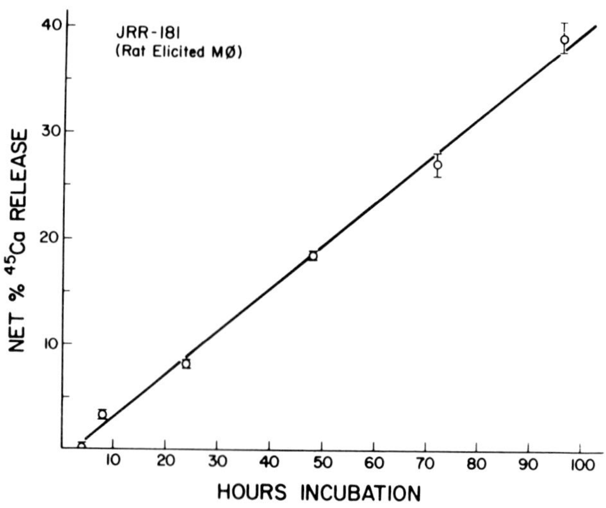

Fig. 3. Typical time course experiment showing the linear relationships between period of incubation and net % ^{45}Ca released from bone by peritoneal macrophages. Values represent mean ± SEM.

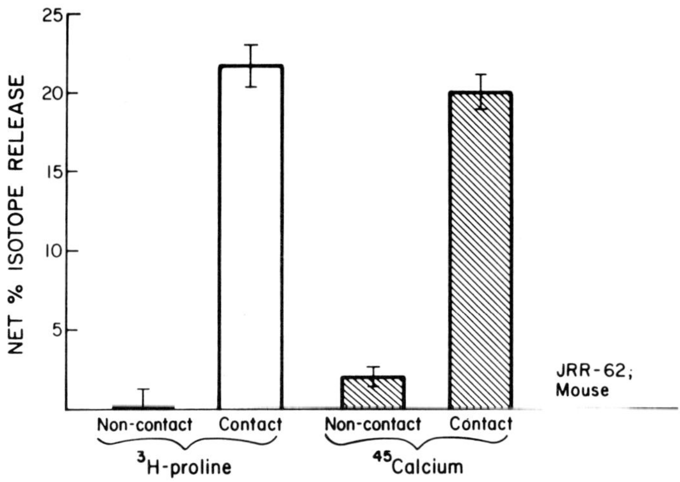

Fig. 4. This experiment demonstrates the capacity of peritoneal macrophages to mobilize the organic (^{3}H-proline labeled) and inorganic (^{45}Ca-labeled) matrices of bone when contact between the cell and bone is permitted. In contrast, inhibition of cell-bone contact by interposition of a polycarbonate filter (non-contact) virtually eliminates resorption.

THE SEQUENCE OF BONE RESORPTION

Bone resorption is in reality a complex process involving 1) recruitment of osteoclast precursors to bone, 2) attachment of these precursors to the matrix, 3) their differentiation into osteoclasts and 4) matrix degradation. All but the last (matrix degradation) is difficult to study using traditional models. On the other hand, we believe isolated cell (macrophages) systems permit one to individualize and quantitate the particular events.

Osteoclast Recruitment

Mundy et al (1978) have shown that human circulating monocytes are chemotactically attracted to products of bone resorption. These observations suggest that osteoclast precursors are recruited to bone by components of the matrix. In fact, our chemotaxis experiments with the isolated bone matrical component, osteocalcin (bone GLA protein), type I collagen fragments and α-2HS glycoprotein supports this hypothesis (Malone et al 1982).

Attachment of Resorptive Cells to Bone

Cell-matrix attachment is clearly essential for both osteoclast differentiation (Krukowski, Kahn 1982) and bone degradation (Holtrop, King 1977). However, the mechanism by which resorptive cells attach to bone has, in the past, remained completely enigmatic, largely because its study requires independent assessment of the relative contributions of matrix and cells to the process. Our models, however, permit such an assessment (Figure 5), and we found the relationship of cell-matrix attachment to subsequent bone degradation is more complex than previously appreciated. Glucocorticoids, for example, stimulate the capacity of macrophages to both bind (Bar-Shavit et al 1983a) and degrade (Teitelbaum et al 1981) bone. On the other hand, macrophages attach poorly to osteomalacic bone (Bar-Shavit et al 1983b), yet once bound, these cells degrade the matrix with increased vigor. This latter observation is in keeping with the clinical observation that osteomalacic bone contains few osteoclasts, but may be degraded at an accelerated rate (Z Bar-Shavit, unpublished observations).

We have also made progress in understanding the biochemistry of resorptive cell-bone attachment. Our experiments indicate that specific sugar residues in both the cell membrane and bone matrix are essential to such binding and that these saccharides function by interacting with specific lectins (receptors) (Bar-Shavit et al 1983c). Furthermore, in circumstances of stimulated cell-bone attachment (e.g., glucocorticoid treatment), specific membrane glycosylation is enhanced (Bar-Shavit et al 1983a), while diminished binding (e.g., in osteomalacia) is associated with decreased matrix oligosaccharide content (Bar-Shavit et al 1983b).

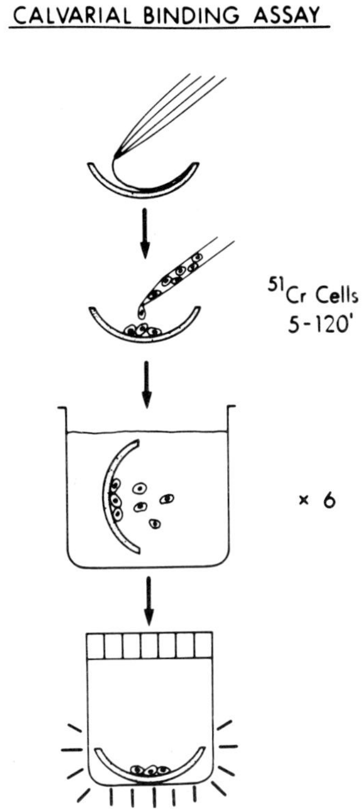

Fig. 5. One of several cell-bone attachment assays developed in this laboratory. In this assay, the endocranial surface of periosteal-free rat pup calvaria serves as the attachment substrate. ^{51}Cr-labeled macrophages are placed on the calvaria, incubated for up to 2 hours, and the calvaria vigorously rinsed to remove non-adherent cells. The number of adherent cells is expressed in terms of the percentage of added radioactivity which remains associated with the calvaria.

Osteoclast Differentiation

A change in the number of osteoclasts reflects either a) alterations of the life span of differentiated osteoclasts or b) the rate of maturation of osteoclast precursors. Distinction between these two events can only be inferred when one uses complex cellular systems and hence the state of differentiation of target cells of bone-seeking hormones has been poorly understood. The use of isolated macrophage-based systems, however, permits study of defined populations of cells at desired stages of differentiation. We found, for example, that 1,25(OH)$_2$D$_3$ fails to directly stimulate the resorptive activity of terminally differentiated macrophages (Kahn et al 1980). However, this metabolite does promote the maturation of an immature, non-resorptive macrophage-like cell line (HL-60) into mature monocytes, and in doing so, converts them into bone resorbing cells (Bar-Shavit et al, in press). These studies, of course, indicate that 1,25(OH)$_2$D$_3$ stimulates osteoclastogenesis by enhancing the rate of precursor cell differentiation.

Glucocorticoid treatment of man (Hahn et al 1979) and other animals (Jee et al 1966) also leads to osteoclast proliferation. In contrast to 1,25(OH)$_2$D$_3$, however, we observed that this family of steroids stimulates fully differentiated macrophages to resorb bone (Teitelbaum et al 1981), but fails to effect immature cells in a similar fashion (Z Bar-Shavit, unpublished observations). These studies suggest that unlike the maturation-enhancing effect of 1,25(OH)$_2$D$_3$, glucocorticoids promote bone resorption by activating differentiated osteoclasts.

Matrix Degradation

The ultimate event in bone resorption is, of course, matrix degradation, which is the component of the resorptive process most easily measured by a variety of experimental models. Macrophage-based resorptive systems do, however, offer significant advantage in studying the mechanisms of bone degradation. For example, as mentioned above, the use of traditional resorption assays precludes identity of the primary target cells of those bone-seeking hormones which ultimately alter matrix resorption. Our studies involving glucocorticoids (Teitelbaum et al 1981) (Figure 6), 1,25-(OH)$_2$D$_3$ (Bar-Shavit et al, in press) and calcitonin (Kahn et al 1980) (Figure 7) demonstrate the feasibility of addressing these issues with macrophage-based models. Furthermore, we have recently shown that parathyroid hormone-treated lymphocytes produce a factor which stimulates macrophage-mediated bone degradation, illustrating that modulation of osteoclastic activity by other cells may be physiologically important (Perry et al, in press). Finally, bone degradation reflects an interaction of cells and matrix and hence,

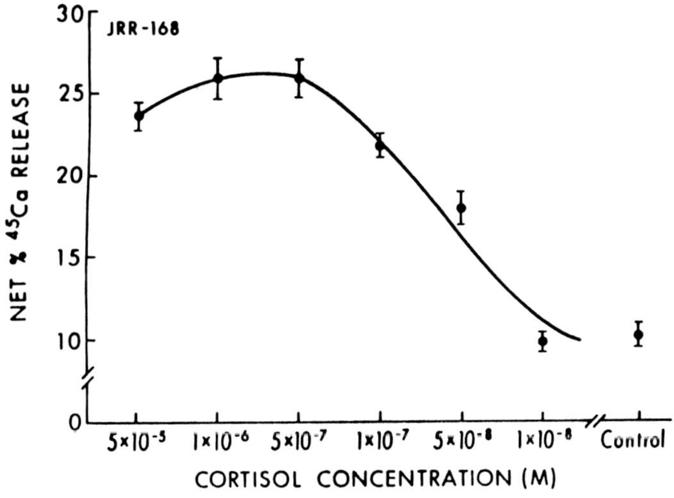

Fig. 6. Macrophage-mediated bone resorption under the influence of cortisol. Stimulated resorption occurs at physiological concentrations of the steroid (5 x 10^{-8}M) and is optimal at levels achieved pharmacologically (10^{-6}M).

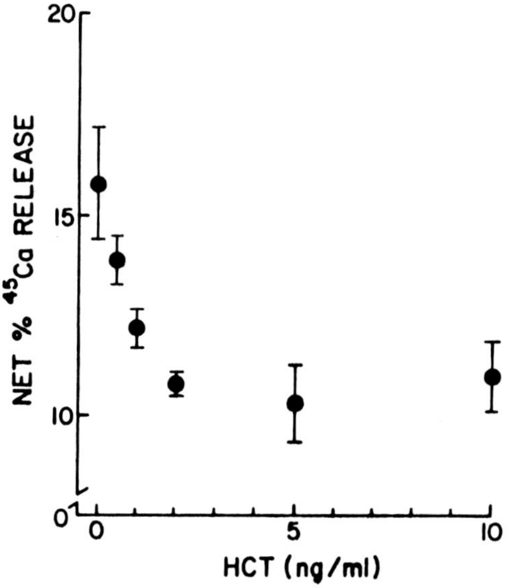

Fig. 7. Suppression of macrophage-mediated resorption by the potent osteoclast inhibitor, human calcitonin (HCT).

alteration of either component may effect the resorptive process. Because of the inherent inability to physically separate cells and matrix in traditional resorption models, the latter are generally not suitable for studies designed to determine whether bone-seeking agents act by modifying one or the other component of bone. In contrast, the separate addition of macrophages and bone in the newer assay systems, permits such individualization and has, for example, enabled us to clarify the means by which diphosphonates inhibit resorption (Reitsma et al 1982).

In this review, we have discussed only a few aspects of the resorptive process that are uniquely amenable to study by the use of isolated cell systems. We believe, however, that these observations represent only the "tip of the iceberg", and that in the near future, systems such as we have described, will be used to study bone resorption at the molecular level, an approach which should shed light on the causes of osteopenia.

ACKNOWLEDGEMENTS

This work was supported by NIH grant DE-05413.

REFERENCES

Bar-Shavit Z, Kahn AJ, Teitelbaum SL (1983a). Glucocorticoids, progesterone and osteoporosis. In Proceedings from the Fifth Annual Meeting of the American Society for Bone and Mineral Research.

Bar-Shavit Z, Kahn AJ, Teitelbaum SL (1983b). Defective binding of macrophages to bone in rodent osteomalacia and vitamin D deficiency: In vitro evidence for a cellular defect and altered saccharides in the bone matrix. J Clin Invest (in press).

Bar-Shavit Z, Teitelbaum SL, Kahn AJ (1983c). Saccharides mediate the attachment of rat macrophages to bone in vitro. J Clin Invest (in press).

Bar-Shavit Z, Teitelbaum SL, Reitsma P, Hall A, Pegg LE, Trial J, Kahn AJ. Induction of monocytic differentiation and bone resorption by 1,25-dihydroxyvitamin D_3. Proc Natl Acad Sci USA (in press).

Brand JS, Raisz LG (1972). Effects of thyrocalcitonin and

phosphate ion on the parathyroid hormone stimulated resorption of bone. Endocrinology 90:479.

Burger EH, Van der Meer JW, van de Gevel JS, Gribnau JC, Thesingh GW, Van Furth R (1982). In vitro formation of osteoclasts from long-term cultures of bone marrow mononuclear phagocytes. J Exp Med 156:1604.

Chambers TJ, Loutit JF (1979). A functional assessment of macrophages from osteopetrotic mice. J Pathol 129:57.

Coccia PF, Krivit W, Cervenka J, Clawson CC, Kersey JH, Kim TH, Nesbit ME, Ramsay NKC, Warkentin PI, Teitelbaum SL, Kahn AJ, Brown DM (1980). Successful bone marrow transplantation for infantile malignant osteopetrosis. N Engl J Med 302:701.

Göthlin G, Ericsson JLE (1976). The osteoclast. Review of ultrastructure. Clin Orthop 120:201.

Hahn TJ, Halstead LR, Teitelbaum SL, Hahn BH (1979). Altered mineral metabolism in glucocorticoid-induced osteopenia: Effect of 25-hydroxyvitamin D administration. J Clin Invest 64:655.

Heath DA, Palmer JS, Aurbach GD (1972). The hypocalcemic action of colchicine. Endocrinology 90:1589.

Holtrop ME, Cox KA, Clark MB, Holick MF, Anast CA (1981). 1,15-dihydroxycholecalciferol stimulates osteoclasts in rat bones in absence of parathyroid hormone. Endocrinology 108:2293

Holtrop ME, King GJ (1977). The ultrastructure of the osteoclast and its functional implications. Clin Orthop 123:177.

Jee WSS, Blackwood EL, Dockum NL, Haslam RK, Kince FA (1966). Bio-assay of responses of growing bones to cortisol. Clin Orthop 49:39.

Kahn AJ, Malone JD, Teitelbaum SL (1980). Mononuclear phagocytes respond to "bone-seeking" hormones and bone matrix constituents. In Cohn DV, Talmage RV, Matthews JL (eds): "Hormonal Control of Calcium Metabolism," Amsterdam: Excerpta Medica, p 182.

Kahn AJ, Stewart CC, Teitelbaum SL (1978). Contact-mediated resorption by human monocytes, _in vitro_. Science 199:988.

Kallio DM, Garant PR, Minkin C (1972). Ultrastructural effects of calcitonin on osteoclasts in tissue culture. J Ultrastruct Res 9:205.

King GJ, Holtrop ME, Raisz LG (1978). The relation of ultrastructural changes in osteoclasts to resorption in bone cultures stimulated with parathyroid hormone. Metabol Bone Dis Rel Res 1:67.

Ko JS, Bernard GW (1981). Osteoclast formation in vitro

from bone marrow mononuclear cells in osteoclast-free bone. Am J Anat 161:415.

Krukowski M, Kahn AJ (1982). The inductive specificity of mineralized bone matrix in ectopic osteoclast differentiation. Calcif Tissue Int 34:474.

Lerner U (1980). Relationship between bone resorption and lysosomal enzyme release as demonstrated by the effect of 1α-hydroxy-vitamin D-3 in an organ culture system. Biochim Biophys Acta 632:204.

Malone JD, Teitelbaum SL, Griffin GL, Senior RM, Kahn AJ (1982). Recruitment of osteoclast precursors by purified bone matrix constituents. J Cell Biol 82:227.

Minkin C (1981). Defective macrophage chemotaxis in osteopetrotic mice. Calcif Tissue Int 33:677.

Mundy GR, Varani J, Orr W, Gondek MD, Ward PA (1978). Resorbing bone is chemotactic for monocytes. Nature 275:132.

Perry HM III, Chappel JC, Bellorin-Font E, Martin KJ, Teitelbaum SL. Parathyroid hormone receptors on circulating mononuclear cells. J Biol Chem (in press).

Reitsma PH, Teitelbaum SL, Bijvoet OLM, Kahn AJ (1982). Differentiation action of the bisphosphonates, APD and Cl_2MDP on rat macrophage-mediated bone resorption in vitro. J Clin Invest 70:927.

Rodan GA, Martin TJ (1981). Role of osteoclasts in hormonal control of bone resorption - a hypothesis. Calcif Tissue Int 33:349.

Schelling SH, Wolfe HJ, Tashjian AH (1980). Role of the osteoclast in prostaglandin E_2-stimulated bone resorption. A correlative morphometric and biochemical analysis. Lab Invest 42:290.

Teitelbaum SL, Malone JD, Kahn AJ (1981). Glucocorticoid enhancement of bone resorption by rat peritoneal macrophages in vitro. Endocrinology 108:795.

Teitelbaum SL, Stewart CC, Kahn AJ (1979). Rodent peritoneal macrophages as bone resorbing cells. Calcif Tissue Int 27:255.

Tinkler SM, Linder JE, Williams DM, Johnson NW (1981). Formation of osteoclasts from blood monocytes during 1α-OH vitamin D-stimulated bone resorption in mice. J Anat 133:389.

Tran Van P, Vignery A, Baron R (1982). An electron microscopic study of the bone remodeling sequence in the rat. Cell Tissue Res 225:283.

Vaes G (1968). On the mechanisms of bone resorption. The action of parathyroid hormone on the enzymes and on the extracellular release of acid by bone cells. J Cell

Biol 39:676.

DISCUSSION

DR. WILLIAMS: What is the time frame in which you could radiographically see cortical reabsorption in your patients when they were treated with cortisol?

DR. TEITELBAUM: It is quite variable. First of all, 30% bone loss is required before you can identify osteopenic changes on radiographs. I have seen patients who will show radiographic evidence of bone loss within a few months, and in others it takes years. It depends upon where they start. In other words, if their initial bone mass is just above the limits of detection of osteopenia by X-ray, they may show radiographic evidence of the lesion very rapidly. There are also new techniques, like computerized tomography and dual photon absorptiometry which are more sensitive indicators of bone loss.

DR. BELL: You didn't say by what mechanism the osteoclast actually dissolves bone samples in your model system.

DR. TEITELBAUM: I didn't comment on this issue because I don't have much information. Let me just tell you about some "old saws" that don't appear to be true. One of the classical hypotheses regarding bone absorption is that lysosomal enzymes play an important role. Glucocorticoids block the release of lysosomal enzymes, and indeed they do so in our system despite a great enhancement of resorption.

The other issue is organic acids. It seems to me, at least teleologically, that organic acids are the most likely agents to remove the bone mineral during resorption. We have been able to manipulate the system with glucocorticoids whereby we can reduce total organic acid concentration in the medium and still enhance resorption. However, if you put a filter between the bone and the glucocorticoid-treated cells, you block organic acid release and shut off resorptiom completely. This indicates that the resorptive events occur at the cell-matrix interface or the microenvironment between the cell and the bone. The use of isolated cell systems offers the potential of probing that microenvironment.

DR. BELL: Have you looked at collagenolytic activity in the system?

DR. TEITELBAUM: Yes, we have. We addressed that question as part of a larger issue, namely, the similarity of resorptive macrophages to osteoclasts. The problem with resolving that issue is that nobody knows how osteoclasts behave. In any event, when we set out to examine the relationship between the two cells we made two assumptions, namely, that osteoclasts must degrade the organic and inorganic matrix of the bone and they must do it in a manner that is dependent on contact with the bone. The experiment we performed involved placing a filter between the cells and the bone particles. Our control was to have the bone in contact with cells and the filter in a non-interfering position. If you inhibit contact between the cells and the bone you block resorption. In addition, if you look at the release of both ^{3}H-proline, which we use to label the organic matrix, and ^{45}Ca which labels the inorganic matrix, they are about the same. So, there is a parallel release of both the organic and inorganic matrix in this system. Moreover, matrix degradation is extracellular. We have done time-lapse cinematography to prove this point. This is not a manifestation of phagocytosis.

DR. SCARPELLI: Hasn't anyone ever looked at either macrophage or osteoclast interface with bone by electron microscopy (EM)?

DR. TEITELBAUM: Those studies have been done many times, and certainly there are lysosomal enzymes at that location. However, no one has quantitated organic acid content cytochemically at that location by EM.

DR. SCARPELLI: What sort of acids are you talking about?

DR. TEITELBAUM: We have looked at lactate and citric acid.

DR. HIGH: In regard to the inhibitory effect (bone-sparing effect) of estrogen on the action of parathyroid hormone on bone, how do you account for those observations where prolonged estrogen therapy in post-menopausal women resulted in a worsened skeletal condition?

DR. TEITELBAUM: That is an excellent question.

DR. HIGH: Is the same thing true for progesterone? With regard to the inhibitory (bone-sparing) effect of progesterones on the skeletal action of glucocorticoids, how do you account for those reported observations where prolonged estrogen-progesterone therapy to normal women resulted (at times) in premature menopause with secondary skeletal effects?

DR. TEITELBAUM: There is very little data on progesterone. Perhaps you know of a study that I haven't seen, but I do not know of a long-term study on progesterone. You are certainly correct about estrogens. The data we have regarding estrogen therapy are that it works for the first ten years after menopause. There are, however, some patients who have a rapid bone loss after the first ten years if they are maintained on estrogens. We have no idea what happens after the first ten years. At present, this problem is a black box.

Comparative Pathobiology of Major Age-Related Diseases: Current Status and Research Frontiers, pages 207–219

A NONHUMAN PRIMATE MODEL FOR THE OSTEOPENIA OF AGING

Darrell D. Williams, Ph.D. and
Douglas M. Bowden, M.D.

Regional Primate Research Center and Department of Psychiatry and Behavioral Sciences, University of Washington, Seattle, WA 98195

INTRODUCTION

Osteopenia of aging is the progressive loss of bone mass, which in humans usually begins in the fourth decade of life. It is generally recognized as a part of the normal aging process. In women, the onset is five to ten years earlier and the rate of bone loss is greater than in men (8-10% vs. 4-5% per decade). For two to five years after menopause, the rate of loss may be accelerated to 1.5-2.2% per year (Giansiracusa, Kantrowitz 1982; Heaney 1976; Skillman 1980). Bone loss that becomes so severe that the integrity of the skeleton is threatened with fracture is considered pathologic and termed osteoporosis. It has been suggested that individuals with osteoporosis may simply represent the extreme of the distribution for the normal osteopenia of aging in individuals who, for one reason or another, have relatively small bone mass as young adults (Skillman 1980).

While the basic mechanism for the osteopenia of aging is unclear, several factors have been identified that can influence the rate of bone loss. Among these factors, the availability of calcium and vitamin D, decline in physical activity, and estrogen withdrawal following menopause have received the most attention (Aloia 1982; Heaney et al 1978; Skillman 1980). These factors and others probably act in concert to produce the normal osteopenia of aging. When the contribution of one or more of them is amplified, as in the abrupt fall in estrogen levels at menopause, the potential for osteoporosis is increased.

Our interest in the osteopenia of aging stems from Comfort's (1969) observation that the metacarpal osteoporotic index (Dequeker et al 1969) is one of the strongest biological correlates of chronological age in man. We have been interested in developing a biological index of aging, based on a battery of noninvasive, independent physiological measurements that show appreciable change with age. We would use such an index to evaluate the effects of nutritional or clinical interventions on the rate of aging in the pig-tailed macaque (*Macaca nemestrina*). The osteoporotic index was one potentially useful measure to evaluate for inclusion in the aging battery.

We have previously reported preliminary evidence for the utility of such a measurement in the pig-tailed macaque (Bowden 1979). We evaluated the percent cortical area (PCA) of the second metacarpal (Garn 1970) in a cross-sectional study of aging in 20 female pig-tailed macaques representing three age groups: 4, 10, and 20 years or older. Age group differences in the cortical thickness of the bone were similar to those reported for humans.

A number of other studies on the same group of animals indicated the utility of this species as a model for man in many aspects of research on aging (Bowden 1979). As an outgrowth of those studies on a relatively small number of animals, a colony of more than 60 pig-tailed macaques was established for multidisciplinary research on the biology of aging. Located at the Primate Field Station of the Washington Regional Primate Research Center, the colony is about equally divided as to sex and contains animals that, in 1981, ranged from 4 to 25 years of age.

This paper presents our first assessment of longitudinal data from the aging colony and focuses on similarities in bone remodeling between this macaque model and man. In the human, observations over at least a decade are necessary to detect significant change in most indices of biological aging. Equating one macaque year to three human years, we did not expect to find significant changes in bone thickness in the two years since the study began. We did expect, however, to replicate findings of our cross-sectional study on females, to establish whether similar findings characterize the male of this species, and to identify trends in bone remodeling. It is instructive even at this early point in the study to examine the trends of bone remodeling in the various age and sex groups and to compare them with changes known to occur in human osteopenia of aging.

METHODS AND PROCEDURES

Sixty-five pig-tailed macaques (*M. nemestrina*) were grouped into four age categories: 4-5 years old (10 males and 9 females), 9 years old (4 males and 4 females), 11-15 years old (8 males and 8 females), and 18+ years old (12 males and 10 females). Placement in a specific age group was based on known birthdate or best estimate of age in 1981. Age estimates for 15 animals that were feral-born, and thus lacked documented birthdates, were established for the males by comparison of body weight six months after introduction into the colony with weights of age-known, colony-born males. Such ages were estimated conservatively in that a maximum age of five years was assigned at entry to animals that entered the colony as full adults. Similar weight comparisons and dates of first pregnancy were used for the females.

Purina Monkey Chow 5083 (15% protein) was fed to all animals from weaning or from entry into the colony until August 1981. At that time, the animals in this study were placed on one of two semipurified, isocaloric diets prepared in-house. One diet duplicated the average United States human diet in contents of cholesterol, salt, and refined sugar, and in the proportions of calories derived from fat and carbohydrates. In the second diet, the proportions of calories derived from fat and refined sugar were reduced by 50%; cholesterol and salt were reduced by 83% and 75%, respectively. The vitamin and mineral content of the special diets either equalled or slightly exceeded those provided by Purina Monkey Chow. All diets were fed *ad libitum*. There was no reason *a priori* to anticipate a differential effect of the two diets on the osteopenia of aging, and preliminary analysis of the data in terms of possible dietary influence have supported that expectation.

Changes in bone mass were estimated by radiography. The animal was anesthetized; the right hand was placed palm down, with fingers spread, on the film cassette, and held in place by a bag of lead pellets. Two radiographs of each hand, taken an average of 1.9 years apart, were used for a paired analysis of within-animal changes in bone mass of the second metacarpal of the right hand. Care was taken to maintain the same source-to-object distance, milliamperage, kilovoltage, film, cassette, and x-ray machine for all films. The measure of bone mass, PCA of the right metacarpal, was calculated according to the method of Garn (1970). Total diameter (T) and medullary or marrow diameter (M) were measured at midshaft to the closest 0.05 mm under 1.75x magnification using a Helios dial caliper with needle-points. Garn found that the cortical changes in tubular bones are best described in terms of the total envelope of tubular bone in cross section. Therefore, by treating the measurements T and M as diameters of concentric circles, we calculated the cross-sectional area of the total bone by the formula $3.14 \times (T/2)^2$ and the cross-sectional area of the marrow cavity by the formula $3.14 \times (M/2)^2$. The cross-sectional area of cortical bone was estimated by subtracting the area of the inner circle from the area of the outer circle. All measurements were made by the same individual (DDW) without knowledge of the age or sex of the animal. The coefficient of variation, $(s.d./\bar{x}) \cdot 100$, based on 10 repeated measurements of five randomly chosen radiographs, was 0.98% for T and 2.10% for M.

Recognizing that the areas bounded by the outer and inner surfaces of the cortical bone are linear functions of T^2 and M^2, respectively, we calculated PCA by the formula:

$$PCA = \frac{T^2 - M^2}{T^2} \times 100,$$

where $(T^2 - M^2)$ = cortical area (CA).

Constant magnification between paired radiographs was confirmed by comparing the measurements of the length of the proximal phalanx of the third finger on the paired films of each animal whose epiphyses had closed. The coefficient of variation for measurements between radiographs was 1.38%, which was similar to the error obtained for the repeated measurement of T and M given above.

The paired analysis for change in PCA was calculated by the formula:

$$(1) \qquad \Delta PCA = \frac{PCA_1 - PCA_2}{t}$$

where the subscripts 1 and 2 represent the first and second radiographs and t equals the time in years between the two radiographs.

The ΔPCA is a measure that combines changes in total diameter and in medullary diameter of the bone. In addition to analyzing this integrated measure, we analyzed the data independently for change in the contributing components. The formulas used were:

$$(2) \qquad \Delta T^2 = \frac{T_1{}^2 - T_2{}^2}{T_1{}^2} \times \frac{100\%}{t},$$

$$(3) \qquad \Delta M^2 = \frac{M_1{}^2 - M_2{}^2}{M_1{}^2} \times \frac{100\%}{t},$$

$$(4) \qquad \Delta CA = \frac{CA_1 - CA_2}{CA_1} \times \frac{100\%}{t}.$$

RESULTS

As expected, few of the differences in measurements taken at the beginning of the study and two years later reached statistical significance (Table 1), although several distinct trends were apparent (Figure 1). For the males the PCA (lower left graph in Figure 1) did not change in the youngest group; it tended to increase in the 9-year-olds and then decreased at an accelerating pace in the older age groups. The females showed a somewhat different pattern of change. The youngest group showed a substantial decrease in PCA, a trend which reversed to an apparent slight gain in the 9-year-old group. Although this direction of change was similar to that of males in the same age group, the extent of change was considerably less in the females. As in the males, there were declines in PCA in the older age groups, but unlike the males, the rate of decline in PCA did not appear to accelerate in the oldest group.

Understanding of the changes in PCA was enhanced by analysis of the component measures comprising that index of cortical bone thickness. Deposition of new bone can take place at both the outer and inner surfaces of cortical

Table 1. Mean annual changes in cortical bone of the right second metacarpal in four age groups of pig-tailed macaque

Change (%/year)		Age Group (Years) Males				Females			
		4-5	9	11-15	18	4-5	9	11-15	18
ΔT^2	Mean	16.4	4.5	3.9	3.0	6.7	10.6	-0.6	7.7
	SEM	3.7	1.9	1.5	1.8	1.6	5.4	4.3	7.0
	n	10	4	7	10	9	4	6	7
	p	< .002	NS	< .05	NS	< .002	NS	NS	NS
ΔM^2	Mean	28.0	9.9	10.5	15.7	26.3	8.4	14.2	13.6
	SEM	9.0	4.4	7.1	6.1	15.9	13.5	16.5	10.9
	n	10	4	7	10	9	4	6	7
	p	< .01	NS	NS	< .05	NS	NS	NS	NS
Δ CA	Mean	17.0	4.1	4.1	1.5	6.0	11.4	-1.3	3.3
	SEM	3.9	1.8	1.9	1.6	1.8	4.8	4.6	3.6
	n	10	4	7	10	9	4	6	7
	p	< .002	NS	NS	NS	< .05	NS	NS	NS
Δ PCA	Mean	-0.01	0.72	-0.47	-1.29	-0.80	0.11	-0.80	-0.54
	SEM	0.40	1.27	0.73	0.63	0.72	1.83	0.86	0.56
	n	10	4	8	12	9	4	8	10
	p	NS	NS	NS	NS	NS	NS	NS	NS

T^2, total cross-sectional area of bone; M^2, medullary cross-sectional area; CA, absolute cross-sectional area of cortical bone; PCA, percent cortical area (Garn 1970). SEM, standard error of the mean; NS, not statistically significant at the $p \leq .05$ level.

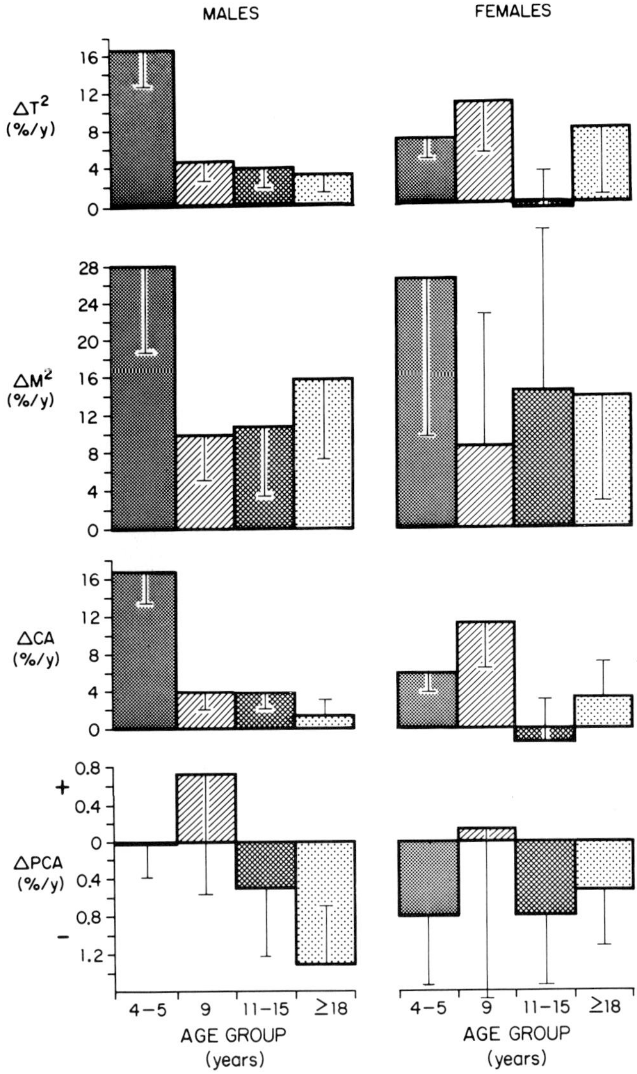

Fig. 1. Mean changes in major indices of bone remodeling for four age groups of male and female _M. nemestrina_. Brackets indicate 1 SEM. For explanation of symbols see legend of Table 1.

bone. Resorption of bone, however, apparently occurs only at the inner, marrow surface. Thus, while an increase in total cross-sectional surface area (T^2) reflects bone deposition on the outer surface, change in medullary area (M^2) reflects the balance of bone deposition and resorption at the inner surface. A decreased M^2 represents net deposition; an increase represents net resorption at the inner surface.

Using these relations, one can see that the virtual absence of change in PCA for the 4- to 5-year-old males (Figure 1) does not reflect a lack of cortical bone growth. This age group actually showed a 17% increase in cortical area due to 17% expansion of T^2, even though there was also a 28% expansion in M^2. All of these changes were statistically significant (Table 1).

In the 9-year-old males, a decline in the rate of expansion of both T^2 and M^2 indicated a reduced rate of growth of cortical bone. From this age on, the males exhibited a continuing decline in the rate of peripheral bone deposition as reflected in T^2 and an increase in the ratio of bone resorption to deposition at the medullary surface as reflected in M^2. As a result of these concomitant changes, cortical bone occupied progressively less of the total cross-sectional area of bone (PCA). It is important to note, however, that even though the rate of decrease in PCA had accelerated to 1.3% per year in the oldest group of males, the total cross-sectional area of cortical bone (CA) continued to increase.

The females showed less consistent trends than the males in their pattern of bone remodeling. The index reflecting the balance of resorption to deposition at the medullary surface (M^2) in the 4- to 5-year-old females was as high as in males, but peripheral deposition, as measured by T^2, failed to increase adequately to prevent a decline in PCA. Consequently, although CA continued to expand, there was a 0.8% decrease in PCA even for this youngest age group. In the 9-year-old group, T^2 tended to increase while the rate of change in M^2 decreased. This resulted in an increase in CA and a slight positive shift in PCA similar to, but smaller than, that of the 9-year-old males. As in the males, the rate of change in M^2 increased in the 11- to 15-year-old females, but the increase was greater than in the males and was matched by an equally sharp decline in T^2. Net cortical bone growth (CA) was nil in this group of females, so that PCA tended to decrease. It appears that in the female, as in the male, the total cross-sectional area of the bone continued to expand even in the oldest age group.

In both the human and the nonhuman primate female, a positive correlation has been shown between cortical bone mass and parity (Garn 1970; Bowden et al 1979). We sought to test that relation in our females using the PCA calculated from their most recent radiographs and their pregnancy records. Only the 21 females whose reproductive records were complete were included in the analysis.

All females in this study had undergone bilateral tubal ligation on entry into the aging colony to prevent disruption of a variety of longitudinal measures by pregnancy. Live births, cesarean sections, and stillbirths were coded as 1 and spontaneous abortions as 0.5. The data were ranked and a Spearman rank correlation coefficient was calculated; since a positive correlation was postulated on the basis of previous reports, a one-tailed test of significance was used. A significant positive correlation between percent cortical area measurements and parity was found: $r_s = 0.77 (p < 0.001)$.

DISCUSSION

Cortical bone remodeling in the pig-tailed macaque, as in the human, is not a process in which bone growth takes place solely in the growing years and bone loss only in the waning years. Deposition of new bone at the endosteal and subperiosteal surfaces and resorption at the endosteal surface are dynamic processes that continue well into the last third of the life span. In humans, the rate of change in cross-sectional CA is known to vary with age. Both deposition and resorption are most rapid during the adolescent years, slow markedly during the adult years up to the fourth decade, and then increase slightly again as resorption outpaces apposition during the second half of the life span (Garn 1970). Consequently, the minimal time interval between measurements required to show significant remodeling changes might be expected to differ between adolescent and adult animals.

The maximal life span of pig-tailed macaques, based on

data from captive animals, is estimated to be 30 to 35 years (Bowden, Jones 1979). Thus in biological terms, one macaque year is approximately equivalent to three human years. According to this estimate, the average span of 1.9 years between paired radiographs would correspond to about six human years.

Our data demonstrated statistically significant changes in bone remodeling in the youngest age group. It appears, therefore, that two years is adequate to demonstrate significant changes in adolescent macaques, in which rapid growth contributes to extensive bone modification. As expected, however, the changes in the adult age groups were not significant and can be viewed only as trends at present. With these considerations in mind, it is of interest to compare the values reported here with those reported for humans.

The average annual decreases in PCA for the two oldest groups (11-15 years and 18+ years) were, respectively, -0.47% and -1.29% per year for males and -0.80% and -0.54% per year for females. Adjusting for the difference in life span, these PCA measurements would be equivalent to -0.15% and -0.43% per year for human males and -0.26% and -0.18% per year for human females. The males' rates were similar to those of -0.4 to -0.5% per year reported for men, while the females' rates were considerably smaller than those reported for women beyond the fourth decade of life (-0.8 to -1.0% per year) (Skillman 1980).

PCA is a useful index for following the relatively slow change in the relation of cortical bone to total bone in the metacarpal, but as a derived variable integrating two components, it can mask the dynamic aspects of bone remodeling. This point is well illustrated by the lack of change in PCA in the 4- to 5-year-old males despite the intense bone remodeling reflected in M^2 and T^2 (Figure 1). Therefore we advocate, as has Garn (1970), that T^2 and M^2 be examined separately to determine their individual contributions to changes in CA and PCA.

Changes in T^2 and M^2 in the different age groups revealed several important similarities and one major contrast in cortical bone remodeling in humans and this simian model. For instance, the high rate of cortical bone resorption in the adolescent animals, which declined during early adulthood and then increased again in the oldest adults, is the same pattern seen in humans. Another similarity is the subperiosteal apposition of new cortical bone producing a continual increase in the total diameter of the bone throughout life in both sexes (Garn 1970). In addition, endosteal resorption, as judged by increasing M^2, began sooner in females (11-15 years) than in males (18+ years), similar to the trend in humans (Skillman 1980).

A difference between the monkey model and the human osteopenia of aging was seen in the oldest group of females. These animals, being in the second half of their life spans, would be postmenopausal if they were humans; their rate of decline in PCA would be accelerated relative to that of the younger females (Heaney 1976; Skillman 1980) and considerably greater than that of males in the same age group. By contrast, the rate of decrease in PCA for macaque females in this age group was less than that of the younger adult females, and the resorption rate, as reflected in ΔM^2, seemed comparable to that of the males in the oldest age group. This difference is probably due to the fact that, while macaque females undergo menopause similar to that of women, they do so considerably later in their life span (Hodgen et al 1977; Graham et al 1979).

Observations at the time of tubal ligation indicated that even the oldest animals (18-20 years old) had healthy, viable ovaries and oviducts with seemingly normal cyclic follicular rupture. The fact that menopause is delayed in macaques may offer the opportunity to follow the advance of osteopenia in the aging primate female without the influence of postmenopausal hormonal changes which seem to contribute substantially to the loss of bone mass in human females.

Our finding of a positive and significant correlation between parity and PCA confirms earlier observations in this species (Bowden et al 1979). This relation suggests either decreased loss or increased apposition of bone during or after pregnancy. Analysis of a similar finding in humans has revealed that the gain in bone mass occurs during pregnancy owing to deposition of bone at the endosteal surface. Although subsequent lactation can reduce this gain, short periods of nursing lead to positive net gains which are potentially additive throughout the childbearing years (Garn 1970). This, of course, provides for a greater bone mass at the time of menopause and, theoretically, greater protection from fractures in later life.

In summary, the trends in direction and magnitude of cortical bone changes in female pig-tailed macaques reported in this two-year longitudinal study were consistent with results of our previous cross-sectional study, which indicated close similarity to the osteopenia of aging in humans. This study also established that the phenomenon exists in male pig-tailed macaques but begins, as in humans, somewhat later than in females. The one important difference from the human condition was the absence of the accelerated loss of cortical bone typical of postmenopausal women. Thus, this simian model may provide an opportunmity to study the osteopenia of aging in senescent primate females uncomplicated by the hormonal changes of menopause.

REFERENCES

Aloia JF (1982). Estrogen and exercise in prevention and treatment of osteoporosis. Geriatrics 37:81.

Bowden DM (1979). "Aging in Nonhuman Primates." New York: Van Nostrand Reinhold.

Bowden DM, Jones ML (1979). Aging research in nonhuman primates. In Bowden DM (ed): "Aging in Nonhuman Primates," New York: Van Nostrand Reinhold, p 1.

Bowden DM, Teets C, Witkin J, Young DM (1979). Long bone calcification and morphology. In Bowden DM (ed): "Aging in Nonhuman Primates," New York: Van Nostrand Reinhold, p 335.

Comfort A (1969). Test-battery to measure ageing-rate in man. Lancet II:1411.

Dequeker JV, Baeyenos JP, Claessens J (1969). The significance of stature as a clinical measurement of ageing. J Am Geriatr Soc 17:169

Garn SM (1970). "The Earlier Gain and the Later Loss of Cortical Bone." Springfield, Illinois: C. C. Thomas.

Giansiracusa DF, Kantrowitz FG (1982). "Rheumatic and Metabolic Bone Diseases in the Elderly." Lexington, Massachusetts: The Collamore Press DC Heath and Co.

Graham CE, Kling OR, Steiner RA (1979). Reproductive senescence in female nonhuman primates. In Bowden DM (ed): "Aging in Nonhuman Primates," New York: Van Nostrand Reinhold, p 183.

Heaney RP (1976). Estrogens and postmenopausal osteoporosis. Clin Obstet Gynecol 19:791.

Heaney RP, Recker RR, Saville PD (1978). Menopausal changes in bone remodeling. J Lab Clin Med 92:964.

Hodgen GD, Goodman AC, O'Conner A, Johnson DK (1977). Menopause in rhesus monkeys: Model for study of disorders in human climacteric. Am J Obstet Gynecol 127:581.

Skillman TG (1980). Can osteoporosis be prevented? Geriatrics 35:95.

DISCUSSION

DR. TEITELBAUM: I think the problem you are having reflects the greatest difficulty that we all have in measuring bone mass. Because of your relatively small number of animals, I can't share your confidence that your data will improve. I think the only way that you may be able to improve your statistics is to use a different technique such as computerized tomography or dual photon absorptiometry.

DR. HIGH: I was wondering the same thing with regard to the sensitivity of your method. What are the precision, accuracy and reproducibility of your methods? If treatment-related changes are within those percentages of error, you won't see an effect. Alternative methods, where the precision, accuracy and reproducibility have been determined to be good, include single photon absorptiometry for appendicular skeletal evaluation and histomorphometric evaluation of (both pre- and post-treatment) biopsies of the rib and iliac crest.

DR. WILLIAMS: The measurements that I have made here were checked for precision of measurement error by selecting at random about five radiographs and then taking ten measurements on each. I then looked at the degree of variance in my measurements. The coefficient of variation was around 1.5%. That is about the only way that I have at present of assessing my error. I am sure you know that when looking at a radiograph in this manner there is a limit to one's ability to identify the cortical bone surfaces, even under magnification.

Comparative Pathobiology of Major Age-Related Diseases:
Current Status and Research Frontiers, pages 221–234

COMPARATIVE PATHOBIOLOGY OF CHRONIC DESTRUCTIVE PERIODONTITIS

Barnet M. Levy, D.D.S., M.S.

The University of Texas Dental Branch,
P.O. Box 20068, Houston, TX 77225

One characteristic of aging in mammals is an increasing incidence of certain progressive diseases (Kohn 1978). There is ample evidence to indicate that one of the diseases associated with aging is chronic destructive periodontal disease. It is apparently a disease of civilization, since it seems to occur only in man and the other animals that live with him. While usually not life threatening, it is a chronic inflammatory disease detrimental to health. It has been calculated that the total area of gingival sulcular ulceration in humans with peridontitis would be equal to an ulcer about the size of a silver dollar (40 mm). Such a chronic ulcerative nonhealing process on any part of the body would be stressful. In addition, chronic destructive periodontal disease is the primary cause of loss of teeth in aging adults and the elderly. To lose all of one's teeth at an age when physical vigor may be waning must have an immeasurable emotional impact. In addition, the loss of vertical dimension, resulting in overclosure of the mandible, a protruding raised chin and wrinkled perioral skin, the characteristic facial picture of senescence, would add additional emotional stress. Masticatory function would also be decreased so that nutritional status, which may have been declining, worsens.

The periodontium is a system of connective tissues composed of cementum, fibrous connective tissue and bone, covered by squamous epithelium. It includes the gingiva. Most of the connective tissues in the system are collagenous. Collagen is a substance which has been studied in great detail with respect to aging. Once growth ceases almost all collagen is in the form of mature insoluble fibrils. In the absence of severe tissue stresses or inflammation, the amount of collagen remains constant and demonstrates very little turnover (Kohn 1978). Current data indicate that following maturity, insoluble collagen throughout the body continues to undergo intermolecular cross-linking, although the types of bonds that form in aging collagen are not known. We do know, however, that old collagen is one of the more insoluble biological substances and small numbers of additional bonds may cause very marked changes in the properties of collagen. Almost no work has been done on the biochemistry of the collagens and other fibrillar proteins of the periodontal membrane with age.

Many of the age changes observed in the periodontal tissues of mice have also been found in man and other animals (Miles 1961). The histological changes associated with the aging mouse periodontal tissues have been carefully worked out by Tonna (1973). The changes associated with aging in the mouse periodontium include extensive gingival recession accompanied by a reduction of the supporting connective tissue, including the gingival and crestal fibers. There was also a reduction in the thickness of the free and attached gingiva. The submucosa was wider in the aged than in the young mouse. The alveolar crest was resorbed resulting in a flattened crest free of osteoid. With resorption of the alveolar bone, many areas of the marrow were exposed to the periodontal fibers. There was also a marked narrowing of the periodontal ligament space with age. The usual arrangement of both the transverse and the oblique fibers was lost as the total fiber mass became significantly reduced. There were massive amounts of cementum which accumulated along the root surfaces and especially at the root apices. Since some of the cementum which formed spurs near the apex of the tooth became detached, cementical formation was prevalent in the older animals. Tonna also reported a consistent mild inflammatory process with aging, which involved areas of the subcrevicular and periapical regions. These inflammatory lesions, however, did not extend into the periodontal ligament. Similar lesions have been described in aged rats.

The periodontium of the nondiseased aging marmoset, a small South American primate which may develop a fulminating chronic destructive periodontitis with age, has been investigated in depth (Levy et al 1972a). In aged marmosets the cribriform plates are narrower than those of mature animals. The crestal bone is reduced in width and the cellularity in the bone marrow spaces is noticeably diminished. Neither the lamellar arrangement of the alveolar bone proper nor the embedded ends of the attachment fibers are demonstrable in aged animals, but they are quite distinct in mature adults.

Within the periodontal ligament there is a perceptible decrease in cellular elements. Some of the ligaments have calcified attachment fibers. The calcifications are manifested as small calcospherites which occasionally coalesce to form masses paralleling the direction of the attachment fibers (Figure 1). There were several notable changes in the periodontal vasculature of the aged marmosets. The arteriole vessels exhibit arteriosclerotic changes which include intimal thickening and elastic hyperplasia (Figure 2). The vessels also show a deposition of periodic acid-Schiff (PAS)-positive material in both the intima and media that give the vessels a hyalinized appearance. The arteries of the

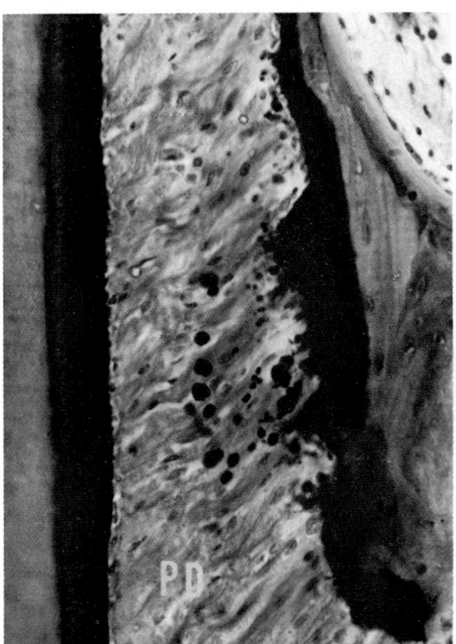

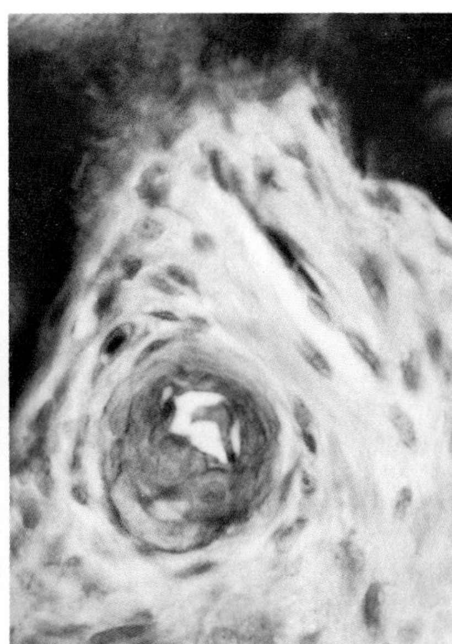

Fig. 1. Photomicrograph illustrating a relatively acellular periodontal ligament (PD) in which there are numerous calcospherites.

Fig. 2. Narrowing of lumen in a small arteriole in the periodontium of an aged marmoset.

gingiva, periodontal ligament, bone and palate exhibit sclerotic changes with the same frequency.

Thus the fibrous, osseous, and vascular compartments of the marmoset periodontium were all histologically affected by the aging process. Some histochemical changes were also evident. In the adult mature marmoset the collagen of the periodontal ligament is mildly PAS-positive, alcianophilic with alcian blue-PAS and argyrophilic with silver impregnation. The fibers of the aged animals are intensely PAS-positive and none are argyrophilic when subjected to the corresponding staining procedures. The tinctorial alterations reflect a loss of acid mucopolysaccharides and either an increase in or an unmasking of neutral carbohydrates.

Age-related changes in the periodontium of the lateral incisors of the pigtail monkey have also been described (Ive et al 1980). With increasing age the roots migrate towards the labial-cortical plate which results in the development of a bony root prominence on the labial periosteal surface. The width and relative area of the periodontal ligament space decreased significantly with age. There was a significant increase in cementum thickness. It was suggested that a relationship may exist between the decrease in the width of the periodontal ligament and a simultaneous decrease in occlusal forces associated with age.

There have not been many in-depth studies of the changes in the human periodontium with age. Most reports in the literature, however, suggest that there is a decrease in the width of the periodontal membrane, an increase in cementum and a recession of the gingiva with age. In a study by Nedelman and Bernick (1978), the alveolar mucosa and bone in edentulous jaws of people ranging in age from 72 to 92 years were studied histologically. The connective tissue of the lamina propria of all the edentulous specimens showed marked changes. The collagenous elements were thick and arranged in dense parallel bundles similar in architecture to dense connective tissue seen in a ligament. The alveolar and gingival arteries exhibited arteriosclerotic changes and in some instances the lumina were nearly occluded. There was osteoporosis of the edentulous maxillae and mandibles in both the men and the women, although the degree of osteoporosis was greater in the women. There is still much to be learned about the normal aging of periodontal tissues of man and other animals.

The inflammatory diseases of the periodontium may vary with the etiologic agent (necrotizing ulcerative gingivitis) as well as with the age and the resistance of the patient (acute marginal gingivitis and/or destructive periodontitis). The most common periodontal disease of man is chronic destructive periodontitis, in which there is not only chronic inflammation of the gingiva but a destructive alteration of the periodontal ligament, alveolar bone and cementum. Chronic destructive periodontitis may occur at any age and in this respect it is not much different from other diseases of the aged and of aging. It occurs most frequently in post reproductive mature adults and progresses either slowly or rapidly as the individual ages.

Where phases of human disease such as chronic destructive periodontitis can only be studied on a histologic basis with difficulty, we must depend on experimental animals. The appropriateness of each animal analogue will have to be judged by its capacity to explain and predict the observed events. Animals used for the study of human disease must meet several rather stringent requirements. If the disease to be compared with the human is destructive periodontitis, the animal must have a dental apparatus analogous to that of man. Such an animal should be susceptible to the development of chronic destructive periodontitis spontaneously. The absolute prerequisite, however, for the search for an animal in which the clinical and pathologic findings can be compared with those of the human is a detailed knowledge of the disease to be studied.

Chronic destructive periodontal disease is a chronic inflammatory lesion. MacKay and Burnet (1964) stated that "chronic inflammation, which is a concept requiring critical reassessment, is characterized by destruction of the specialized elements of the tissue, and a cellular infiltration composed predominantly of cells concerned in the mediation of immune responses -- lymphocytes and plasma cells." There is considerable evidence to indicate that chronic destructive periodontitis is an immunologically mediated chronic inflammatory disease of the gingiva and periodontal tissues. The pathogenesis of the disease is not understood although strict adherence to a program of oral hygiene reduces the incidence of gingivitis and of periodontitis.

Disease does not exist except as a reaction to injury. It has been suggested that autoimmunization should be considered in persistently active and recurring chronic inflammatory processes such as chronic destructive periodontitis (Levy 1973). It has been pointed out by Glynn and Halbarow (1965) that autoimmune reactions play a major role in the pathogenesis of chronic inflammatory diseases. There is considerable debate in the literature as to exactly how autoimmune processes enhance chronic inflammatory diseases and whether, in fact, there is an autoimmune compartment to chronic inflammation. There are, of course, accepted markers of autoimmune disease, two of the most important of which are the accumulation of lymphocytes and plasma cells in tissues and a significant transient or lasting benefit from treatment with corticosteroid drugs.

There has been substantial investigation into the immunological markers of aging. Space does not permit a thorough review of this important and interesting subject here. Evidence is accumulating that there is an increase in the average immunological reaction as we grow older. The gammaglobulins increase steadily with age (Das, Bhattacharya, 1961) and the average spleen weight relative to body weight increases with age (Walford, Hildemann 1964). In addition, Walford (1962) has pointed out that skin grafts between mice having minor histocompatibility differences were about 75% successful between young mice but that when old mice were used as both donors and recipients almost no grafts were successful.

In addition to the above implications of a B-cell derived immunopathy in the aged, there is considerable evidence that the T-cell limb of the immune system is also involved. The cellular mass of the thymus declines progressively following sexual maturity, so that by midlife, it is only 10 to 15% of its maximal mass. By age 60 it is a small shriveled tissue, frequently difficult or impossible to locate. One of the age-related effects of "normal" aging on the immune system is a decrease in thymus-derived or T-cell functional capacity. In addition, a subpopulation of T cells, the T-suppressor cells, are also depressed.

There is also evidence for an age-associated hyperglobulinemia with an increase in normal autoantibody titers, indicating a superactivity of the B cells. This may be a reflection of the depression of the T-suppressor inhibition of B lymphocytes allowing the B cells an increase in functional response. These observations, coupled with the finding that there is an increase in autoimmune diseases with aging (diabetes, rheumatoid arthritis, etc.) led us to examine in detail the immunologic parameters of patients with and without periodontitis and to study the animal analogues of destructive periodontitis from an immunologic standpoint. We have demonstrated (Mackler et al 1977) that T cells play an active role in gingivitis but that B cells play a major role in the pathogenesis of destructive periodontitis. Gingivitis seems to be a disease of younger people while periodontitis is a disease of older individuals. In addition we have shown (Robertson et al 1978) that patients with primary humoral defects have less periodontal inflammation than age and plaque matched immunocompetent subjects. Since destructive periodontitis appears to be more active in the older age groups, an understanding of the relationship between immunocompetency and aging becomes imperative if we are to adequately prevent and/or treat the disease.

As stated earlier, it is the response to injury, not the injury itself, that produces the manifestations of disease. If we don't have the appropriate complement of cells with which to react, we cannot react appropriately.

The usual laboratory animals such as mice, rats, hamsters, guinea pigs, and rabbits do not fit the criteria for an analogue of human periodontal disease. Their dentitions are quite different from that of man. They do not develop "spontaneous" chronic destructive periodontitis. The oral flora of rodents differs greatly from that of humans. In addition, mice, rats, and hamsters have a tendency to recover from infection acquiring little hypersensitivity. On the other hand, guinea pigs and humans often develop a high degree of hypersensitivity following infection.

Spontaneous periodontitis has not been reported in hamsters although periodontitis can be induced in older animals on a specific high carbohydrate diet. Hamster periodontitis is characterized by a large accumulation of microbial plaque in the gingival crevice. The gingiva recedes and there is a change in the contour of its margin. Deep periodontal pockets are formed as the disease progresses. Subepithelial inflammatory responses, so characteristic of human gingivitis, have not been described for periodontal disease in the hamster.

The dog is an animal that develops severe chronic destructive periodontitis as it ages. Epidemiologic investigations indicate that the etiology of their periodontitis is plaque and calculus, as it is in man (Hull et al 1974). A careful study of the histopathology of spontaneous periodontitis in dogs has been reported by Hamp and Lindberg (1977). Almost all of the animals with severe periodontitis were over 10 years of age. Histologically, there was a dense subepithelial infiltrate of plasma cells intermingled with lymphocytes. There was a marked loss of alveolar bone and the crevicular or "attachment" epithelium migrated beyond the cementoenamel junction. The lesions were very similar to those described in man.

Although cats do develop destructive periodontitis with age, very little in the way of either epidemiologic and/or histologic evaluation has been reported for that species.

The nonhuman primate has a dentition similar to that of man but most old world monkeys are large, expensive and difficult to handle and they require considerable space for housing and maintenance. The marmoset is a small, relatively inexpensive South American primate with none of the disadvantages of its larger family members. The marmoset periodontium is capable of demonstrating the degenerative reactions spontaneously. In addition, the degenerative changes of osteomalacia and hyperparathyroidism are radiologically and histologically similar to those seen in people with those diseases. Changes in the periodontium of aged marmosets are almost identical with those seen in aged men (Levy et al 1970).

Periodontal disease in the marmoset is associated with bacterial plaque on the teeth. The plaque usually calcifies and is histologically similar to human calculus. The periodontal lesion is a chronic destructive inflammatory lesion whose cellular exudate is predominantly lymphocytic and monocytic. (The marmoset does not produce plasma cells.) As the disease progresses, alveolar bone loss is obvious (Figures 3, 4). The marmoset may also be treated by the usual therapeutic measures of scaling, curettage and maintenance of good oral hygiene which leads to clinical improvement of the periodontitis.

Chronic destructive periodontitis in the marmoset, like other known autoimmune diseases, is remarkably sensitive to cortisone therapy. Injections of cortisone into the marmoset with marked gingivitis and periodontitis reduces the chronic inflammatory reaction associated with plaque and calculus

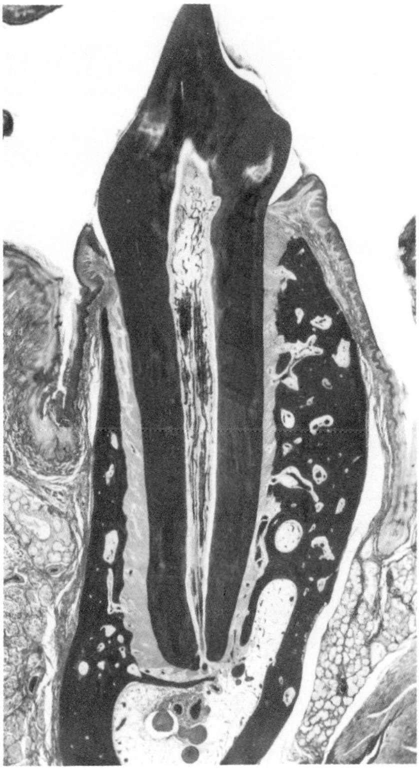

Fig. 3. Photomicrograph of B-L section of lst lower premolar of mature adult marmoset demonstrating a "normal" or disease-free gingiva and periodontium.

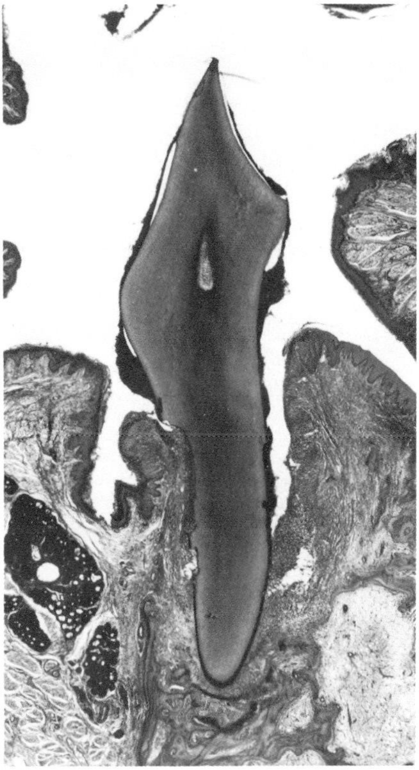

Fig. 4. Photograph of B-L section of lower lst premolar of an aged (15+ years) marmoset, demonstrating the ravages of chronic destructive periodontitis.

(Levy et al 1972a). In addition, the marmoset is highly susceptible to the atherosclerotic stimulus of high fat diets (Dreizen et al 1973). It reacts rapidly to adjuvant injections in the periodontium so that within a very short period of time there is almost total destruction of the periodontal supporting tissues (Levy et al 1972b).

The marmoset thus seems to be an ideal animal analogue in

which to study diseases of aging, especially those chronic destructive diseases associated with dental microbial plaque.

ACKNOWLEDGEMENTS

The original research reported was supported in part by Grant AG00118 from the National Institute on Aging, National Institutes of Health, Bethesda, Maryland.

REFERENCES

Das BC, Bhattacharya SK (1961). Changes in human serum protein fractions with age and weight. Can J Biochem Physiol 39:569.

Dreizen S, Levy B, Bernick S (1973). Diet-induced atherosclerosis in the marmoset. Proc Soc Exp Biol Med 143:1218.

Glynn LE, Halbarow EJ (1965). "Autoimmunity and Disease." Philadelphia: E. A. Davis.

Hamp S-E, Lindberg R (1977). Histopathology of spontaneous periodontitis in dogs. J Periodont Res 12:46.

Hull PS, Soames JV, Davis RM (1974). Periodontal disease in a Beagle dog colony. J Comp Pathol 84:143.

Ive JC, Shapiro PA, Ivey JL (1980). Age related changes in the periodontium of pigtail monkeys. J Periodont Res 15:402.

Kohn RR (1978). "Principles of Mammalian Aging." 2nd edition. Englewood Cliffs, New Jersey: Prentice Hall, p 7, 37.

Levy B (1973). Prevention of periodontal disease -- a pathologist's view. Int Dent J 23:476.

Levy BM, Dreizen S, Bernick S (1972a). "The Marmoset Periodontium in Health and Disease." Monographs in Oral Science, Vol I, Basel: S. Karger.

Levy B, Dreizen S, Bernick S, Grant D (1970). Comparative study of periodontium of aged marmosets and humans. J Dent Res 49: Abst #604.

Levy B, Nelms DC, Dreizen S, Bernick S (1972b). Delayed hypersensitivity reaction in the periodontium of the marmoset. A preliminary report. In Goldsmith EI, Moor-Jankowski J (eds): "Medical Primatology," Basel: S. Karger, p 191.

MacKay IR, Burnet FM (1964). "Autoimmune Diseases. Pathogenesis, Chemistry and Therapy." Springfield, Illinois: C. C. Thomas.

Mackler BF, Frostad KB, Robertson PB, Levy B (1977). Immuno-

globulin bearing lymphocytes and plasma cells in human periodontal disease. J Periodont Res 12:37.
Miles AEW (1961). Aging in the teeth and oral tissues. In Bourne GH (ed): "Structural Aspects of Ageing." New York: Hafner, p 352.
Nedelman CI, Bernick S (1978). The significance of age changes in human alveolar mucosa and bone. J Prosthet Dent 39:495.
Robertson PB, Wright TE, Mackler BF, Lenertz DM, Levy B (1978). Periodontal status of patients with abnormalities of the immune system. J Periodont Res 13:37.
Tonna EA (1973). Histological age changes associated with mouse parodontal tissues. J Gerontol 28:1.
Walford RL (1962). Auto-immunity and aging. J Gerontol 17:281.
Walford RL, Hildemann WH (1964). Chronic and subacute parabiotic reactions in the Syrian hamster: Significance with regard to transplantation immunity, experimental amyloidosis, and an immunologic theory of aging. Transplantation 2:87.

DISCUSSION

DR. REAVEN: I am very curious to know whether the cortisone treatment consisted of a single injection. Is it given systemically or locally? Is it possible to treat humans?

DR. LEVY: We used systemic injections of cortisone. It is not recommended as a form of treatment. It is an experimental tool. When I reported this finding to a dental group, I made it quite clear that I was not proposing a new form of treatment. In humans and in the marmoset, if the bacterial plaque is removed from the teeth of a young adult and kept off either by personal oral hygiene or through the activities of a dental hygienist, the disease is arrested and doesn't progress.

DR. REAVEN: Is that all? I know someone who suffers from this problem, and in this case it is not so easily solved. I am wondering whether there are recalcitrant situations that you know of?

DR. LEVY: I think chronic periodontitis is a disease of aging. Aging starts at, I don't know, whatever we decided yesterday, at age 40 or 30. Those who objected swear it starts at 60.

DR. HACKEL: I believe old age has been defined to be present in "people who are ten years older than I am."

DR. LEVY: The point that I want to make is that most people over the age of 35 have some form of this disease. I would say about 90% of the people do. Now, 95% of those are treatable by the method I mentioned. There are about 5% of the people who do not respond to that kind of treatment. I think they are the same 5% who do not respond to other forms of treatment for chronic inflammatory diseases such as, for example, chronic bronchitis. I don't know the answer to Dr. Reaven's question.

DR. BERENSON: Can you separate the effect of bacterial infection from that of the aging process? Is chronic bacterial infection initiating all of the changes?

DR. LEVY: I think that reactions to bacterial infection in young people are different from reactions to bacterial infection in old people. I think it is different in all young animals as compared to old ones. I don't believe you can separate clearly and precisely the effect of bacterial infection from aging. If you isolate lymphocytes from the gingiva of young people with gingivitis, the predominant cell is a non-B cell (mostly T cells). In persons over 60 with marked periodontal disease, the lymphocytes are mostly B cells.

DR. BERENSON: You are suggesting that the immunologic phenomena have been altered, and that, in turn, alters the response to a trauma of some sort.

DR. LEVY: Yes, that is what I am suggesting.

DR. BERENSON: The second question is, if we are on a high-fat, high-carbohydrate diet, and if we advocate a lower fat diet and increase carbohydrates, will other changes occur? You show changes with a high-fat diet in a small artery and also changes at the arteriolar level. Do you think that a high-carbohydrate diet will contribute to this type of disease?

DR. LEVY: The data are that if you feed a high-sucrose diet, that is, one much higher than normal, to rodents, you have a good opportunity to elicit destructive periodontitis, especially in hamsters and rats. I don't think there are any data on high-sucrose diets with relation to periodontal disease in primates. There is a relationship between high-sucrose diets and dental caries in human and nonhuman primates.

DR. TERRY: I would simply like to know the expected life span and the age of sexual maturity in these animals.

DR. LEVY: The age of sexual maturity of the marmoset is, I think, 18 months, plus or minus a few months, and the life span is not really documented, but I believe it is about about 15 years, plus or minus a year or two.

DR. TEITELBAUM: Dr. Roy Page has described a group of individuals with periodontal disease who have defects in chemotaxis of their polymorphonuclear leukocytes. This would suggest that there is a subpopulation of individuals who are susceptible to periodontal disease. Would you comment on that please?

DR. LEVY: There is a subpopulation of individuals who are hypersusceptible to periodontal disease, but that is not the disease I was describing, although it looks very similar to it. It is a disease which occurs in young people and is called juvenile periodontitis because it begins before the age of 12 or 13, and is almost impossible to control because there is a defect in the polymorphonuclear leukocytes.

DR. TEITELBAUM: Do the older individuals that you have described have defects in chemotaxis of polymorphonuclear leukocytes?

DR. LEVY: I do not have that data. Data are just being accumulated because of the work with juvenile periodontitis patients. I think that Dr. Page is doing this, and we are doing it in our laboratory also. The older people that we have examined do not have, as far as we now know, a defect in the chemotactic activity of their polymorphonuclear leukocytes.

DR. SCARPELLI: To what extent does the hard calcareous mass contribute to this disease by way of trauma?

DR. LEVY: I don't think it contributes by way of trauma. It carries the microbial plaque on its surface. Once the plaque calcifies, the organisms, of course, are dead and calcified. It just acts as a good base on which the microbial plaque can live.

DR. WISSLER: I would like to go back to the altered small arteries which you showed; not the ones in the tongue but those in the periodontal region. Are these reasonably constant in the human and in the marmoset, or are they variable, and if so, are they correlated with anything? It is unusual, I think, to see this kind of arteriolar medial change just as a part of aging and, of course, it frequently goes with hypertension and diabetes. I wonder if there is any knowledge or any work on what these changes in small blood vessels might be due to.

DR. LEVY: In humans it is found quite frequently. We found it in all of our animals over ten or 11 years of age. It has never been associated with a disease process, and I believe it is reversible. By that I mean it comes and goes. We did a study of these changes in the tongue which seems to be very susceptible to vascular change. It is found in newborn children and in aged people. In some cases, the blood vessels seem to be practically occluded, and yet there are no infarcts distal to it in the tongue or gingiva. It is a very interesting lesion, as you pointed out, and I don't think it contributes to any disease process.

DR. WISSLER: We have also been interested in the tongue arteries, and my impression is that their changes, which are mostly intimal, really are present in quite small arteries and are associated with diet more than anything else. Spontaneous lesions in the tongue arteries of the macaques which we have studied are not very frequent. We have studied rhesus monkey arteries over almost their total natural life span. I don't think that the tongue artery lesions you showed are similar to the ones you showed in the periodontal disease lesions. Both are very interesting types of lesions and deserve more study.

Comparative Pathobiology of Major Age-Related Diseases: Current Status and Research Frontiers, pages 235–249

ESSENTIAL HYPERTENSION: A DISEASE OF THE REGULATION OF MEMBRANE Na TRANSPORT

Mitzy Canessa, Ph.D., Carlo Brugnara, M.D., and Alan Kopin, M.D.

Department of Physiology and Biophysics, Harvard Medical School, Boston, MA 02115

Inherited biochemical differences among individuals and among populations have been related to differences in susceptibility to disease as well as to differential human survival.

As an attempt to define susceptibility to hypertension in the human population, we have proposed to investigate the polymorphism of red cell Na transport systems. This can be instrumental in explaining why, in the same habitat, two or more discontinuous forms of Na transport traits may have different susceptibility to elevated blood pressure. Three systems which transport Na in red cells display large inter-individual variance: the Na pump, the Na/Na exchange, and the Na-K cotransport (Canessa et al 1980; Garay et al 1980). The Na pump seems to be controlled directly or indirectly by several hormones such as aldosterone, thyroid, vasopressin and a natriuretic hormone. The Na_i/Na_o exchange and the Na-K cotransport appear to be under genetic control. Alterations of these three transport systems can be found in individuals with essential hypertension.

The polymorphism of these two red cell Na transport systems (the Na/Na exchange and the Na-K cotransport) might help to (1) investigate inherited differences in distinct populations to provide answers to the questions of epidemiologists about the prevalence of hypertension in certain populations; (2) unravel the causes of family resemblance in blood pressure; (3) provide an estimate of hypertensive risk early in life; (4) design adequate preventive nonpharmacological management at the individual level.

Several observations have indicated that heredity is involved in the pathogenesis of hypertension in man. Population and family studies in relatives, young siblings, newborns, twins, adoptees, and spouses (Pickering 1968; the Report of the Hypertension Task Force 1979; Yamori 1980) have emphasized human hypertension as a distinct genetic trait. However, the controversy initiated by the work of Pickering (1968) and Platt (1963) about the mode of inheritance and the number of genes involved remains unsolved.

Several epidemiological studies have contributed to establish risk factors such as age, weight, sex, and race (Paul 1980). The investigation of the relationship between the polymorphism of red cell Na transport systems and susceptibility to essential hypertension can fill the existing gap between human genetics and the epidemiology of essential hypertension (MacMahon 1978).

Two ouabain-insensitive systems, the Na/Na exchange and the Na-K cotransport, translocate Na across the red cell membrane, and they are both altered in individuals and in families with essential hypertension. The two transport systems can be distinguished operationally by their different properties (Canessa et al 1981; 1982). In agreement with this finding, the Na/Na exchange system appears altered in certain individuals and the Na-K cotransport in others. Notably, both disturbances seem to have strong familial aggregation as well as different ethnic and geographic distribution. These three properties are characteristic of genetic traits. It is not clear whether they represent different forms of hypertension (mild, severe) and/or different physiopathological entities such as vasoconstrictive or volume-dependent hypertension.

Since essential hypertension is an age-dependent disease, we would like to discuss the age dependence of red cell Na transport systems and their possible role in the pathophysiology of this disease.

CLINICAL AND PATHOPHYSIOLOGICAL HETEROGENEITY OF ESSENTIAL HYPERTENSION

Several studies have demonstrated the heterogeneity of the hypertensive disease in terms of clinical forms, cardiovascular hemodynamics, neurohumoral mechanisms, salt, and water balance (Genest et al 1977). Recently, our studies have documented the heterogeneity of the alterations of Na transport across the red cell membrane in this syndrome (Table 1).

From the clinical point of view, the distinction between mild, labile, and severe hypertension has been a matter of discussion (Genest et al 1977). Mild hypertension has been defined taking into account the levels of diastolic and systolic blood pressure, and the presence or absence of target organ damage. However, recent studies using non-invasive techniques such as the echocardiogram (to measure cardiac output) have indicated that a large fraction of the mild and labile hypertensive population may have a decreased aortic distensibility as is the case in severe hypertension (Perry, Smith 1978).

From the point of view of cardiovascular hemodynamics, the patients with essential hypertension have been divided into two groups: those with hyper- and hypodynamic circulation. In subjects with hyperdynamic circulation, the elevated cardiac output and left ventricular hypertrophy observed seem to be more than a simple consequence of the elevated arterial pressure.

These hypertensive phenomena can be analyzed by assessing the relative contribution of vasoconstrictive and volume components. The major determinant of long-term changes in the volume component is the state of Na balance. The relative Na intake determines the degree of activation of humoral factors promoting Na retention (renin-angiotensin-aldosterone axis) or Na excretion (natriuretic hormone and kallikrein hormone). The volume expansion might be caused by Na intake relatively high for the cell's extruding ability. The volume-dependent hypertension is characterized by the reduced activity of the renin-angiotensin system and quite possibly by an increased level of the natriuretic hormone. The vasoconstrictive form of hypertension is characterized by decreased activity of the renin-angiotensin system, low plasma volume, and elevated peripheral resistance.

The elevation of the peripheral resistance in patients might be related to inadequate activity of the sympathetic nervous system. Arteriolar hypersensitivity or hyperresponse to pressor agents such as norepinephrine or angiotensin II (AII) might be related to alterations in the Na or K gradient

Table 1

HETEROGENEITY OF ESSENTIAL HYPERTENSION

Category		Parameter	Variants	
CLINICAL	1.	Mild		
	2.	Labile		
	3.	Severe, Accelerated		
CARDIOVASCULAR HEMODYNAMIC	1.	Increased Vascular Peripheral Resistance		
	2.	Cardiac Output	Normal Increased	Blood Volume Inotropism
NEUROHUMORAL REGULATION	1.	Renin-Angiotensin-Aldosterone	Normal Low High	
	2.	β-Adrenergic System	Hyperadrenergic Hypoadrenergic	
	3.	Natriuretic Hormone	High Normal	
Na TRANSPORT SYSTEMS	1.	Na/Na Countertransport	Elevated Normal	
	2.	Na-K Cotransport	Normal Reduced	
	3.	Na Pump	Elevated Reduced	

across the smooth muscle and endothelial cells. The operation of the ouabain-sensitive Na pump in vascular smooth muscle (VSM) cells hyperpolarizes the cell and keeps the membrane potential away from the threshold of contraction. The modulation of the Na pump in VSM by inhibitory factors such as the natriuretic hormone can bring about a significant reduction in membrane potential and contribute to the hypersensitivity to pressor agents.

Several subgroups have been classified according to their abnormalities in plasma renin activity or catecholamines. These abnormalities seem to be age dependent. Gavras et al (1982) have recently examined the humoral characteristics of young (under 40 years) vs. old (older than 60) patients with essential hypertension. The young patients have normal levels of plasma renin activity and low levels of norepinephrine, while in older patients the response of the renin-angiotensin-aldosterone axis to acute volume changes is decreased and the norepinephrine levels are increased.

HETEROGENEITY OF ALTERATIONS OF RED CELL Na AND K TRANSPORT IN ESSENTIAL HYPERTENSION

In studying red cell Na transport in hypertension, we have uncovered a high degree of heterogeneity in the human population affected by essential hypertension and in the members of their families (Canessa et al 1980, 1981, 1983b; Adragna et al 1982a). The degree of heterogeneity in red cell cation transport expressed in essential hypertension is in agreement with the epidemiological and clinical finding that hypertension is not homogeneous in different populations. It is not yet clear how many of these subtypes are related to some clinical forms of hypertension such as mild, labile, or severe or to different pathophysiological origin.

Measurements of red cell Na and K transport pathways have uncovered various derangements in essential hypertension. Since it is not one system that is altered in hypertensive patients and their offspring, in looking for a predictor of the pre-hypertensive state, it is important to study the K_m or the V_{max} of these three transport systems that regulate the Na and K gradient: The Na pump, the Na-K cotransport and the Na-Li countertransport. Several studies published on this matter have not met this criterion thereby introducing a great deal of confusion into this new area of research.

The V_{max} of Li_i-Na_o countertransport is found elevated in red cells of Caucasian hypertensives (Canessa et al 1980; Adragna et al 1982a) (Subset I). The fraction of affected patients in case-controlled studies varies from 20 to 90% in different parts of the world. In an unselected male population, this fraction has been determined to be 35-40% (Trevisan et al 1983). Notably, in black hypertensives (Canessa et al 1983b), the Na exchange system is not elevated. The V_{max} of the Na-K cotransport system has been measured as the furosemide-sensitive Na and K fluxes into Na-free and K-free medium. This transport system appears normal in hypertensive subjects with elevated countertransport. In contrast, Na-K cotransport is significantly reduced in patients with normal Na countertransport (black) (Canessa et al 1983b) and mild hypertensives (Caucasian) (Adragna et al 1982b). In many of these individuals (Subset II) there is also a significant reduction of the K_m for internal Na. The alteration of this kinetic parameter makes the Na-K cotransport system inoperative for Na extrusion in the physiological range of cellular Na concentrations. We have finished a complete study of the Na and K fluxes through the Na-K cotransport system in order to understand its regulation by internal Na and external K. Our results indicate that at steady-state physiological ion concentrations, the Na-K cotransport system operates in the direction of net Na extrusion. The transport reaction seems to have a stoichiometry of $2\ Na_i + 3\ K_i = 2\ Na_o + 3\ K_o$ and a $K_{eq} = 20$. The alterations in the V_{max} or the K_m for Na_i in this transport system will determine a lower capacity to regulate the Na gradient (Canessa et al 1983a).

The V_{max} of the ouabain-sensitive Na pump is also reduced in some subjects (Langford et al 1983; Hamlin et al 1982) and markedly elevated in young hypertensives with accelerated hypertension (Garay et al 1980). Most likely, the cause of these disturbances is the level of circulating inhibitor of the Na pump (Hamlin et al 1982), the natriuretic hormone.

We would like to discuss the significance of the different subsets of alterations of Na and K transport in the physiopathology of hypertension. An interpretation, probably too premature at this stage of our research, is that the elevated countertransport (Subset I) found in some subjects and certain populations reflects the turning on of a protective trait which controls Na extrusion in VSM in response to early vasoconstrictive changes. The elevation of the Na exchange might be a good predictor of early vasoconstrictive changes or of severe hypertension. The subset of patients with low values of the V_{max} and K_m for Na_i of the Na-K cotransport (Subset II) is found with higher frequency in the black hypertensive subjects. Many of these subjects also have a reduced V_{max} of the Na pump and elevated cellular Na (Langford et al 1983). Their overall capacity to regulate the Na gradient with a similar Na intake is lower than in subjects with normal Na pump, Na-K cotransport and elevated Na countertransport. We have tentatively identified this group as salt-sensitive (or volume dependent hypertensive). These individuals may behave as salt-loaded while having a similar Na intake to that of the Subset I subjects. The physiological response to salt loading requires a turning off of the renin-angiotensin-aldosterone axis and a turning on of the natriuretic hormone. Several studies have documented that hypertension in blacks is more frequently the low-renin type. However, it remains to be determined whether the humoral and membrane alterations of Na transport are present in the same subjects.

FAMILIAL RESEMBLANCE IN Li-Na COUNTERTRANSPORT AND Na-K COTRANSPORT

Family resemblance is in the middle ground of genetics and epidemiology and can be used to identify environmental causes of human diseases. Familial aggregation of blood pressure has been adequately documented by several studies (Miall et al 1967; Annest et al 1979; Rose et al 1979). The heritability of blood pressure has been estimated at 50% in twin studies (Rose et al 1979).

We have studied 23 Caucasian families comprising two parents and a minimum of two offspring. The age of the offspring varied between 10 and 20 years. The families were classified into three groups: Group 1: the parents were documented normotensives. The family history of the grandparents was negative for hypertension as established by records of their age, age of death, cause of death, treatment for hypertension, stroke, and heart trouble. Group 2: the parents were normotensive but the grandparents had family history of hypertension. Group 3: one or both parents were hypertensive.

Several intrafamilial correlation coefficients for Li_i-Na_o countertransport and Na-K cotransport are statistically significant in the 23 Caucasian families studied (Adragna et al 1982b). All of them are close to the maximal value expected for one-half the genes in common ($r = 0.5$). These data, however, do not clarify what proportion of the familial aggregation can be ascribed to heritability or environmental factors such as common household, similar caloric intake, and salt intake. We hope to obtain an accurate estimation of the heritability for Na countertransport, Na-K cotransport and the Na pump from an on-going study on twins carried out in collaboration with Dr. Francis Lewitter from the Channing Laboratory of Harvard Medical School. Preliminary results estimate the heritability of the Na countertransport and Na-K cotransport at 50% and at zero for the Na pump.

AGE DEPENDENCE OF RED CELL Na TRANSPORT SYSTEMS

It is well known that hypertension in men has an onset at 40 years and in women at 50 years (Paul 1980). However, as early as 15 to 20 years, we can observe that some of the offspring of hypertensive patients have an elevated Na countertransport or a significantly reduced Na-K cotransport. If both transport systems are genetically determined, they should both be present at birth in the red cells. The Na pump and Na-K cotransport are present at birth, but the Na countertransport is absent.

During the first week of life, important volume redistribution and blood pressure changes take place. We do not know whether Li_i-Na_o countertransport appears in red cells one week or three months after birth. In the first case, this will indicate which humoral factors may control the expression of countertransport. In the second case, it will indicate that a developmental gene switch controls its expression.

Two different groups have reported that Li_i-Na_o countertransport decreases with age in normotensive but not in hypertensive subjects. Brugnara et al (1983) studied normotensive subjects ($n = 31$) between 10 and 80 years of age. Countertransport correlated negatively (r = 0.65; p >0.001) with age. Burke et al (1983) studied normotensive subjects (n = 120) between 20 and 80 years of age and found a similar decrease of countertransport with age. Brugnara also showed that the elevation of countertransport correlated with high response of plasma renin activity to volume depletion elicited by the diuretic furosemide. Since the activity of the renin-angiotensin-aldosterone axis also decreases with age, a possible hypothesis linking these findings would be that elevated countertransport in the offspring of hypertensive patients reflects an early response in the turnover rate of this Na transport system triggered by early changes in the cardiovascular hemodynamic and humoral control of Na balance. Since similar elevations of the countertransport system are found in the third trimester of pregnancy (Worley 1982), this disturbance of Na transport may be more likely an expression of the ability to turn on the system to regulate the Na gradient. We have no data available yet on the age dependence of Na-K cotransport and the Na pump. The assay of the V_{max} of outward Na-K cotransport and of the Na pump in nystatin loaded cells has adequate reproducibility to undertake such a study. The age dependence of the Na pump should be studied particularly in women before and after the menarche and menopause. Such studies may help to clarify the hormonal control of the Na pump and the factors influencing its age dependence.

ACKNOWLEDGEMENTS

This work was supported by NIH grants GM-25686 and HL-25064. Our thanks to Marianita Sanchez for excellent secretarial assistance.

REFERENCES

Adragna N, Canessa M, Solomon H, Slater E, Tosteson DC (1982a). Red cell Li-Na countertransport and Na-K cotransport in patients with essential hypertension. Hypertension 4:795.

Adragna N, Ellison C, Solomon H, Matthysse S, Tosteson DC, Canessa M (1982b). Intrafamilial correlation coefficients for Na countertransport and cotransport in essential hypertension. Clin Res 30:334.

Annest JL, Sing ChF, Biron P, Mongeau J (1979). Familial aggregation of blood pressure and weight in adoptive families. Am J Epidemiol 110:479.

Brugnara C, Corrocher R, Foroni L, Steinmayr M, Bonfanti F, Sandre GD (1983). Li-Na countertransport in erythrocytes of normal and hypertensive subjects: Relationship with age and plasma renin activity. Hypertension 5:529.

Burke W, Hornung S, Copeland BR, Furlong CE, Motulsky AG (1983). Red cell sodium-lithium countertransport in hypertension. Recent Advances in Hypertension Mechanisms, Int Symp, Acapulco, Mexico (in press).

Canessa M, Adragna N, Solomon H, Connolly T, Tosteson DC (1980). Increased Li-Na countertransport in patients with essential hypertension. N Engl J Med 302:772.

Canessa M, Bize I, Adragna N, Tosteson DC (1982). Cotransport of lithium and potassium in human red cells. J Gen Physiol 80:149.

Canessa M, Bize I, Solomon H, Adragna N, Tosteson DC, Dagher G, Garay R, Meyer P (1981). Na countertransport and cotransport in human red cells: Function, dysfunction and genes in essential hypertension. Clin Exp Hypertens 3:783.

Canessa M, Brugnara C, Cusi D, Tosteson DC (1983a). Net Na extrusion and equilibrium of Na fluxes through the Na-K cotransport system. J Gen Physiol (in press).

Canessa M, Spalvins A, Adragna N, Falkner B (1983b). Red cell Na countertransport and cotransport in normotensive and hypertensive blacks. Hypertension (in press).

Garay RP, Dagher G, Pernollet G, Devinck M, Meyer P (1980). Inherited defect in Na-K cotransport system in erythrocytes from essential hypertensive patients. Nature 284:281.

Gavras I, Gavras H, Chobanian AV, Tiffts CD, Melby JC, Jicks H (1982). Hypertension and age, clinical and biochemical correlates. Clin Exp Hypertens A4 7:1097.

Genest J, Koiw E, Kuchel O (1977). "Hypertension, Physiopathology and Treatment." New York: McGraw Hill.

Hamlin JM, Ringel R, Schaeffer J, Levinson PD, Hamilton BP, Kowarski AA, Blaustein M (1982). A circulating inhibitor of Na-K ATPase associated with essential hypertension. Nature 300:650.

Langford HG, Canessa M, Watson RL (1983). A salt-sensitive population subset with distinct red blood cell Na and K fluxes. Clin Res (in press).

MacMahon B (1978). Epidemiological approaches to family resemblance. In Morton NE, Chung CS (eds): "Genetic Epidemiology," New York: Academic Press, p 3.

Miall WE, Heneage P, Khosla T, Lovell HG, Moore F (1967). Factors influencing the degree of resemblance in arterial pressure of close relatives. Clin Sci 32:271.

Paul O (1980). Epidemiology of hypertension. In Gross F, Robertson JS (eds): "Arterial Hypertension," Boston: G. K. Hall Medical Publishers, p 15.

Perry MH, Smith FW (1978). Mild hypertension: To treat or not to treat. Ann NY Acad Sci 304:1.

Pickering G (1968). "High Blood Pressure." London: J. A. Churchill, Ltd.

Platt R (1963). Heredity in hypertension. Lancet I:899.

Report of the Hypertension Task Force (1979). "Pediatric and Genetic Subgroup," Vol 6 (NIH Publication No. 79-1628), Bethesda, Maryland.

Rose RJ, Miller JZ, Gunn CE, Christian JC (1979). Aggregation of blood pressure in the families of identical twins. Am J Epidemiol 109:503.

Trevisan M, Ostrow D, Cooper R, Liu K, Sparks S, Okonek A, Stevens E, Marquardt J, Stamler J (1983). Abnormal red blood cell ion transport and hypertension. The people's gas company study. Hypertension 5:363.

Worley RJ, Hentschel WM, Cormier C, Nutting S, Pead G, Zelenkov K, Smith JB, Ash KO, Williams RR (1982). Increased sodium-lithium countertransport in erythrocytes of pregnant women. N Engl J Med 307:412.

Yamori Y (1980). Heredity of hypertension. In Gross F, Robertson JS (eds): "Arterial Hypertension," Boston: G. K. Hall Medical Publishers, p 28.

DISCUSSION

DR. TEITELBAUM: As you pointed out, there are a number of mechanisms by which one can account for Na and K transport in red cells, particularly a ouabain-sensitive and -insensitive pump. Have you been able to determine whether or not the red cells from hypertensive patients are ouabain-sensitive or -insensitive insofar as the increased countertransport mechanism is concerned?

DR. CANESSA: Excuse me if I didn't make myself very clear. There are several types of sodium transport systems. One is a gradient generator, which is a Na-K pump, ouabain-sensitive. The other transport systems such as the Na-K cotransport and Na countertransport, use the Na and K gradients, generated by the Na-K pump. Both transport systems, the Na-K cotransport and the Na countertransport, are ouabain-insensitive, that is to say they can operate in the presence of ouabain.

Both transport systems can operate in red cells because the red cell is a very peculiar cell. It has a very low cation permeability, and when the Na-K pump is inhibited by ouabain, the Na and K gradients are very slowly dissipated. So even when the pump is ouabain-inhibited, the Na and K gradients are still maintained during the time that we measure Na-K cotransport and Na countertransport. In other cells it might not be true, because the gradient generated by the Na pump is balancing a higher passive permeability.

DR. TEITELBAUM: Can you block the countertransport system you are studying with amiloride?

DR. CANESSA: The Li_i-Na_o countertransport system is amiloride-insensitive. The foregoing suggests that this is not a sodium-proton exchange system which is very sensitive to amiloride. Some investigators have suggested that the Li-Na countertransport system can operate as a Na-H^+ exchange.

DR. BERENSON: These are beautiful studies. It is interesting that you find this type of difference in black hypertensives in comparison to whites. Do race differences carry over into other cells, for example, the kidney tubules perhaps? We know that there are other differences that occur in the races related to hypertension. We found, for example, that in black children renin values are low, and I suspect aldosterone is also low. We know that black children, presumably on the same diet as whites, excrete less potassium in urine.

DR. CANESSA: You have asked me many questions. It is well known that hypertension in blacks has been characterized as low renin hypertension or volume-dependent hypertension in contrast to vasoconstrictive hypertension. I think that our picture of sodium transport in the red cells of black hypertensives supports the hypothesis that hypertension in blacks is related to a lower capacity of their cell membrane to transport sodium. Many of these subjects have very elevated cellular sodium. The reason why the sodium pump activity of the red cell membrane is low raises the question of whether this is related to modulatory factors such as the "natriuretic hormone". I didn't mention this matter in my presentation because this hormone has been very elusive to isolate. However, this is a matter of recent active research.

DR. BERENSON: You are suggesting that this might be due to proteins contained within the red blood cells or on the surface membrane.

DR. CANESSA: Yes.

DR. BERENSON: The natriuretic hormone, a circulating hormone, may have an effect.

DR. CANESSA: The natriuretic hormone may control renal Na excretion by modulation of the activity of the ouabain-sensitive Na pump. I am not saying that all the Na transport systems are genetically determined. Some of them, such as the ouabain-sensitive Na pump, are humorally regulated by Na retaining factors such as aldosterone, or a Na excretion factor such as the natriuretic hormone.

DR. LEE: Did you look at the effect of calcium on the sodium transport system in your studies?

DR. CANESSA: Yes. Dr. Garay has looked at the effect of calcium in Na-K cotransport, and he has reported that calcium inhibits Na-K cotransport, so it could be that in some subjects the low Na-K cotransport might be caused by high calcium, but we have not studied it. We are studying the effect of calcium in the sodium exchange system, and we have to wait for more data on this.

DR. BOHR: Can you tell us what is known about the endocrine influence on these transport systems?

DR. CANESSA: I think I can tell very little, and I think our findings raised the point of hormonal regulation of Na-K cotransport and Na countertransport. The only thing we know is that the ouabain-sensitive Na pump might be modulated by a plasma factor which is called "natriuretic hormone".

DR. BOHR: Isn't there a study of pregnancy related to these transport systems?

DR. CANESSA: Yes. It has been reported that countertransport is elevated in the third trimester of pregnancy (Williams et al). Logan et al in Toronto have reported that the elevation of countertransport might be different in normal pregnancy as compared to eclampsia. So these findings raise the question of whether or not there is humoral control of Li-Na countertransport. Since there are many humoral changes in pregnancy we do not know which hormone is responsible for the increased countertransport. We have found that in pregnant black women there is not such a significant elevation of their transport system.

I forgot to answer Dr. Berenson's question about the presence of the system in cells other than red cells. The Na-K cotransport is present in the distal tubules and also in the smooth muscle and endothelial cells of arteries. We are studying the function of Na-K cotransport in these cells.

DR. WISSLER: What the world needs, obviously, is a quick and easy test to detect people who are susceptible to essential hypertension. It is clear that there are no quick and easy answers to the development of such tests for most disease processes. It seems to me that you and your group have come a long way in opening the door to developing an approach for detecting persons who will be hypertension susceptible to sodium imbalance in their diet. Do you think there are proteins and/or enzymes in the red cell wall which can be used as probes or measures of transport in red cells which might offer a better opportunity for identifying groups which have an essential defect and are therefore more susceptible to sodium overload and hypertension?

DR. CANESSA: The problem is complicated, as I pointed out, and there are different Na transport systems altered in different individuals, and probably in different populations. Our view is that you have to measure at least the three Na transport systems. The Na pump has been studied for several decades, so we may soon have the necessary antibodies to measure them in a simple and rapid fashion.

However, as I mentioned, Na-K cotransport and countertransport have recently been discovered in human red cells. We didn't know how they functioned a few years ago. At present we have established how they function *in vivo*. I think we have established some approaches to isolate them now, and then when we have isolated them, we can probably find some procedures to detect them in a simpler manner than at present. Before we do that we have to know if it is really useful to screen the family of hypertensive patients, as well as for screening in epidemiological studies. I think for the meantime, we have to measure these systems under kinetic conditions for V_{max} and K_m.

DR. BERENSON: You are to be congratulated for making an advance in this area. I think people deny that hypertension exists in children, for example. We have been attempting to show that it does exist, and I think this is evidence with another marker that it does.

DR. CANESSA: Thank you very much for your stimulating comments. As you know, we just started our research with the thought that these systems would be good genetic markers. I would say now, at least they are good markers of the prehypertensive state in early life; at least between 15 years and 40 years of age in around 30-40% of the total hypertensive population. It is not clear in the case of countertransport if this will be useful at an earlier age. People are not born with countertransport, and we don't know when this appears. We are born with the Na pump and Na-K cotransport. We do not know what happens in the red cell membrane to the Na transport systems between birth and adolescence.

Comparative Pathobiology of Major Age-Related Diseases: Current Status and Research Frontiers, pages 251–267

VASCULAR SMOOTH MUSCLE DYSFUNCTION IN HYPERTENSION

Alex L. Harris, Ph.D., R. Clinton Webb, Ph.D., and David F. Bohr, M.D.

Department of Physiology, University of Michigan Medical School, Ann Arbor, MI 48109

INTRODUCTION

Arterial hypertension, whether clinical or experimental, is characterized by an increased total peripheral vascular resistance. This increase in resistance is initiated by a variety of events; however, regardless of the initiating event, the common denominator in all types of hypertension is a vascular change. Even in situations where the initiating factor, such as genetic predisposition, renal ischemia, or mineralocorticoid excess, is known, the sequences of events leading from the initiating factor to the alteration of the vasculature are not known. Little insight into the nature of the vascular change can be made from the study of the initiating factors or of the sequence of events leading to the vascular change. Instead, examination of the structural, functional and cellular differences that lead to and maintain the increased arterial pressure must be made. For a more complete overview of research on nature of the vascular change, readers are referred to recent reviews (Webb, Bohr 1981; Winquist et al 1982; Folkow 1982). This current chapter deals only with the most recent research contributing information about some factors responsible for the increased vascular resistance seen in hypertension.

STRUCTURAL ALTERATIONS OF THE BLOOD VESSELS

The heart and systemic arteries hypertrophy in hypertension (Folkow 1982). The microvasculature also undergoes structural changes in hypertension, exhibiting both wall thickening and rarefaction.

In a recent review article, Folkow (1982) presented evidence that increased vascular wall thickness in hypertension could account for the increased total peripheral vascular resistance associated with a rise in arterial pressure. He has hypothesized that medial hypertrophy or hyperplasia of the resistance vessels increases the wall-to-lumen ratio in such a way that the wall encroaches upon the lumen even when the vascular smooth muscle is relaxed and to a greater extent when it contracts. With smooth muscle contraction the thick wall is forced into the lumen decreasing its cross-sectional area and increasing resistance to flow.

Recent morphological studies have examined the changes responsible for the wall thickening with reference to cellular hypertrophy, hyperplasia and polyploidy. Yamori et al (1981) have analyzed cultured aortic vascular smooth muscle cells from spontaneously hypertensive rats (SHR), SHR-stroke prone (SHR-SP) and normotensive WKY rats. They observed that the rate of growth of smooth muscle cultures from SHR and SHR-SP, was greater than that from age matched WKY rats. The incorporation of [^{3}H]thymidine and [^{14}C]leucine and the ornithine decarboxylase activity of smooth muscle cells were also greater in both SHR and SHR-SP when compared to WKY rats. They interpreted the differences in these indices as indicating that cells from rats with genetic hypertension are intrinsically different from those of normotensive rats, independent of the elevated arterial blood pressure. These investigators also observed that alpha-adrenergic but not beta-adrenergic stimulation of these cells resulted in a dose-related increase in ornithine decarboxylase activity. These observations suggest that sympathetic tone may play a role in the structural vascular change. In keeping with these studies, Bevan and Tsuru (1979) have observed that sympathetic denervation of the ear artery in the growing rabbit is associated with a decreased smooth muscle DNA synthesis and vessel growth.

Greenberg et al (1981) have presented evidence that a circulating factor may exist as a mediator of hypertrophy observed in portal vein from SHR. In this study, SHR were parabiosed with WKY rats, matched for age and sex. Blood pressure rose in WKY parabiosed with SHR (WKY/SHR) over a 3-week to 5-month period. In the portal veins of the WKY/SHR pairs the wet and dry weight and protein content increased and structural and functional changes were observed, similar to those in SHR/SHR pairs. However, WKY/WKY pairs exhibited none of these alterations. These data suggest that a circulating factor in SHR may initiate the venous smooth muscle derangements observed during the development of spontaneous hypertension. These data also support the conclusion of Bell and Overbeck (1979) and Nilsson and Folkow (1980) who found that structural alterations occur in the low pressure side of the circulation in coarctation and spontaneous hypertension, respectively.

Whether the increase in vessel wall thickness in hypertension is due to hypertrophy or hyperplasia, or both, has been a hotly debated subject. Observations of a greater number of vascular smooth muscle cells labeled with [^{3}H]-thymidine (Yamori et al 1981) or a greater DNA content per unit vessel length or weight (Mangiarua et al 1981) indicate that hyperplasia may be the principal change responsible for medial thickening. However, morphological (Olivetti et al 1980) and biochemical (Owens et al 1981) measurements have suggested that the increase in smooth muscle mass may be accounted for solely by cellular hypertrophy. Most recently Lee et al (1983a,b) have conducted extensive light and electron microscopic studies indicating that both hypertrophy and hyperplasia are involved in the medial thickening in the SHR compared to the WKY rat. They also made the observation that with the completely relaxed arteriole the thicker wall of the SHR vessel did not encroach on the size of the lumen (compared to that of the WKY). Although this observation does not agree with earlier interpretations by Folkow (1982) it does not dispute the importance of a greater wall thickness in amplifying the magnitude of constrictor response effected by vascular smooth muscle contraction.

Owens and Schwartz (1982) have presented interesting new evidence indicating that aortic smooth muscle hypertrophy in SHR is accompanied by an increase in the frequency of polyploid cells. They reported that the largest portion of the increment in vascular smooth muscle cell mass is due to a 2-3-fold increase in the frequency of tetraploid and octaploid cells. The cells have 2-5 times the mass of a normal WKY diploid cell. These cells incorporate an increased amount of [^{3}H]thymidine proportional to the nuclear ploidy. These findings could account for an increase in DNA synthesis and content without a parallel increase in vascular smooth muscle number.

A recent study by Brayden et al (1983) investigated the biochemical and mechanical properties of resistance vessels from SHR and normotensive WKY rats. They measured the DNA, contractile protein and connective tissue protein composition of small (approximately 170 μm I.D.) mesenteric and cerebral resistance vessels. The DNA content of these arteries was elevated by nearly 30% in the SHR compared to that of the WKY rats. The amounts of actin and myosin, when normalized to DNA content, were not different in SHR mesenteric arteries compared to control, but were greatly decreased in the SHR cerebral arteries compared to control. The functional implications of the contractile protein measurements agreed with determinations of active smooth muscle cell stress-generating capabilities, which is not different in SHR mesenteric arteries and decreased in the SHR cerebral arteries.

FUNCTIONAL CHANGES IN BLOOD VESSELS

In an earlier review (Webb, Bohr 1981) dealing with vascular smooth muscle in hypertension, we presented extensive evidence indicating that in hypertension this muscle undergoes an increase in sensitivity based on changes in the plasma membrane. These changes are not secondary to the increase in wall stress caused by the arterial hypertension, as they may actually precede the hypertension. Evidence developed since that review was written will be presented here. It continues to support the primacy of functional vascular lesions in the pathogenesis of hypertension. First, recent evidence will be reviewed that further characterizes the nature and consequences of differences in the vascular smooth muscle cell membrane in hypertension. Finally, new evidence will be cited indicating that the nervous system may play as important role in the functional changes.

Membrane Abnormalities

Increased vascular sensitivity to serotonin and catecholamines in hypertension appears to be associated with an increased plasma membrane permeability to monovalent ions (Garwitz, Jones 1982a,b; Jones et al 1981; Friedman et al 1982). Passive fluxes of monovalent ions (sodium, potassium, chloride), as well as norepinephrine- and serotonin-stimulated potassium turnover are increased in vascular smooth muscle from hypertensive animals. These alterations in monovalent ion handling precede the development of elevated blood pressure (Jones 1982). An increased permeability to monovalent ions may act to decrease membrane potential and results in an increased vascular contractile response in hypertension.

Recent studies have demonstrated that the leakage of sodium into a cold lithium solution is much more rapid from SHR aortas than that observed from WKY aortas (Ito et al 1981; Koike et al 1982). Interestingly, long term administration of captopril in the SHR suppressed the increased sodium leak in the aorta, whereas treatment with hydralazine had no effect. Both drugs reduced the blood pressure. These findings of the ability of captopril to suppress the leakiness of vascular smooth muscle membranes suggest the involvement of the renin-angiotensin-aldosterone system in the genesis of the abnormal ion permeability seen in hypertension.

Recent unpublished studies from our laboratory have developed two additional types of evidence that indicate that there is altered membrane permeability in vascular smooth muscle from hypertensive animals: 1) increased responsiveness to ouabain; and 2) contractile responses to calcium following treatment with EGTA. Isolated vascular segments from SHR and DOCA hypertensive rats contract to a greater level in response to ouabain, an inhibitor of Na-K ATPase than do those from normotensive control rats (WKY). Threshold responses in aortic strips occur at approximately 10^{-6} M ouabain in hypertensive rats, compared to 10^{-4} M in normotensive controls. Monensin, a sodium ionophore, potentiates contractile responses to ouabain in aortic strips from both hypertensive and control rats, but the magnitude of potentiation is greater in the normotensive animals. Amiloride, a blocker of sodium channels, causes a greater inhibition of contractile responses to ouabain in aortic strips from DOCA hypertensive rats compared to that in normotensive controls. These observations suggest that the altered responsiveness to ouabain in arteries from hypertensive animals is related to a greater membrane permeability to sodium ions in vascular smooth muscle from these animals.

Treatment of vascular smooth muscle from hypertensive rats with the calcium chelator, EGTA, makes the membrane unstable so that it leaks calcium upon subsequent exposure to the cation. Vascular smooth muscle from normotensive rats does not contract in response to elevated calcium when it has been previously treated with EGTA. Further observations have indicated that the cell membrane of vascular smooth muscle from the hypertensive animal is not as readily stabilized by high concentrations of calcium as is that of the control animal (Webb, Bohr 1980; Winquist et al 1982). This membrane leakiness to calcium and this failure of calcium to produce stabilization may be associated with the decreased ability of plasma membranes from hypertensive rats to bind calcium (Kwan et al 1980). This inadequate calcium binding may also be responsible for the greater monovalent ion leak and for the increase in vascular smooth muscle sensitivity in hypertension.

Devynck et al (1981) studied the calcium binding properties of plasma membrane enriched fractions from various tissues (heart, liver, nerve endings, and erythrocytes) in young hypertensive rats and their normotensive controls. They found that whatever the tissue, plasma membrane from SHR exhibited a reduced calcium binding capacity. It appears that this deficient calcium binding is a generalized membrane defect in hypertension.

A change in the electrogenic sodium pump is another cell membrane abnormality that may contribute to altered vascular responsiveness in hypertension. Experimental evidence suggesting that the activity of the electrogenic pump is increased in hypertension is based on the following evidence: 1) a decreased membrane potential at 16°C which inactivates Na-K ATPase (Hermsmeyer 1976; Hermsmeyer et al 1982); 2) an increased ouabain-sensitive uptake of rubidium (Brock et al 1982); 3) an increased relaxation to potassium ion (Webb et al 1983a); 4) an increased ouabain potentiation of norepinephrine, vasopressin and $BaCl_2$-induced constrictor responses (Gothberg et al 1980); and 5) an increased Na-K ATPase activity based on measurements of inorganic phosphate cleaved from ATP (Allen, Seidel 1977). It has been proposed that an increased pump activity may result in a greater membrane depolarization during cell activation by vasoactive agents which cause a short circuit of the potential generated by the pump (Hermsmeyer 1976).

In contrast, a depressed pump activity has been documented in low-renin volume expanded forms of hypertension (Pamnani et al 1981). This depressed pump activity is thought to be caused by a circulating ouabain-like factor that binds to digoxin antibodies (Gruber et al 1982; De Wardener, Clarkson 1982). Because of the increased passive leak of sodium and potassium through the cell membrane of vascular smooth muscle in the hypertensive animal, this tissue should be particularly vulnerable to pump inhibition. Pump inhibition should depolarize the vascular smooth muscle and thereby increase its sensitivity in responding to vasoactive agents.

The Role of Neurogenic Control on the Functional Vascular Changes in Hypertension

Abel and Hermsmeyer (1981) have extended their earlier observations indicating that the increased vascular smooth muscle sensitivity to norepinephrine is caused by altered membrane electrical properties. They have now transplanted tail arteries from young SHR to the anterior eye chamber of adult WKY rats and found that the smooth muscle of the transplanted vessel took on the normal membrane electrical properties of the vasculature of the host. However, if, prior to the transplant, the host animal was subjected to a surgical sympathectomy of the region of the eye, the transplanted vessel retained the membrane properties of the hypertensive donor animal. The sympathetic nervous system seemed to be a determinant of the membrane characteristics of both the normotensive and hypertensive vessels.

In another electrophysiological study, Willems et al (1982) observed that the membrane potential of the mesenteric vein *in vivo* was lower in the SHR than in the WKY rat. They presented evidence indicating that this low membrane potential of the SHR was due to an altered autonomic nervous system control that involved both alpha- and beta-adrenergic systems. They concluded that in the hypertensive animal the alpha-adrenergic activity exerts a depolarizing influence by interfering with the expression of the beta-adrenergic hyperpolarization.

Several other studies suggest that increased vascular responsiveness in hypertension may be related to an altered interaction between the adrenergic nerve endings and vascular smooth muscle cells. This junctional complex provides the mechanism for sympathetic control of vascular function. Both the catecholamine content (Crabb et al 1980; Webb et al 1983b) and catecholamine histofluorescence (Fink, Brody 1978; Ljungqvist 1974) have been found to be decreased in vascular beds of hypertensive animals. Ultrastructural studies (Azevedo et al 1981) indicate a decrease in the number of dense core vesicles in adrenergic nerve endings of arteries from renal hypertensive rats and dogs. Interpretation of the significance of this catecholamine depletion in terms of vascular function has been speculative. Based on recent observations (described below), we hypothesize that there is an altered neurotrophic activity to vascular smooth muscle in hypertension.

Table 1 summarizes the effects of innervation and hypertension on vascular smooth muscle. The hypothesis that adrenergic nerves exert a neurotrophic influence on vascular function is based on the observation that contractile responses in several experimental conditions correlate with the naturally occurring variability in catecholamine content among different blood vessels in the rat (tail artery > mesenteric artery > aorta). Furthermore, vascular responses to these experimental conditions are increased in arteries from normotensive rats following either surgical or chemical denervation procedures.

In each case, the vascular response of the artery from the hypertensive rat (SHR, unilateral renal artery constricted rat, DOCA-induced hypertension) responds in a manner similar to the artery with the less dense adrenergic innervation. These observations offer strong support to the hypothesis that vascular changes in hypertensive animals may be related to an altered neurotrophic influence.

SUMMARY

Because most forms of clinical and experimental hypertension are caused by an increase in total peripheral resistance, the investigator must study the blood vessel in order to understand the reason that the arterial pressure goes up. In established hypertension the walls of the arteries and resistance vessels are thickened largely as an adaptive change in response to the elevated arterial pressure. This wall thickening serves to amplify the vasoconstrictor effect of vascular smooth muscle contraction and thereby exaggerate any tendency for pressure to rise. Recent studies have indicated that the wall thickening reflects both hypertrophy and hyperplasia of the smooth muscle cell. Interesting new observations reveal that there is a high incidence of multi-

Table 1
Innervation and hypertension in vascular smooth muscle

Experimental Condition	Artery type Tail (T) Mesenteric (M) Aorta (A)	Innervated (I) or Denervated (D)	Normotensive (N) or Hypertensive (H)
Catecholamine content	T > M > A	I > D	N > H
Norepinephrine sensitivity	T < M < A	I < D	N < H
Phasic contraction to norepinephrine in calcium-free physiological salt solution	T > M > A	?	N > H
K-free contraction	T > M > A	I > D	N > H
Spontaneous activity	T < M < A	I < D	N < H
Methysergide sensitivity	T < M < A	I < D	N < H
Ouabain suspense	T < M < A	I < D	N < H
Arachidonate response	T < M < A	?	N < H
EGTA treatment (response to calcium, calcium leak)	T < M < A	?	N < H

(See legend next page)

First column: experimental conditions compared. Second column: normal arteries with different degrees of innervation. Third column: chemical or surgical denervation. Fourth column: normotensive vs. hypertensive rats. Responses of vascular smooth muscle from hypertensive rats resemble those of a poorly innervated muscle. From Webb et al (1983b); Webb, Bohr (1983); Bohr et al (1983); Moreland et al (1983).

---

nucleated smooth muscle cells in the media of the blood vessel in hypertension.

Increases in vascular smooth muscle sensitivity and membrane permeability may precede the arterial pressure elevation or occur early in the development of hypertension. These observations argue that these functional changes may be the cause of the hypertension. Recent literature has contained extensive evidence supporting both humoral and neurogenic regulators as being responsible for these functional vascular changes.

ACKNOWLEDGEMENTS

Studies reported in this review were supported by grants from the National Institutes of Health (HL-18575, HL-27020). R.C.W. is a recipient of a Research Career Development Award from the National Institutes of Health (HL-00813).

REFERENCES

Abel PW, Hermsmeyer K (1981). Sympathetic cross-innervation of SHR and genetic controls suggests a trophic influence on vascular muscle membranes. Circ Res 49:1311.

Allen JC, Seidel C (1977). EGTA stimulated and ouabain inhibited ATPase of vascular smooth muscle. In Casteels R, Godfraind T, Ruegg JC (eds): "Excitation-Contraction Coupling in Smooth Muscle," Amsterdam: Elsevier/North Holland Biomedical Press, p 211.

Azevedo I, Castro-Tavares J, Garret J (1981). Ultrastructural changes in blood vessels of perinephritic hypertensive dogs. Blood Vessels 18:110.

Bell DR, Overbeck HW (1979). Increased resistance and impaired maximal vasodilation in normotensive vascular beds of rats with coarctation hypertension. Hypertension 1:78.

Bevan RD, Tsuru H (1979). Long-term denervation of vascular smooth muscle causes not only functional but structural change. Blood Vessels 16:109.

Bohr DF, Harris AL, Guthe CC, Webb RC (1983). Hypertension: Multiple membrane malfunctions. In Sambhi MP (ed): "Recent Advances in Hypertension Mechanisms," Amsterdam: Martinus Nijholt. In press.

Brayden JE, Halpern W, Brann LR (1983). Biochemical and mechanical properties of resistance arteries from normotensive and hypertensive rats. Hypertension 5:17.

Brock TA, Smith JB, Overbeck HW (1982). Relationship of vascular sodium-potassium pump activity to intracellular sodium in hypertensive rats. Hypertension 4(Suppl II): II-43.

Crabb GA, Head RJ, Hempstead J, Berkowitz BA (1980). Altered disposition of vascular catecholamines in hypertensive (DOCA-salt) rats. Clin Exp Hypertens 2:129.

Devynck MA, Pernollet MG, Nunez AM, Meyer P (1981). Calcium binding alteration in plasma membrane from various tissues of SHR. Clin Exp Hypertens 3:797.

De Wardener HE, Clarkson EM (1982). The natriuretic hormone: Recent developments. Clin Sci 63:415.

Fink GD, Brody MF (1978). Neurogenic control of the renal circulation in hypertension. Fed Proc 37:1202.

Folkow B (1982). Physiological aspects of primary hypertension. Physiol Rev 62:342.

Friedman SM, McIndoe RA, Spieckerman G (1982). Ion-selective electrode studies of cell Na^+ components in vascular smooth muscle of WKY and SHR. Am J Physiol 242:H751.

Garwitz ET, Jones AW (1982a). Aldosterone infusion into the rat and dose-dependent changes in blood pressure and arterial ionic transport. Hypertension 4:374.

Garwitz ET, Jones AW (1982b). Altered ion transport and its reversal in aldosterone hypertensive rats. Am J Physiol 243:H527.

Gothberg O, Jandhyala B, Folkow B (1980). Studies on the role of sodium-potassium-activated ATPase as determinant of vascular reactivity in Wistar-Kyoto and spontaneously hypertensive rats. Clin Sci 59:187s.

Greenberg S, Gaines K, Sweatt D (1981). Evidence for circulating factors as a cause of venous hypertrophy in SHR. Am J Physiol 241:H421.

Gruber KA, Rudel LL, Bullock BC (1982). Increased circulating

levels of an endogenous digoxin-like factor in hypertensive monkeys. Hypertension 4:348.
Hermsmeyer K (1976). Cellular basis for increased sensitivity of vascular smooth muscle in spontaneously hypertensive rats. Circ Res 38(Suppl I):53.
Hermsmeyer K, Abel PW, Trapani AJ (1982). Norepinephrine sensitivity and membrane potentials of caudal (tail) arterial muscle in DOCA-salt, Dahl and SHR hypertension in the rat. Hypertension 4(Suppl II):II-49.
Ito K, Koike H, Miyamoto M, Ozaki H, Kishimoto T, Rakawa N (1981). Long-term effects of captopril on cellular sodium content and mechanical properties of aortic smooth muscle from SHR. J Pharmacol Exp Ther 219:520.
Jones AW (1982). Ionic dysfunction and hypertension. Adv Microcirc 11:134.
Jones AW, Heidlage JF, Maeyer R, Day B, Freeland A (1981). Non-specific supersensitivity of aortic ^{42}K fluxes during DOCA hypertension in the rat, and the effects of anti-hypertensive therapy. In Worcel M, Bonvalet JP, Langer SZ, Menard J, Sassard J (eds): "New Trends in Arterial Hyper-tension," Amsterdam: Elsevier/North Holland Biomedical Press, p 163.
Koike H, Miyamoto M, Ito K (1982). Long-term effects of captopril on passive sodium permeability and contractility in vascular smooth muscles of spontaneously hypertensive rats. Am J Cardiol 49:1505.
Kwan CY, Belbeck L, Daniel EE (1980). Abnormal biochemistry of vascular smooth muscle plasma membrane isolated from hypertensive rats. Mol Pharmacol 17:137.
Lee RMKW, Forrest JB, Garfield RE, Daniel EE (1983a). Ultra-structural changes in mesenteric arteries from spontaneously hypertensive rats. Blood Vessels 20:72.
Lee RMKW, Garfield RE, Forrest JB, Daniel EE (1983b). Morpho-metric study of structural changes in the mesenteric blood vessels of spontaneously hypertensive rats. Blood Vessels 20:57.
Ljungqvist A (1974). The role of the intrarenal sympathetic innervation in the development of renal hypertension. Acta Pathol Microbiol Scand 82:450.
Mangiarua E, Basso N, Ruiz P, Tanquini AC (1981). Vascular structural changes in DOC-salt hypertensive rats. Hyper-tension 3(Suppl II):183.
Moreland RS, Major T, Webb RC (1983). Monensin and increased responsiveness to ouabain and K^+-free solution on aortae from spontaneously hypertensive rats. Fed Proc 42:743.
Nilsson M, Folkow B (1980). Structurally reduced compliance

of the venous capacitance vessels in the spontaneously hypertensive rat. Acta Physiol Scand 110:215.

Olivetti G, Anversa P, Melissari M, Loud A (1980). Morphometry of medial hypertrophy in the rat thoracic aorta. Lab Invest 42:559.

Owens GK, Rabinovitch PS, Schwartz SM (1981). Smooth muscle cell hypertrophy versus hyperplasia in hypertension. Proc Natl Acad Sci USA 78:7759.

Owens GK, Schwartz SM (1982). Alterations in vascular smooth muscle mass in the spontaneously hypertensive rat. Role of cellular hypertrophy, hyperploidy, and hyperplasia. Circ Res 51:280.

Pamnani MB, Clough DL, Huot DL, Haddy FJ (1981). Sodium-potassium pump activity in experimental hypertension. In Vanhoutte PM, Leusen I (eds): "Vasodilatation," New York: Raven Press, p 391.

Webb RC, Bohr DF (1980). Vascular reactivity in hypertension: Altered effect of ouabain. Experientia 36:220.

Webb RC, Bohr DF (1981). Recent advances in the pathogenesis of hypertension: Consideration of structural, functional and metabolic vascular abnormalities resulting in elevated arterial resistance. Am Heart J 102:251.

Webb RC, Bohr DF (1983). The membrane of the vascular smooth muscle cell in experimental hypertension and its response to serotonin. In Stephens N (ed): "Smooth Muscle Contractions," New York: Marcel Dekker. In press.

Webb RC, Cohen DM, Bohr DF (1983a). Potassium-induced vascular relaxation in two kidney-one clip, renal hypertensive rats. Pflug Arch 396:72.

Webb RC, Johnson JC, Bohr DF (1983b). Adrenergic neurotransmission in tail arteries from two kidney-one clip, renal hypertensive rats. Hypertension (in press).

Willems WJ, Harder DR, Cortney SJ, McCubbin JW, Stekiel WJ (1982). Sympathetic supraspinal control of venous membrane potential in spontaneous hypertension in vivo. Am J Physiol 243 (Cell Physiol 12):C101.

Winquist RJ, Webb RC, Bohr DF (1982). Vascular smooth muscle in hypertension. Fed Proc 41:2387.

Yamori Y, Igawa T, Kanbe T, Kihara M, Nara Y, Horie R (1981). Mechanisms of structural vascular changes in genetic hypertension: Analysis of cultured vascular smooth muscle cells from SHR. Clin Sci 61:121s.

DISCUSSION

DR. SCARPELLI: I want to congratulate you on an absolutely outstanding presentation. I am impressed by the rapidity with which the change occurs after you implant desoxycorticosterone acetate (DOCA). To me it suggests the changes follow a mechanical stretching or as you call it, increased vessel wall stress. I am reminded of some experiments done some years ago in which mechanically stretched muscle led to an increase in ion flux that occurred very rapidly, which was then followed by augmented protein synthesis. These are considered to be the cellular events that presage muscle hypertrophy, and I am wondering to what extent you have something here that is similar.

DR. BOHR: That is an excellent description of Sidney Friedman's original observation. The question really gets into the sequence of events that make the membrane become leakier. Once it gets leakier more pump activity is called for because the sodium that leaks in drives the pump, and also maybe more pump sites are built. Presumably that is what happens when the mineralocorticoid acts on the renal tubular cell causing an increase in sodium leak. It is the increased sodium leak that stimulates more pump sites to develop. I didn't answer your question.

DR. SCARPELLI: I don't know that anybody can at this point, but it suggests that simple mechanical stretching of membrane can lead to some rather profound changes in its function and, perhaps, chemical structure.

DR. BOHR: I agree with you on the stretch, but you still are faced with what causes the initial stretch, what causes the pressure to go up in the first place. You have to have another mechanism to make it go up in the first place to stretch it to cause the leak, and this is where the puzzle is.

DR. WISSLER: I think both of the last two presentations have been remarkable. They indicate that we might be getting close to the point where we can take some of the essential or idiopathic nature out of the essential hypertension, and I think they fit together very well. I was glad you opened with some indication of how hypertension becomes more of a problem with age. I think that is one reason for including it as a topic in this symposium. I wonder whether there have been any studies done, that you know of, comparing smooth muscle from old versus young individuals, or are we dealing, really, with Dr. Canessa's defect in the countertransport or sodium-potassium cotransport system, which gets worse with age in the smooth muscle cell as well as in the red cell? Is there any evidence, so far, about age effects on the kinds of things you were describing or the kinds of things that Dr. Canessa was describing?

DR. BOHR: I don't know of any major studies of the effects of age *per se*. There are some minor age-related observations. The receptor population on the membrane changes with age. Beta-adrenergic receptors decrease with age. Mineralocorticoid hypertension is much harder to produce in an old rat than a young rat. I do not know of major studies of the membrane lability in old and young, and that would be an interesting thing to look at.

DR. BELL: My question is like Dr. Scarpelli's. I would like to know what happens at the cellular level in response to pressure changes. Since smooth muscle cells are under pressure constantly in a blood vessel, a qualitative change must occur as a function of some quantitative difference in pressure. It is the time sequence of the appearance of the changes at the cellular level in response to the pressure increase that I ask about. Specifically, how soon do cell proliferation and cell secretory activity increase or change under these conditions?

DR. BOHR: I interpret your question as concerning the hyperplasia and hypertrophy and the increases in extracellular products that occur. These are responses of the cell to increases in wall stress, and they reflect the length of time that the pressure has been up and how high it has been. To me, the interesting question is, what initiates the change in sensitivity of the smooth muscle cell that makes the pressure increase in the first instance, and why does this happen so fast?

Let me tell you one thing that happens between the initiating factor such as desoxycorticosterone acetate (DOCA) administration, and the final common pathway, the vascular change. If a lesion is placed in a certain place in the hypothalamus, mineralocorticoid administration will not cause hypertension and will not induce the vascular change. These hypothalamic centers are involved in some way in producing the vascular change. It is not known whether the efferent regulator is a ouabain-like circulating factor or neurogenic. This efferent control system can act within 48 hours on the vascular muscle cell. This is in a much faster time frame than is necessary for the structural change.

DR. BELL: What is the time interval between the application of elevated pressure and the measurable response in resistance to that pressure?

DR. BOHR: We have looked for increased structural resistance as early as two weeks after the DOCA administration, and the change is there already. These changes are reversible.

DR. BELL: Within that short period of time have there been noticeable cytological changes?

DR. BOHR: Dr. Friedman has seen noticeable cytologic changes within two weeks in the laboratory.

DR. LEE: Thank you very much for your presentation. A group from Oregon recently suggested that hypertension in the elderly is related to decreased dietary calcium because high dietary calcium intake reduces blood pressure in the elderly. I would like your comment on that.

DR. BOHR: Dr. David McCarren in Oregon has been looking at plasma levels of calcium, and there is a tendency for these to be low in hypertension, and he has postulated an etiologic relationship between the low plasma calcium level and hypertension. I have not studied this relationship. The low plasma calcium level is hypothesized as making the smooth muscle cell membrane more labile.

DR. LEE: Have you changed the diet in your pig model? We used a spontaneous hypertensive turkey model. We doubled the calcium concentration in their diets and reduced their blood pressures by 30 mm Hg, but their serum calcium concentration did not change.

DR. BOHR. We have not studied calcium in the pig. We have reduced the sodium intake from 150 down to 20 mEq and that reverses the pressure elevation. Calcium could very well be important also. I am glad to learn that it is important in the turkey.

DR. TERRY: In regard to the increased difficulty of inducing hypertension in the older animals and in regard to the hypothalamic lesion preventing the lesion, one might point out that there are only 50% of the dexamethasone binding sites in the 26-month-old Fischer rat as compared with the 5- or 14-month-old Fischer rat. Binding affinity remains unchanged. Furthermore, there are only about 50% as many hypothalamic neurons in several of the nuclei in these aged rats.

DR. BOHR: That was beautiful. Thank you.

Comparative Pathobiology of Major Age-Related Diseases: Current Status and Research Frontiers, pages 269–288

EXTRACELLULAR MATRIX CHANGES IN DIABETES MELLITUS

Joseph R. Williamson, M.D. and Charles Kilo, M.D.

Washington University School of Medicine,
St. Louis, MO 63110

INTRODUCTION

Increased quantities of extracellular matrix have long been recognized, in the form of scar tissue, in the vasculature of diabetics. Indeed, the markedly increased mortality and morbidity due to cardiovascular disease in the diabetic is strongly associated with accumulation of collagenous components of scar tissue in the large arteries, in the glomerular capillaries of the kidney, and in the eye. The excess scar tissue accumulates in the innermost layers (intima) of the arteries, eventually occluding them, and in the outermost layer of capillaries throughout the body. In recent years there has been a growing interest in qualitative as well as quantitative changes in collagen of skin, joints, lungs, heart, and kidney and in components of extracellular matrix in the blood and urine.

The increased quantity of collagen in tissues is consistent with the view that it is the product of a proliferative response (of the involved tissues) to injury (Williamson, Kilo 1980) or that degradation of collagen is impaired. Although the qualitative changes described in collagen could account for its accumulation on the basis of impaired degradation, the nature of the injury (stimulus) which might cause increased synthesis of collagen is not known.

In contrast to the increased tissue content of collagens, glycosaminoglycans appear to be decreased in amount and/or extent of sulfation, suggesting decreased synthesis and rate of sulfation and/or increased rates of degradation.

Virtually nothing is known regarding changes in elastin or in the fibronectin family of extracellular matrix constituents in diabetes.

In this review we will consider the nature of the changes in collagens and glycosaminoglycans in diabetes, candidate mechanisms responsible for them, and their pathophysiological consequences.

COLLAGEN AND GLYCOSAMINOGLYCAN CHANGES

Changes in Cardiovascular Collagens

Although type III collagen is the most common form of collagen in normal arteries, type I is the major form accumulating in atherosclerotic plaques in the nondiabetic (McCullagh, Balian 1975; McCullagh et al 1980). While the type of collagen accumulating in plaques of diabetics is presumed to be the same as that in the nondiabetic, this has not been documented to our knowledge.

On the other hand, collagen accumulating in small vessels of the diabetic is type IV. Although morphologic techniques applied at the level of the electron microscope have documented excess accumulation of capillary basement membrane in many tissues throughout the body (Williamson, Kilo 1981), the only tissue in which sufficient amounts of purified basement membrane have been obtained for biochemical analysis is the kidney. Reports from several investigators have confirmed that the collagen accumulating in glomerular basement membrane (GBM) of diabetic humans is type IV (Beisswenger, Spiro 1970; Klein et al 1975). Studies by Brownlee and Spiro, (1979) and by Cohen et al (1982) in rats with diabetes induced by injection of streptozotocin indicate that glomerular synthesis of type IV collagen is increased and the observations of Cohen et al (1982) suggest that degradation is also impaired.

Haider et al (1978) reported that the acid soluble fraction of collagen extracted from monkey hearts was significantly reduced while the collagen content was increased. Regan et al (1981) reported that the collagen content of diabetic dog hearts was increased also. In contrast, Modrak (1980) reported that the collagen content of hearts of rats with streptozotocin induced diabetes of 26 weeks duration was not increased. The absence of collagen accumulation in Modrak's animals may be related to the much shorter duration of diabetes in the rats relative to that in the monkeys and dogs.

Recent studies by several groups of investigators have documented an increase in hexose bound to collagen by non-enzymatic reactions. Nonenzymatic glucosylation of proteins was first described in hemoglobin but has since been documented in a large number of proteins which have relatively slow turnover rates and are exposed to ambient glucose levels over extended time periods. Increased glucosylation of collagen has been observed in rat aorta (Rosenberg et al 1979), human GBM (Uitto et al 1982; LePape et al 1981a), and rat GBM (Cohen et al 1980; LePape et al 1981a). Recent investigations of Uitto et al (1982) demonstrated a 2.5-fold increase in nonenzymatically mediated glucosylation of type IV collagen isolated from human GBM with no change in enzymatically mediated hydroxylysine-0-glycosides. This finding differs from the small increase in enzymatic glycosylation of collagen reported by Beisswenger and Spiro (1970) but is in agreement with the findings of Westberg and Michael (1973) and of Kefalides (1974).

Earlier controversies regarding whether increased glycosylation of type IV collagen occurs in diabetes are probably attributable to differences in methods employed to isolate and purify GBM which yielded preparations containing varying proportions of type IV collagen and other basement membrane constituents such as laminin and the proteoglycan heparan sulfate.

In addition to the increased quantity and glucosylation of vascular collagen, increased cross-linking has been reported for GBM collagen (LePape et al 1981a) and for myocardial collagen (Haider et al 1978).

Changes in Nonvascular Collagen

Type I collagen in diabetes has been examined most extensively in skin and tendon. Francis et al (1974) reported that skin collagen from diabetic subjects was less soluble in neutral salt solutions than collagen from control subjects. Skin collagen solubility in acid solution was reduced, degradation by pepsin was impaired, and high molecular weight components were increased in diabetic subjects examined by Schnider and Kohn (1981). Buckingham et al (1981) reported that solubility of skin collagen in 0.5 m acetic acid was reduced in 2 of 3 subjects with limited joint mobility. Fleischmajer et al (1970) reported that total collagen content was increased 3 to 4 times normal in skin biopsies of diabetics with scleredema.

The only investigators reporting increased solubility of skin collagen in animals with experimentally induced diabetes are Berenson et al (1972). These investigators also reported that skin collagen solubility of hyperinsulinemic animals was decreased. The explanation for the apparent discrepancy in the observations of Berenson et al (1972) and other investigators is not clear but may be related to differences in collagen extraction conditions.

Hamlin et al (1975) reported that tendon collagen obtained from human diabetics at autopsy was less readily digested by collagenase than collagen from controls. Golub et al (1978) subsequently also demonstrated a substantial decrease in solubility of rat tail tendon collagen in diabetic animals.

It is unclear at the present time whether rates of collagen formation and degradation are significantly altered in skin and tendon of human diabetics. Certainly in human diabetics with scleredema there is marked thickening of the skin with proportionate increases in collagen and proteoglycans (Fleischmajer et al 1970). On the other hand, in diabetic rats which are losing weight, total skin collagen decreases (Schneir et al 1982) although collagen content per unit dry weight of tissue remains constant. It is unclear, however, whether skin collagen is lost in diabetic animals not losing weight or who are gaining weight albeit at a slower rate than nondiabetic controls.

An increase in collagen content has also been reported in a variety of other tissues from diabetics including rat lung (Madia et al 1979), human nucleus pulposus (Aufdermaur et al 1980) and human bone (Silberberg et al 1981). Aufdermaur et al (1980) also found that the acid soluble fraction of collagen extracted from nucleus pulposus was decreased by 20% compared to nondiabetics. In these studies the precise type of collagen was not ascertained.

Schneir et al (1979) have reported that total collagen content of intestinal tracts of diabetic rats is increased 60%, consistent with the marked hypertrophy of the gut induced by diabetes. The collagen content per unit dry weight of tissue, however, is not increased.

In all of these studies of collagen solubility in vascular and nonvascular tissues, increased cross-linking has been inferred on the basis of previous investigations documenting that an increase in collagen cross-links reduces collagen solubility in neutral salt solutions and weak acids (Bailey et al 1974; Uitto 1971) and renders it more resistant to proteolytic degradation (Vater et al 1979). The studies of Chang et al (1980) provide further evidence that the decreased solubility of type I collagen in diabetic animals results from increased cross-linking mediated by the enzyme lysyl oxidase. Those investigators found that D-penicillinase and ß-aminopropionitrile (inhibitors of cross-link formation induced by lysyl oxidase), in doses that did not affect overall collagen production, completely prevented the decreased solubility of collagen observed in diabetic rats. Their findings as well as those of Golub et al (1978) also provided evidence for increased intramolecular cross-linking of collagen in diabetic rats.

Increased glucosylation of collagen in nonvascular tissues has been described in human skin (Buckingham et al 1981; Schnider, Kohn 1981), human tendon (Schnider, Kohn 1980), and rat tail tendon (LePape et al 1981b).

While many investigators have likened the late complications of diabetes to an acceleration of the normal aging process, LePape et al (1981b) and Bailey (1981) have concluded that type I collagen changes associated with diabetes differ from those observed in "normal" aging. Aging changes in collagen from nondiabetics include an increase in nonreducible cross-links and a slight increase in (nonenzymatic) N-glucosylation of collagen with a concomitant decrease in reducible cross-links. In diabetics, on the other hand, the marked increase in N-glucosylated collagen is not accompanied by a decrease in reducible cross-links. This finding that reducible cross-links are not reduced in the diabetic may be explained by the additional finding of Stevens et al (1978) that glucosylated proteins are more susceptible to sulfhydryl oxidation leading to formation of disulfide cross-links. The precise nature of the differences in collagen changes in the diabetic and the nondiabetic remain to be determined.

Glycosaminoglycan Changes

Although much attention has been focused on collagen changes in diabetes, it would appear that glycosaminoglycan (GAG) changes are equally ubiquitous and possibly as important. Substantial changes, generally reductions, in GAG content, synthesis and/or sulfation have been reported in virtually every tissue examined in the diabetic. These tissues include skin, cornea, cartilage, bone, and vertebral disc as well as GBM, coronary arteries, and aorta. Schiller and Dorfman (1957) reported that the turnover rate of mucopolysaccharides in rat skin is decreased in diabetic animals and that this decrease is reversed by insulin treatment. They have also shown that hyaluronic acid is reduced by 38% and chondroitin sulfate by 27% with no change in heparan sulfate in skin from diabetic rats (Schiller, Dorfman 1963). The latter findings have been confirmed by Berenson et al (1972).

Cohen and Foglia (1970) reported a biphasic change in GAG content of aortas of pancreatectomized rats. Chondroitin-4-sulfate, chondroitin-6-sulfate, and dermatan sulfate were increased 3 months after pancreatectomy when diabetes was relatively mild. However, both chondroitin sulfates were reduced by 25% at 6 months after pancreatectomy. Brosnan et al (1973) demonstrated a 20% decrease in heparan sulfate and chondroitin sulfate but no change in hyaluronic acid or dermatan sulfate content of dog aortas five weeks after pancreatectomy. More recently, Sirek et al (1981) have reported differences in GAG levels in different arteries of insulin treated dogs. Of particular interest was the increased level of dermatan sulfate in coronary arteries which they attributed to intermittent hyperinsulinemia. Brown et al (1982) reported a decrease in $^{35}SO_4$ incorporation into GAGs of aortas of rats with streptozotocin diabetes.

Aufdermaur et al (1980) reported that the hexosamine content (an index of GAGs) was reduced by 30% in vertebral discs of human diabetics. Several investigators have documented decreased incorporation of $^{35}SO_4$ into GAGs of developing bone and/or cartilage in rats with experimentally induced diabetes (Brown et al 1982; Weiss et al 1981; Weiss, Reddi 1980; Axelsson et al 1983; Phillips, Young 1976).

Likewise, decreased *in vivo* incorporation of $^{35}SO_4$ into rat GBM has been reported by Cohen and Surma (1981), Brown et al (1982), and LePape et al (1981a). Parthasarathy and Spiro (1982) have recently reported a 40% reduction in hexuronic acid content (another index of GAGs) of GBM isolated from human diabetics. This observation would appear to differ from that of Berenson et al (1970) who reported 2-fold increases in hyaluronic acid and heparan sulfate and a 3-fold increase in chondroitin sulfate B in whole renal cortex of kidneys from diabetics with nodular diabetic glomerulosclerosis. They reported a 4-fold increase in hyaluronic acid with only small increases in heparan sulfate (1.1 x normal) and chondroitin sulfate B (1.5 x normal) in kidneys from diabetics with diffuse glomerulosclerosis. Since Berenson's observations were based on whole renal cortex which would include interstitium as well as glomeruli, they are not directly comparable to those of Parthasarathy and Spiro (1982) which were based on purified GBM. On the other hand, in view of the fact that the yield of GBM from diabetic kidneys was 2x that of controls in the study of Parthasarathy and Spiro (1982), the 40% reduction in hexuronic acid relative to GBM may not represent an absolute decrease in GAG content per kidney or per unit of glomerular filtration surface area.

Recent experiments by Rohrbach et al (1982a,b) and by Kjellen et al (1983) are also of considerable interest. Rohrbach et al (1982a) have grown the EHS tumor (a tumor which produces large amounts of basement membrane material) in genetically diabetic (db/db) mice and in mice with diabetes induced by streptozotocin. In both groups of diabetic mice, synthesis of the major GAG, heparan sulfate, is reduced by 25% relative to controls. When the tumor is grown in genetically diabetic mice, but not in streptozotocin diabetic mice, laminin synthesis is increased 2-fold. Kjellen et al (1983) have recently demonstrated a reduction in the sulfate content of heparan sulfate isolated from liver cell plasma membranes of diabetic rats. Since heparan sulfate is a common proteoglycan in cell membranes, this finding indicates that proteoglycan and GAG changes in diabetes are not restricted to extracellular matrix.

PATHOGENESIS OF EXTRACELLULAR MATRIX CHANGES

Nonenzymatic Glucosylation of Collagen

It now seems clear that the increased number of sugar residues associated with collagen from diabetic subjects results from nonenzymatic glucosylation. This reaction involves the addition of a glucose molecule to a protein via a ketoamine linkage with the N-terminal amino acid or an ε-amino group of lysine and hydroxylysine moieties. The ketoamine linkage is accomplished in 2 steps, the first being formation of a labile Schiff base intermediate. This Schiff base is slowly converted to the stable ketoamine form by an Amadori rearrangement (see reviews by Monnier, Cerami (1982); Perejda, Uitto (1982)). The extent of glucosylation is a function of glucose concentration and duration of exposure of protein to glucose. Since collagen turns over very slowly and contains relatively large numbers of lysine and hydroxylysine residues, it is highly susceptible to non-enzymatically mediated glucosylation.

In view of the fact that cross-link formation induced by the enzyme lysyl oxidase also involves lysine and hydroxylysine residues, one might anticipate that lysyl oxidase mediated collagen cross-links would be reduced in diabetes and the collagen might be more soluble than normal. The finding that this does not occur may be explained by the increase in lysyl oxidase activity in tissues observed by Madia et al (1979). A relatively small increase in the number of lysyl oxidase mediated cross-links may markedly reduce collagen solubility and increase its resistance to proteolytic digestion. In addition, glucosylated proteins appear to be more susceptible to oxidation and formation of disulfide cross-links (Stevens et al, 1978).

Increased Collagen Cross-links

That increased cross-linking of collagen associated with diabetes is mediated, in large part, by the enzyme lysyl oxidase would appear to be reasonably well established by the studies of Chang et al (1980) and of Madia et al (1979) as described above. Further studies are needed to determine whether the increase in lysyl oxidase mediated cross-links is due to decreased insulin levels or to hyperglycemia. The possibility that insulin levels *per se* may modulate lysyl oxidase activity is suggested by the fact that the enzyme is susceptible to modulation by other hormones and endocrine perturbations. Glucocorticoids inhibit lysyl oxidase activity (Benson, LuValle 1981) as does hypophysectomy (Shoshan, Finkelstein 1976) while estrogens increase its activity (Sanada et al 1978; Ozasa et al 1981); fasting has no effect (Madia et al 1979).

Increased Accumulation of Collagen

The tissues in which increased accumulation of collagen has been demonstrated in diabetes are the vasculature, including major arteries as well as glomerular capillaries and small vessels throughout the body, the intestinal tract, heart, lung, bone, vertebral disc, and the skin in subjects with scleredema. Although the mechanism(s) responsible for these increases has not been clearly elucidated, the evidence available suggests a multifactorial pathogenesis with increased synthesis and/or decreased degradation induced by different mechanisms in different tissues. For example, the increase in total collagen content of the intestinal tract (Schneir et al 1979) is proportional to the increase in total weight of that organ which is probably a hypertrophic response to the increased work load imposed by hyperphagia.

Renal hypertrophy is also a well documented phenomenon developing early after the onset of diabetes both in man and in experimental animals. Hemodynamic changes in the kidney with increased blood flow and increased glomerular filtration are evident immediately after the onset of diabetes. The mechanical effects of increased blood flow and filtration and the increased work load imposed on the kidney may constitute the stimulus for generalized renal hypertrophy including the increase in glomerular collagen content.

The increased collagen content of the coronary arteries and aorta associated with more rapidly progressive and ultimately advanced atherosclerosis in the diabetic is consistent with increased scar tissue formation in response to vascular injury, the precise nature of which is not known. Potential candidate mechanisms that may contribute to vascular injury and/or stimulate smooth muscle proliferative responses ultimately responsible for collagen production are increased platelet aggregability (with release of platelet growth factors) and increased utilization of glucose by alternate pathways, e.g., the polyol pathway (see review by Williamson et al 1983).

The mechanism(s) responsible for the regional hypertrophy of the skin observed in scleredema with proportional increases in collagen and glycosaminoglycans (Fleischmajer et al 1970), is not known.

The increased collagen content observed in the heart, lung, bone, and vertebral disc may reflect a proliferative response of connective tissue cells to injury-stimulus mediated by the diabetic milieu and/or impaired degradation related to increased glucosylation and cross-linking of diabetic collagen. Clearly, impaired degradation could contribute to collagen accumulation in all tissues of the diabetic.

Glycosaminoglycan Changes

The numerous studies documenting markedly decreased incorporation of $^{35}SO_4$ into GAGs of virtually every tissue examined in animals with experimental diabetes strongly suggests that GAG synthesis and/or sulfation are impaired in the severely insulin deficient diabetic. Since somatomedin plays such an important regulatory role in GAG metabolism and since serum somatomedin activity is reduced in insulin deficient animals and in human diabetics, it seems likely that reduced GAG synthesis in diabetic animals is mediated by decreased somatomedin levels (Phillips, Young 1976). The elevated levels of dermatan sulfate in coronary arteries of insulin treated diabetic dogs with intermittent hyperinsulinemia reported by Sirek et al (1981) are consistent with this hypothesis and suggest the potential importance of achieving normal insulin levels as well as normal glucose levels in the treatment of the diabetic.

Pathophysiological Consequences of Extracellular Matrix Changes

Changes in type I and type IV collagen. Increased cross-linking and increased glucosylation of collagen make it more resistant to degradation by proteolytic enzymes (Bailey et al 1974; Uitto 1971; Lubec, Pollack 1980). These changes would of course favor the accumulation of collagen and progression of macro- and microangiopathy. Increased cross-linking would also be expected to increase the stiffness of collagen. Both the increased amount of collagen and the increased number of cross-links could contribute to decreased myocardial compliance, increased pulse wave velocity, and systolic hypertension observed in diabetics. These collagen changes could also contribute to skin and joint stiffness and contractures which are being recognized with increased frequency in the diabetic and which may be associated with diabetic microangiopathy (Rosenbloom et al 1981). The increased thickening of capillary basement membranes, reflecting accumulation of type IV collagen, might be expected to interfere with emigration of leukocytes into sites of inflammation and injury favoring increased susceptibility to infections.

Glycosaminoglycan Changes

Changes in GAG content and extent of sulfation may have surprisingly diverse consequences in different tissues. GAGs are strongly negatively charged, highly hydrated molecules. Since the density of negative charges in glomerular capillaries appears to be an important determinant of permeation of glomerular capillaries by albumin, there is considerable interest in the possibility that a decrease in glomerular GAG content and/or extent of sulfation might contribute to increased vascular permeability and albuminuria.

In view of the elastic properties and lubricating qualities of GAGs (Bollet 1967), GAG changes in cartilage of diabetics might be expected to accelerate degenerative changes leading to osteoarthritis, the frequency of which is reported to be increased in diabetics (Waine et al 1961).

In light of their physical properties and the demonstration that GAGs associated with type I collagen bind at or near intraperiod D bands (Laros, Cooper 1972), a reduction in the amount and/or charge of GAGs could reduce the spacing and alter the nature of the physical interaction between collagen fibers resulting in stiffening of skin and joints. In view of the very slow turnover of collagen, a recent report (Lieberman et al 1980) that improved glucose control achieved with insulin pumps resulted in a rapid improvement in joint mobility raises the possibility that GAG changes may play an important role in the pathogenesis of skin and joint contractures associated with diabetes. It is of interest in this regard, that in dogs, marked reductions in hyaluronic acid and in chondroitin sulfate, but not in dermatan sulfate, occur in joints which develop contractures after being immobilized for 9 weeks (Akeson et al 1967).

The affinity of GAGs in the aorta for lipoproteins is well known (Vijayagopal et al 1981); however, the physiological significance of the interaction is not understood. If the association is important, then changes in GAGs observed in aortas and coronary arteries of diabetics might be predicted to contribute to accelerated progression of atherosclerotic vascular disease.

CONCLUSIONS

Extracellular matrix changes in diabetes described to date affect collagens and glycosaminoglycans in a wide variety of tissues and appear to be intimately involved in the pathogenesis of late complications of diabetes. These extracellular matrix changes appear to be produced by direct or indirect consequences of insulin deficiency, hyperinsulinemia, and hyperglycemia. They should, therefore, be preventable by therapeutic regimens which normalize plasma glucose and insulin levels.

ACKNOWLEDGEMENTS

This work was supported by USPHS Grant HL13694 and by the Kilo Diabetes and Vascular Research Foundation.

REFERENCES

Akeson WH, Amiel D, LaViolette D (1967). The connective-tissue response to immobility: A study of the chondroitin-4 and 6-sulfate and dermatan sulfate changes in periarticular connective tissue of control and immobilized knees of dogs. Clin Orthop 51:183.

Aufdermaur M, Fehr K, Lesker P, Silberberg R (1980). Quantitative histochemical changes in intervertebral discs in diabetes. Exp Cell Biol 48:89.

Axelsson I, Lorentzon R, Pita JC (1983). Biosynthesis of rat growth plate proteoglycans in diabetes and malnutrition. Calcif Tissue Int 35:237.

Bailey AJ (1981). The nonenzymatic glycosylation of proteins. In Standl E, Mehnert H (eds): "Pathogenetic Concepts of Diabetic Microangiopathy," Hormone and Metabolic Research Supplement Series Vol II, New York: Georg Thieme Verlag, Thieme-Stratton Inc., p 90.

Bailey AJ, Robins SP, Balian G (1974). Biological significance of the intermolecular crosslinks of collagen. Nature 251:105.

Beisswenger PJ, Spiro RG (1970). Human glomerular basement membrane: Chemical alteration in diabetes mellitus. Science 168:596.

Benson SC, LuValle PA (1981). Inhibition of lysyl oxidase and prolyl hydroxylase activity in glucocorticoid treated rats. Biochem Biophys Res Comm 99:557.

Berenson GS, Radhakrishnamurthy B, Dalferes ER, Ruiz H, Srinivasan SR, Plavidal F, Brickman F (1972). Connective tissue macromolecular changes in rats with experimentally induced diabetes and hyperinsulinism. Diabetes 21:733.

Berenson GS, Ruiz H, Dalferes ER, Dugan FA, Radhakrishnamurthy B (1970). Acid mucopolysaccharide changes in diabetic kidneys. Diabetes 19:161.

Bollet AJ (1967). Connective tissue polysaccharide metabolism and the pathogenesis of osteoarthritis. Adv Intern Med 13:33.

Brosnan ME, Sirek OV, Sirek A, Przbylska K (1973). Effect of pancreatectomy, with and without hypophysectomy, and of insulin treatment on the composition of canine aorta. Diabetes 22:397.

Brown DM, Klein DJ, Michael AF, Oegema TR (1982). ^{35}S-Glycosaminoglycan and ^{35}S-glycopeptide metabolism by diabetic glomeruli and aorta. Diabetes 31:418.

Brownlee M, Spiro RG (1979). Glomerular basement membrane metabolism in the diabetic rat. In vivo studies. Diabetes 28:121.

Buckingham BA, Uitto J, Sandborg C, Keens T, Kaufman F, Landing B (1981). Scleroderma-like syndrome and nonenzymatic glucosylation of collagen in children with poorly controlled insulin dependent diabetes (IDDM). Pediatr Res 15:626.

Chang K, Uitto J, Rowold EA, Grant GA, Kilo C, Williamson JR (1980). Increased collagen cross-linkages in experimental diabetes. Reversal by ß-aminopropionitrile and D-penicillamine. Diabetes 29:778.

Cohen MP, Foglia VG (1970). Aortic mucopolysaccharides in experimental diabetes. Diabetes 19:639.

Cohen MP, Surma ML (1981). [^{35}S]Sulfate incorporation into glomerular basement membrane glycosaminoglycans is decreased on experimental diabetes. J Lab Clin Med 98:715.
Cohen MP, Surma ML, Wu V-Y (1982). In vivo biosynthesis and turnover of glomerular basement membrane in diabetic rats. Am J Physiol 242:F385.
Cohen MP, Urdanivia E, Surma M, Wu V-Y (1980). Increased glycosylation of glomerular basement membrane collagen in diabetes. Biochem Biophys Res Comm 95:765.
Fleischmajer R, Faludi G, Krol S (1970). Scleredema and diabetes mellitus. Arch Derm 101:21.
Francis MJO, Ellis JP, Hockaday TDR (1974). Skin collagen in diabetes mellitus in relation to treatment. Proc R Soc Med 67:35.
Golub LM, Greenwald RA, Zebrowski EJ, Ramamurthy NS (1978). The effect of experimental diabetes on the molecular characteristics of soluble rat-tail tendon collagen. Biochim Biophys Acta 534:73.
Haider B, Yeh C-K, Thomas G, Oldewurtel HA, Lyons MM, Regan TJ (1978). Altered myocardial function and collagen in diabetic Rhesus monkeys on atherogenic diet. Trans Assoc Am Physicians 91:197.
Hamlin CR, Kohn RR, Luschin JH (1975). Apparent accelerated aging of human collagen in diabetes mellitus. Diabetes 24:902.
Kefalides NA (1974). Biochemical properties of human glomerular basement membrane in normal and diabetic kidneys. J Clin Invest 53:403.
Kjellen L, Bielefeld D, Hook M (1983). Reduced sulfation of liver heparan sulfate in experimentally diabetic rats. Diabetes 32:337.
Klein L, Butcher DL, Sudilovsky O, Kikkawa R, Miller M (1975). Quantification of collagen in renal glomeruli isolated from human nondiabetic and diabetic kidneys. Diabetes 24:1057.
Laros GS, Cooper RR (1972). Electron microscopic visualization of proteinpolysaccharides. Clin Orthop 84:179.
LePape A, Guitton J-D, Muh J-P (1981a). Modifications of glomerular basement membrane cross-links in experimental diabetic rats. Biochem Biophys Res Comm 100:1214.
LePape A, Muh J-P, Bailey AJ (1981b). Characterization of N-glycosylated type I collagen in streptozotocin-induced diabetes. Biochem J 197:405.
Lieberman LS, Rosenbloom AL, Riley WJ, Silverstein JH (1980). Reduced skin thickness with pump administration of insulin. N Engl J Med 303:940.
Lubec G, Pollack A (1980). Reduced susceptibility of non-

enzymatically glycosylated glomerular basement membrane to proteases. Is thickening of diabetic glomerular basement membranes due to reduced proteolytic degradation? In Lubec G (ed): "The Glomerular Basement Membrane. Renal Physiology," Basel: S. Karger, p 4.

Madia AM, Rozovski SJ, Kagan HM (1979). Changes in lung lysyl oxidase activity in streptozotocin-diabetes and in starvation. Biochim Biophys Acta 585:481.

McCullagh KG, Balian G (1975). Collagen characterisation and cell transformation in human atherosclerosis. Nature 258:73.

McCullagh KG, Duance VC, Bishop KA (1980). The distribution of collagen types I, III and V (AB) in normal and atherosclerotic human aorta. J Pathol 130:45.

Modrak J (1980). Collagen metabolism in the myocardium from streptozotocin-diabetic rats. Diabetes 29:547.

Monnier VM, Cerami A (1982). Non-enzymatic glycosylation and browning of proteins in diabetes. Clin Endocrinol Metab 11:431.

Ozasa H, Tominaga T, Nishimura T, Takeda T (1981). Lysyl oxidase activity in the mouse uterine cervix is physiologically regulated by estrogen. Endocrinology 109:618.

Parthasarathy N, Spiro RG (1982). Effect of diabetes on the glycosaminoglycan component of the human glomerular basement membrane. Diabetes 31:738.

Perejda AJ, Uitto J (1982). Nonenzymatic glycosylation of collagen and other proteins: Relationship to development of diabetic complications. Coll Relat Res 2:81.

Phillips LS, Young HS (1976). Nutrition and somatomedin. II. Serum somatomedin activity and cartilage growth activity in streptozotocin-diabetic rats. Diabetes 25:516.

Regan TJ, Wu CF, Yeh CK, Oldewurtel HA, Haider B (1981). Myocardial composition and function in diabetes. The effects of chronic insulin use. Circ Res 49:1268.

Rohrbach DH, Hassell JR, Kleinman H, Martin GR (1982a). Alterations in the basement membrane (heparan sulfate) proteoglycan in diabetic mice. Diabetes 31:185.

Rohrbach DH, Wagner CW, Star V, Martin GR (1982b). Decreased synthesis of basement membrane (heparan sulfate) proteoglycan in diabetic mice. Diabetes 31 (Suppl 2):28a.

Rosenberg H, Modrak JB, Hassing JM, Al-Turk WA, Stohs SJ (1979). Glycosylated collagen. Biochem Biophys Res Comm 91:498.

Rosenbloom AL, Silverstein JH, Lerotte DC, Richardson K, McCallum M (1981). Limited joint mobility in childhood diabetes mellitus indicates increased risk for microvascular disease. N Engl J Med 305:191.

Sanada H, Shikata J, Hamamoto H, Ueba Y, Yamamuro T, Takeda T (1978). Changes in collagen cross-linking and lysyl oxidase by estrogen. Biochim Biophys Acta 541:408.

Schiller S, Dorfman A (1957). Metabolism of mucopolysaccharides in animals: Influence of insulin. J Biol Chem 227:625.

Schiller S, Dorfman A (1963). The distribution of acid mucopolysaccharides in the skin of diabetic rats. Biochim Biophys Acta 78:371.

Schneir M, Bowersox J, Ramamurthy N, Yavelow J, Murray J, Edlin-Folz E, Golub L (1979). Response of rat connective tissues to streptozotocin-diabetes. Tissue specific effects on collagen metabolism. Biochim Biophys Acta 583:95.

Schneir M, Ramamurthy N, Golub L (1982). Skin collagen metabolism in the streptozotocin-induced diabetic rat: Enhanced catabolism of collagen formed both before and during the diabetic state. Diabetes 31:426.

Schnider SL, Kohn RR (1980). Glucosylation of human collagen in aging and diabetes mellitus. J Clin Invest 66:1179.

Schnider SL, Kohn RR (1981). Effects of age and diabetes mellitus on the solubility and nonenzymatic glucosylation of human skin collagen. J Clin Invest 67:1630.

Shoshan S, Finkelstein S (1976). Lysyl oxidase: A pituitary hormone-dependent enzyme. Biochim Biophys Acta 438:358.

Silberberg R, Scharp DW, Lesker PA (1981). Biochemical studies of bone from diabetic rats and rats bearing transplanted pancreatic islets. Exp Cell Biol 49:61.

Sirek OV, Sirek A, Cukerman E (1981). Intermittent hyperinsulinaemia and arterial glycosaminoglycans in dogs. Diabetologia 21:154.

Stevens VJ, Rouzer CA, Monnier VM, Cerami A (1978). Potential role of glycosylation of lens crystallins. Proc Natl Acad Sci USA 75:2918.

Uitto J (1971). Collagen biosynthesis in human skin. Ann Clin Res 3:250.

Uitto J, Perejda AJ, Grant GA, Rowold EA, Kilo C, Williamson JR (1982). Glycosylation of human glomerular basement membrane collagen: Increased content of hexose in ketoamine linkage and unaltered hydroxylysine-O-glycosides in patients with diabetes. Connect Tissue Res 10:45.

Vater CA, Harris ED, Siegel RC (1979). Native crosslinks in collagen fibrils induce resistance to human synovial collagenase. Biochem J 181:639.

Vijayagopal P, Srinivasan SR, Radhakrishnamurthy B, Berenson GS (1981). Interaction of serum lipoproteins and a proteo-

glycan from bovine aorta. J Biol Chem 256:8234.
Waine H, Nevinny D, Rosenthal J, Joffe IB (1961). Association of osteoarthritis and diabetes mellitus. Tufts Folia Med 7:13.
Weiss RE, Gorn AH, Nimni ME (1981). Abnormalities in the biosynthesis of cartilage and bone proteoglycans in experimental diabetes. Diabetes 30:670.
Weiss RE, Reddi AH (1980). Influence of experimental diabetes and insulin on matrix-induced cartilage and bone differentiation. Am J Physiol 238:E200.
Westberg NG, Michael AF (1973). Human glomerular basement membrane: Chemical composition in diabetes mellitus. Acta Med Scand 194:39.
Williamson JR, Kilo C (1980). Vascular complications in diabetes mellitus. N Engl J Med 302:399.
Williamson JR, Kilo C (1981). The present status of basement membrane thickening in diabetes. In Effros R, Schmid-Schonbein H, Ditzel J (eds): "Microcirculation," New York: Academic Press, p 191.
Williamson JR, Kilo C, Crespin SR (1983). Vascular disease. In Levin ME, O'Neal LW (eds): "The Diabetic Foot," 3rd edition, St. Louis: C. V. Mosby, p 85.

DISCUSSION

DR. KOSIK: I wonder if you have any evidence that the quantity of collagen might regulate the lysyl oxidase levels, and what is known about the regulation of lysyl oxidase?

DR. WILLIAMSON: I am not aware of any evidence that collagen itself regulates lysyl oxidase activity. The only factors I am aware of which influence lysyl oxidase synthesis are the hormones already mentioned and copper. Lysyl oxidase activity of tissues from copper-deficient chicks is very low.

DR. KOSIK: Is it a calcium-activated enzyme?

DR. WILLIAMSON: Not to my knowledge.

DR. REGELSON: Everitt, Denckla, Harrison and others have shown that hypophysectomy has an age-rejuvenating or age-delaying effect, and there is some evidence that collagen returns to the more youthful state. Johnson and Cutler have shown changes in the glomerulus with aging that can be reversed by hypophysectomy. We know that hypophysectomy has been used to treat diabetic retinopathy, and obviously growth hormone has been invoked in relation to much of the pathology of diabetes. You mention this in regard to lysyl oxidase. What is your feeling concerning growth hormone as a factor in the pathology, either directly or through some effect on somatomedin?

DR. WILLIAMSON: I know there has been a lot of interest in the potential importance of growth hormone as a major factor in vascular complications in diabetes. My own personal feeling is that its role and importance in vascular complications of diabetes are unclear. Since both insulin and growth hormone modulate somatomedin levels, the balance between the two hormones, as well as other factors that modulate somatomedin activity, is probably important.

DR. POTTENGER: Would you like to comment as to how sorbitol may affect extracellular matrix?

DR. WILLIAMSON: There is evidence to suggest that accumulation of sorbitol and/or associated phenomena may play an important role in the pathogenesis of cataract formation and in neuropathy in diabetes. Since the enzymes responsible for sorbitol accumulation are present in virtually all tissues, it would be a candidate mechanism for injury to all cells which do not require insulin for glucose uptake and are therefore exposed to ambient glucose levels. Indeed those are the very cell types and tissues affected by the complications of diabetes. It is conceivable that cells injured by sorbitol pathway mechanisms might be stimulated to synthesize more collagen, or their capacity to produce proteases responsible for degradation might be impaired.

DR. BERENSON: I mentioned in our discussions that we actually found an increase of heparan sulfate in diabetic kidneys, and you are showing a decrease based on Spiro's studies. I think I can see how to explain the differences. He is relating the decrease of heparan sulfate to the concentration of basement membrane, but you might note that there is a great proliferation in the basement membrane material in the diabetic kidneys, as you illustrated. Consequently, if you express the result to the total weight of the kidney, you will find that there is an increase of the total polysaccharide present.

Also, I would mention that we find an increase of the

heparan sulfate glycosaminoglycan in Kimmensteil-Wilson lesions, but increases of hyaluronic acid and chondroitin sulfates occur in diffuse glomerulosclerosis in human diabetic kidneys.

You stated that the defect might be one of degradation. I would suggest that the problem in human diabetes may be different from what we see in an experimental model like streptozotocin, which would be a true insulin deficient disease. In studying the tissues from human diabetics we are giving exogenous insulin. In a sense, insulin is present and stimulates production of connective tissues. The two pictures may be different.

DR. WILLIAMSON: I think those are very interesting and important points. I would point out, however, that many of the diabetic animals are not absolutely insulin deficient. It is of particular interest that insulin-treated animals, as well as humans, can have transient periods of hyperinsulinemia, even though they are poorly controlled, which may lead to extracellular matrix changes different from those observed in the absence of insulin treatment.

DR. LORIA: I want to compliment Dr. Williamson for an interesting presentation of this special topic. The point made by Dr. Berenson, concerning the conclusions drawn from the data of Rohrbach et al, who used diabetic mutant animals, should be further emphasized. It is important to know at which stage of clinical diabetes the particular diabetic mutant animals were. The clinical conditions in these mutants will vary from an obesity-maturity type, in the initial stages, to a clinical diabetes which resembles more the juvenile (type I) diabetes. The host responses will differ considerably at the various stages. In our laboratory, we have seen that heterozygote diabetic mutants C57BL/KsJdb+/+m without diabetes mellitus, when challenged with virus could not make an adequate antibody response. In contrast, homozygous diabetic mutants C57BL/KsJdb+/db+ with overt disease, did produce antibodies when challenged with the same virus. Caution should be exercised before final conclusions are made using diabetic mutant animals. The particular diabetic genotype, and the form of its phenotypic expression as diabetes mellitus, should be included in the final conclusions.

DR. WILLIAMSON: I would agree with you completely and

would point out that perhaps the biphasic nature of the changes in glycosaminoglycans reported by Cohen and Foglia reflect a progressive increase in the severity of diabetes in the pancreatectomized rat. Likewise, it is of interest that in the experiments of Rohrbach et al, heparan sulfate production was impaired in the relatively hyperinsulinemic mutant mice as well as in the insulinipenic mice with diabetes produced by streptozotocin. On the other hand, laminin production was increased in the mutant but not in the streptozotocin diabetic mice.

Comparative Pathobiology of Major Age-Related Diseases: Current Status and Research Frontiers, pages 289–305

MICROANGIOPATHY AND ATHEROSCLEROSIS IN DIABETIC CELEBES BLACK MACAQUES (*Macaca nigra*)

Charles Howard, Jr., Ph.D.

Oregon Regional Primate Research Center,
505 N. W. 185th Avenue, Beaverton, OR 97006

INTRODUCTION

The severity of vascular disease increases with age and is exacerbated by diabetes mellitus (Ledet 1976; Pirat 1978; Keen, Jarrett 1979; Kannel, McGee 1979; Ganda 1980). Enhanced vascular sclerosis occurs at numerous anatomical sites. Diabetic human beings have a well-documented microangiopathic triad of basal lamina thickening, retinopathies, and glomerulosclerosis; although these are not found exclusively in diabetics, they are characteristic manifestations of the disease. Macrovascular disease has been most commonly studied in the cerebral, peripheral, and coronary arteries because of their involvement in morbidity and mortality.

There are a number of proposals and some evidence that diabetes *per se* is responsible for some of the macrovascular disease, exclusive of any other contributing factor (Lundbaek 1954; Jarrett, Keen 1975; Danowski et al 1980; Lundbaek 1974). Such a contention cannot be proved or disproved in humans or in animal models in which atherosclerosis is induced by diet. *Macaca nigra* provides one model for studying effects of diabetic aggravation on vascular disease.

Some aspects of carbohydrate impairment develop in most of the mature individuals of the monkey species *Macaca nigra* (Howard 1972). Although only 10 to 15% of the monkeys progress to overt diabetes, if the monkeys live long enough, hormonal and metabolic abnormalities indicative of metabolic deterioration develop in over 70%. The recognizable hormonal changes are increased levels of glucagon and an impaired insulin response to glucose in a tolerance test (Howard, Van Bueren 1981; Howard 1982). Glycemic changes are less noticeable in the early stages, but monkeys eventually have increased postprandial fasting glucose and impaired glucose clearance. The development of diabetes results from a lesion in the islets of Langerhans, in which there is gradual deterioration of all secretory cells and deposition of amyloid (Howard 1978). With increasing islet cell loss, the monkeys become hypoinsulinemic and hyperglycemic, and glucose is minimal. Monkeys are then overtly diabetic by all accepted clinical standards.

Several of the secondary manifestations of diabetes are evident. Cataracts develop in hyperglycemic monkeys; these are removed by discission and aspiration. Both micro- and macrovascular pathologic changes have been documented. The basal lamina surrounding the muscle capillaries becomes significantly thickened with increasing severity of diabetes (Howard 1975). Involvement of the aortic surface in sudanophilia and raised lesions increase with severity of diabetes (Howard 1979); histological changes parallel gross aortic changes.

The purpose of this report is to comment on data obtained from examinations of capillaries and aortas in *Macaca nigra*, and to relate these to the metabolic conditions and ages of the monkeys.

METHODS

Metabolites and Hormones

Food was withheld from sexually mature monkeys of both sexes overnight. For the intravenous glucose tolerance test (iv-GTT), each monkey received a glucose infusion of 0.5 g/kg of body weight. Blood samples were drawn at 15, 30, and 60 minutes. Serum glucose was assayed with a Beckman glucose oxidase analyzer, insulin with an Amersham/Searle kit, and plasma glucagon with 30K antibody. Glucose clearance (K) was calculated from the glucose concentrations at 15, 30, and 60 minutes. The insulin reponse to glucose (ΔIRI) was calculated as the insulin level in the 15-minute sample minus that in the 0-minute sample.

Capillary Assessment

The retinal vasculature was mounted after trypsin digestion and was stained with periodic acid-Schiff. Muscle biopsy samples were removed from a standard site in the left femoral quadriceps, fixed immediately in osmium tetroxide, embedded in Araldite, and sectioned. The basal lamina thickness was measured by the overlay technique; both the average (Siperstein et al 1966) and the minimal (Williamson et al 1969) measurements were recorded.

Macrovascular Assessment

Aortas removed at autopsy were fixed in 10% neutral buffered formalin and stained with Sudan IV. Each was mounted in a flat plastic specimen envelope, and an overlay point count technique was used to assess the surface involvement. The percentage of aortic atherosclerosis was the sum of sudanophilia plus areas of raised plaques (Howard 1979). For histological evaluation, sections removed at standardized sites were stained with Gomori trichrome aldehyde fuchsin for connective tissue elements and with oil red O for visualization of lipid (Howard et al 1980).

RESULTS

Metabolic and Hormonal Measurements

The criteria for judgment of metabolic status of the monkeys are presented in Table 1. Glucose clearance was $>$ 2%/minute in nondiabetic (ND) monkeys and $<$ 1%/minute in diabetic (D) monkeys; an intermediate group, designated as borderline diabetic (BD), had K values intermediate between those of ND and D monkeys. Fasting concentrations of insulin diminished with increasing severity of diabetes. The response of insulin to a glucose bolus is a sensitive indicator of metabolic abnormalities; ND monkeys had ΔIRI values of 150 μU/ml, BD monkeys had 25 to 100 μU/ml, and D monkeys had minimal insulin responses. Fasting concentrations of glucagon also indicated early changes; the increases in glucagon from $<$ 1,000 pg/ml in ND monkeys to $>$ 2,000 pg/ml in the BD group, and diminution to levels in the D group below that in the ND monkeys, were characteristic.

Table 1

Metabolic and hormonal characteristics of *Macaca nigra*[a]

	iv-GTT		Fasting		
	K %/min	ΔIRI (μU/ml)	Glucose (mg/dl)	IRI (μU/ml)	HbA_{Ic} (%)
Nondiabetic	3.2±0.2	153±22	66±4	38±7	2.6±0.2
Borderline diabetic	1.6±0.2	25±5	87±8	26±3	3.5±0.2
Diabetic	0.5±0.3	4±1	363±68	14±2	7.9±0.3

[a]see text for abbreviations; values are mean ± S.E.M.; each category contained at least 12 monkeys.

Changes probably indicated loss of controls on alpha-cell secretion eventually followed by a reduction in the number of alpha cells. Fasting glucose increased with hormonal deterioration but became significantly greater only when monkeys were overtly diabetic. The levels of glycosylated hemoglobin (HbA_{Ic} are much greater in D than in ND monkeys; the slight increase in BD monkeys is significant and reflects increased fasting and postprandial glucose levels.

Microangiopathies

Although a number of retinal vasculature mounts from monkeys of varying metabolic status have been examined, the characteristic retinopathy has not yet been found. The extent of the changes in metabolically impaired monkeys was primarily loss of nuclei and development of atrophic capillaries. Ophthalmic examination and fluorescein angiography revealed occasional possible retinopathies, but abnormalities could not be related to metabolic status.

The average and minimal thicknesses of the basal lamina muscle capillaries in ND, BD, and D monkeys are presented in

Table 2 (Howard 1975).

Table 2

Comparisons of average and minimum basal lamina thicknesses *Macaca nigra*[a]

Metabolic Status	n	ABLT (Å)	MBLT (Å)
Nondiabetic	8	696 ± 16[b]	524 ± 12[b]
Borderline diabetic	4	786 ± 45	599 ± 44
Diabetic	5	837 ± 26[b]	634 ± 32[b]

[a]Abbreviations: ABLT, average basal lamina thickness; MBLT, minimum basal lamina thickness.

[b]$p \lesssim 0.01$ for nondiabetic vs. diabetic groups.

Although values for BD monkeys were intermediate between those of the ND and D monkeys, only the ND and D monkeys were significantly different. The average basal lamina thickness correlated with several metabolic parameters, including K, fasting glucose, and fasting insulin i.e., basal lamina thickness increased with deterioration in metabolic and hormonal states.

Macrovascular Disease

The percentage of surface involvement of the aorta correlated with the severity of diabetes (Howard 1979). An aorta from an aged ND monkey is pictured in Figure 1A. There was occasional sudanophilia, some generalized sudanophilic blush, but no raised lesions; involvement of the aortic surface was < 1.0%. The aorta from an aged D monkey is shown

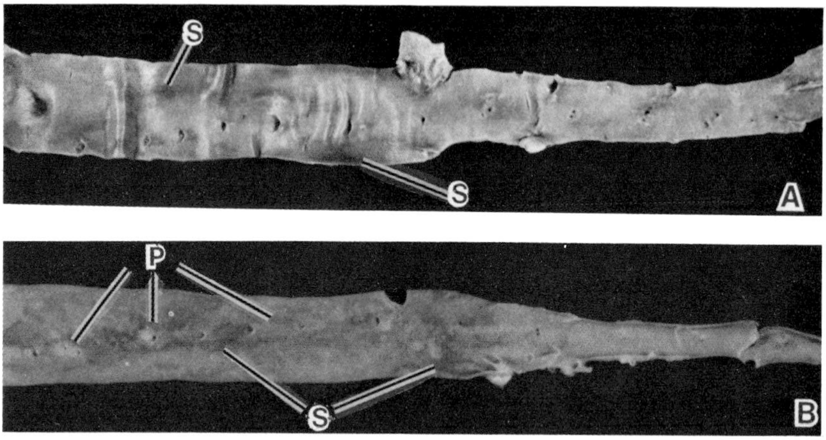

Fig. 1. Aortas from an aged nondiabetic (A) and diabetic (B) monkey. S indicates sudanophilia and P indicates raised plaques.

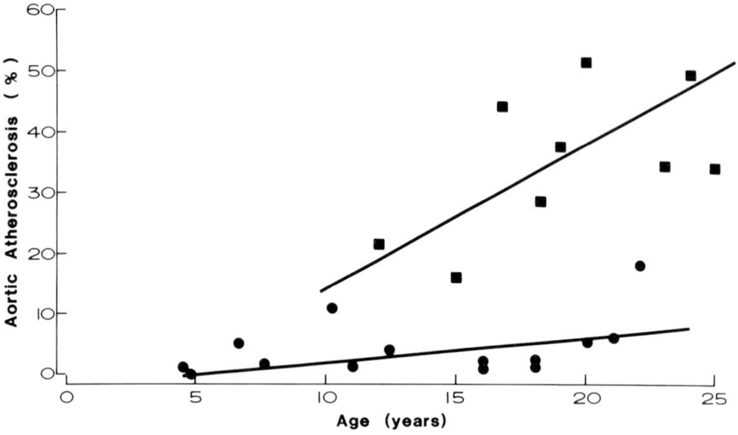

Fig. 2. Relationships of aortic atherosclerosis to age in nondiabetic monkeys (●) and to age plus the effects of diabetes in diabetic monkeys (■). Large variation precluded statistically significant differences.

in Figure 1B. There was extensive sudanophilia and a few areas of raised plaques; surface involvement was > 30%.

Figure 2 illustrates the general effects of aging and diabetes. Monkeys were grouped as severely metabolically impaired, including diabetic, or as nondiabetics; monkey age has been plotted against the percentage of atherosclerosis. The percentage of aortic surface involvement increased slightly with age; the increase with diabetes was dramatically greater, but began only after sexual maturity.

Aortas were examined histologically. Three parameters are compared in Table 3.

Table 3

Comparisons of histological features of *Macaca nigra* aortas[a]

Group	n	Intimal thickness (μm)	Lesion/media ratio	Intimal[b] +media lipid
ND	8	31 ± 6	6.6 ± 0.6	0.09 ± 0.03
BD	9	65 ± 15	12.2 ± 2.4	0.35 ± 0.05
D	7	122 ± 18	20.4 ± 2.6	1.13 ± 0.15

[a]Abbreviations: ND, nondiabetic; BD, borderline diabetic; and D, diabetic. Values are mean ± S.E.M.; all means differed at $p \lesssim 0.05$.

[b]Lipid was measured on a scale in which 1 = < 25% and 2 = 25 to 50% of the area as positive.

The intimal thickness, the ratio of the lesion thickness to that of the media, and the appearance of lipid increased significantly in BD monkeys and were even greater in D monkeys. The lipid deposition was primarily extracellular in the intima, and appeared oriented in association with connective tissue collagen and elastin (Howard et al 1980) (Figure 3A). Lipid-filled foam cells were not a common feature.

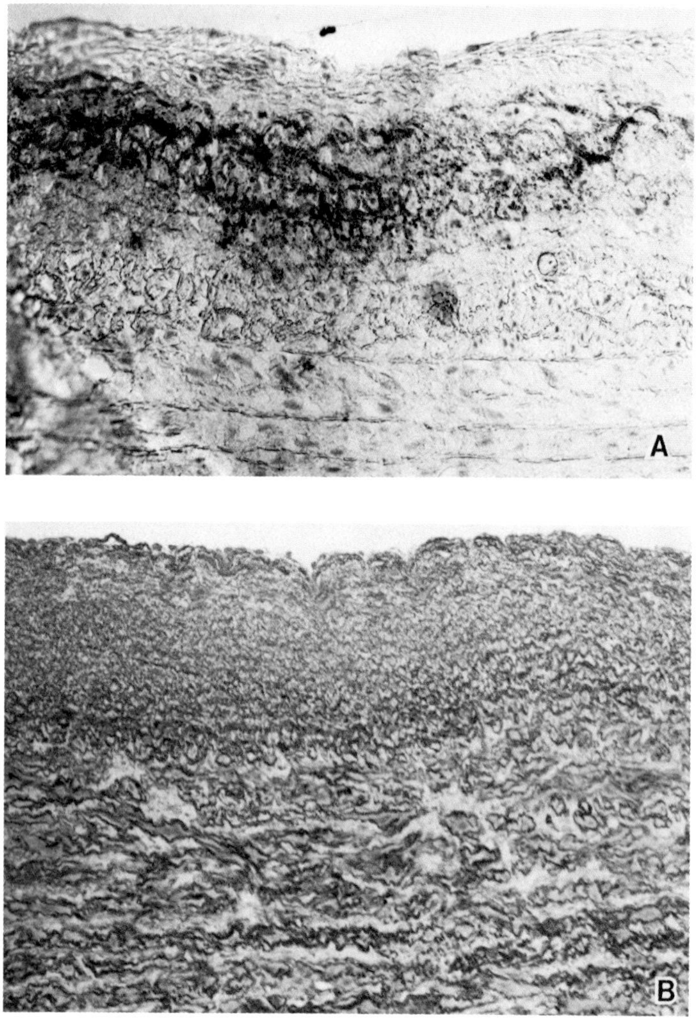

Fig. 3. Aortic sections stained with oil red O to visualize lipid (A) and with Verhoff-Van Giesen to visualize connective tissue (B). Both sections are from a monkey with recent onset of overt diabetes.

Moderate duplication of intimal cells and connective tissue is shown in Figure 3B; some disruption of the inner media is evident. More severe, raised lesions (not pictured) showed extensive duplication and medial disruption.

DISCUSSION

Macaca nigra exhibit vascular problems as they age, but the changes are severely worsened by diabetes. Since their diabetes arises spontaneously, results of the metabolic and hormonal changes can be used to understand similar phenomena in humans. Dietary aggravation and many of the other compounding factors contributing to vascular disease in humans, such as stress, smoking, or hypertension, are missing in this model. Results can be related to aging phenomena and to aging plus the effects of diabetes.

There is only mild to moderate development of microangiopathies. Comprehensive data have been collected only on muscle basal lamina thickness in these monkeys (Howard 1975). Although the thickness increase relative to the severity of diabetes is statistically significant, it is still less than in nondiabetic and diabetic humans. Changes in monkeys may resemble changes in humans only qualitatively. Retinopathies have not been a major feature of these diabetic monkeys; there have been no nonhuman primate models in which retinopathies have been a prominent development associated with diabetes (Howard 1975). Glomerulosclerosis does appear in most diabetic animal models (Brown et al 1982); in the nonhuman primates it requires many years for development. Nonhuman primates do have value as models, but development of microangiopathic lesions is so slow that maintenance of monkeys in a diabetic condition for a long time to allow progression of the various lesions may not be practical. However, the lesions do seem to closely resemble those in human beings (Engerman et al 1982).

Aortic atherosclerosis has been readily produced in nonhuman primates by dietary aggravation (Robison et al 1971; Wissler, Vesselinovitch 1977; Wagner et al 1980; Kritchevsky et al 1977). The characteristic lesions resemble those seen in human aortas.

The development of atherosclerosis in *Macaca nigra* (Howard 1979) can be directly related to the diabetes rather than to the diet since monkeys are fed moderate amounts of a nonatherogenic ration. There is greater thoracic athero-sclerosis than in the abdominal segments, an observation consistent with data on other animal models, yet unlike the data on human atherosclerosis. Extensive macrovascular sclerosis develops slowly and is usually found only in those monkeys that have been severely diabetic for several years. Quantitatively, lesions in monkeys do not get as severe as those in humans. However, monkeys will develop markedly raised plaques with extensive lipid infiltration, fibrous caps, and occasional foci of necrosis. Some sudanophilia and occasional plaques do appear in monkeys with little or no indications of hormonal or glycemic abnormalities. This phenomenon would indicate some contribution of the usual aging changes, i.e., moderate changes in hormones and metabolites would be sufficient to bring about at least minimal amounts of vascular sclerosis.

The histological features of atherosclerosis in these monkeys differ significantly from those seen in other animal models in which atherosclerosis has been induced by dietary aggravation. Dietarily aggravated models usually have in-creases in the lipid-filled foam cells, and the lesion often extends into the media. Macaca nigra aortas show enhanced lipid deposition, but it is confined almost exclusively to the intima. Furthermore, the majority of the lipid is extra-cellular and is associated with the connective tissue (Howard et al 1980; Kramsch et al 1971; Kramsch, Hollander 1973).

If results in Macaca nigra can be taken to reflect the direct effects of diabetes on vascular tissue, then lipid deposited extracellularly in the intima may be one of the diabetes characteristics. Although exact causes are not known, contributing factors in Macaca nigra would include: hypoinsulinemia and impaired insulin secretion in BD and D monkeys; both fasting and postprandial mild to severe hyper-glycemia; and moderately increased levels of the atherogenic very-low-, low-, and intermediate-density lipoproteins. Data obtained from human aortas may be difficult to interpret because there has often been overconsumption of food high in fat for a long period of time; other factors, such as obesity, hypertension, and smoking, can contribute to atherosclerosis. Macaca nigra may give insight into the characteristics of a diabetic micro- and macroangiopathy.

SUMMARY

Macaca nigra can be used to study numerous aspects of the vascular pathology analogous to that which occurs in diabetic human beings. Both micro- and macrovascular sclerosis develop slightly in nondiabetic monkeys with increasing age, and their development is exacerbated by diabetes in most monkeys. Progression of the lesions is slow; they are best studied only after a substantial duration of diabetes. The spontaneous development of diabetes and secondary manifestations in *Macaca nigra* is analogous to the spontaneous development of pathologic changes in aging and diabetic human beings.

ACKNOWLEDGEMENTS

It is a pleasure to acknowledge the technical support of Lynne Bonnet, Joann Wolff, and Tonya Van Bueren, and the cooperation of Dr. James L. Palotay, pathologist, Dr. John Hill, surgeon, and Dr. W. H. Fahrenbach, electron microscopist. This is publication no. 1263 from the Oregon Regional Primate Research Center, supported by General Research Support grant RR-05969 and Animal Resources Branch grant RR-00163, both from the Division of Research Resources, National Institutes of Health (NIH). Work in my laboratory has been supported by NIH grants HL-16661, RR-05969, and AM-21982, and by grants from The Eli Lilly Company, The Murdock Medical Trust, and The Kroc Foundation.

REFERENCES

Brown DM, Andres GA, Hostetter TH, Mauer SM, Price R, Venkatachalam MA (1982). Kidney complications. Diabetes 31(Suppl 1):71.

Danowski TS, Ohlsen P, Fisher ER (1980). Diabetic complications and their prevention or reversal. Diabetes Care 3:94.

Engerman R, Finkelstein D, Aguirre G, Diddie KR, Fox RR, Frank RN, Varma SD (1982). Ocular complications. Diabetes 31(Suppl 1):82.

Ganda OP (1980). Pathogenesis of macrovascular disease in the human diabetic. Diabetes 29:931.

Howard CF Jr (1972). Spontaneous diabetes in *Macaca nigra*. Diabetes 21:1077.

Howard CF Jr (1975). Basement membrane thickness in muscle capillaries of normal and spontaneously diabetic *Macaca nigra*. Diabetes 24:201.

Howard CF Jr (1978). Insular amyloidosis and diabetes mellitus in *Macaca nigra*. Diabetes 17:357.

Howard CF Jr (1979). Aortic atherosclerosis in normal and spontaneously diabetic *Macaca nigra*. Atherosclerosis 33:479.

Howard CF Jr (1982). Correlations of hemoglobin A_{Ic} and metabolic status in nondiabetic, borderline diabetic, and diabetic *Macaca nigra*. Diabetes 31:1105.

Howard CF Jr, Van Bueren A (1981). Immunoreactive glucagon in nondiabetic and diabetic *Macaca nigra*. Horm Metab Res 13:203.

Howard CF Jr, Vesselinovitch D, Wissler RW (1980). Aortic histology in nondiabetic and diabetic *Macaca nigra*. Abstr Circulation 62:III-227.

Jarrett RJ, Keen H (1975). Diabetes and atherosclerosis. In Keen H, Jarrett J (eds): "Complications of Diabetes," Chicago: Yearbook of Medical Publications, p 179.

Kannel WB, McGee DL (1979). Diabetes and cardiovascular risk factors: The Framingham study. Circulation 59:8.

Keen H, Jarrett RJ (1979). The WHO multinational study of vascular disease in diabetes: 2. Macrovascular disease prevalence. Diabetes Care 2:187.

Kramsch DM, Franzblau C, Hollander W (1971). The protein and lipid composition of arterial elastin and its relationship to lipid accumulation in the atherosclerotic plaque. J Clin Invest 50:1666.

Kramsch DM, Hollander W (1973). The interaction of serum and arterial lipoproteins with elastin of the arterial intima and its role in the lipid accumulation in atherosclerotic plaques. J Clin Invest 52:236.

Kritchevshy D, Davidson LM, Kim HK, Krendel DA, Malhotra S (1977). Influence of semipurified diets on atherosclerosis in African green monkeys. Exp Mol Pathol 26:28.

Ledet T (1976). Diabetic cardiopathy. Quantitative histological studies of the heart from young juvenile diabetics. Acta Pathol Microbiol Scand Sect A 84:421.

Lundbaek K (1954). Diabetic angiopathy. A specific vascular disease. Lancet I:377.

Lundbaek K (1974). The special role of diabetic angiopathy. Horm Metab Res (Suppl Series)4:158.

Pirat J (1978). Diabetes mellitus and its degenerative complications: A prospective study of 4400 patients observed between 1947 and 1973. Diabetes Care 1:168, 252.

Robison RL, Hayes KC, McCombs HL, Faherty TP (1971). Effect of dietary fat and cholesterol on circulating lipids and aortic ultrastructure of squirrel monkeys. Exp Mol Pathol 15:281.

Siperstein MD, Norton W, Unger RH, Madison LL (1966). Muscle capillary basement membrane width in normal, diabetic and prediabetic patients. Trans Assoc Am Physicians 79:330.

Wagner WD, St Clair RW, Clarkson TB, Connor JR (1980). A study of atherosclerosis regression in *Macaca mulatta*. Am J Pathol 100:633.

Williamson JR, Vogler NJ, Kilo C (1969). Estimation of vascular basement membrane thickness. Theoretical and practical considerations. Diabetes 18:567.

Wissler RW, Vesselinovitch D (1977). Atherosclerosis in nonhuman primates. Adv Vet Sci Comp Med 21:351.

DISCUSSION

DR. WILLIAMSON: I think this is a beautiful animal model of diabetes, Dr. Howard. Have you done any studies on vascular permeability changes in these animals, and do you have any evidence of proteinuria? Also, could you comment on the type of amyloid in the islets? Finally, do you have any information on whether it is AA-amyloid or IG-derived, or is it perhaps insulin products?

DR. HOWARD: To answer the first question, we have not done studies on vascular permeability. We seldom see protein in the urine unless the monkeys are severely diabetic and often moribund.

As to the type of amyloid, it stains as expected histochemically; it is Congo red positive with birefringence when viewed with polarized light, and it stains blue-green with sulfated alcian blue (SAB). When we isolate the amyloid, the fibrils look similar to those isolated from systemic (primary and secondary) amyloid. We have been trying to isolate islet amyloid for the last several years. One of the problems is solubility. When you homogenize a spleen or a liver or some other organ that contains systemic amyloid, that amyloid remains soluble and appears as a band midway up the tube after centrifugation. However, the islet amyloid pellets with the collagen at the bottom of the centrifuge tube. Our first problem in solubilizing and purifying the amyloid has been to get rid of the collagen. We have gone through a series of steps with acetic acid and with collagenase, and we are now getting a purer preparation of amyloid.

One of the interesting questions is, what is the source of islet amyloid? Some investigators have postulated that the protein source is insulin or proinsulin or a prohormone; this evidence is based mainly on immunocytochemical techniques in which islet amyloid also stained with insulin antibodies. We have not found positive immunocytochemical reactions with anti-insulin antibodies on the amyloid portions of amyloidotic islets or with isolated amyloid.

We have succeeded in isolating amyloid fibrils to a fair degree of purity, and have done some amino acid analyses. We were surprised to find that the closest homology is with type A amyloid. We cannot explain these results at this point because we are not sure why the islet amyloid is insoluble, yet the amino acid composition resembles some of the soluble amyloids. Is it aggregating; is it bound to something else; is it chemically different; and if so, what makes it different? Is the source perhaps an antigen-antibody complex; does the protein arise from the secretory cells; or is the protein totally from the circulation? At this point, we really don't know.

DR. WILLIAMSON: Have you done just a simple permanganate digestion of the tissue?

DR. HOWARD: Yes.

DR. WILLIAMSON: Does the amyloid lose its Congo red affinity?

DR. HOWARD: No.

DR. WILLIAMSON: It doesn't? And have you measured serum amyloid A protein levels?

DR. HOWARD: Yes, we have.

DR. WILLIAMSON: If those are not elevated, and if it is resistant to permanganate digestion, then it would seem unlikely that it would be amyloid A, derived from the serum amyloid A.

DR. HOWARD: We had Dr. Nels Eriksen from Dr. Benditt's

laboratory (University of Washington) measure blood samples from a few monkeys. Serum amyloid A was present and was associated with metabolic impairment.

DR. BERENSON: The amyloid purists say that amyloid is all protein. Whenever we have looked at amyloid tissue we find a high concentration of heparan sulfate. I would just like to suggest that this might be associated with basement membrane material and be generated by proliferation of capillaries. I think your story of antibodies to islet tissue is quite interesting. Maybe a glycoprotein that is present in the kidney is the antigen.

DR. HOWARD: Well, they may be purists as far as the protein is concerned, but historically the A-M-Y of the word amyloid comes from the fact that the material is positive to a carbohydrate stain. So, carbohydrate has always been associated with the protein. Whether carbohydrate is bound to a core of protein, as with the proteoglycans, or whether carbohydrate is merely associated with the protein is not known. We have monitored our isolation procedures with SAB and Congo red. We get a positive carbohydrate reaction (SAB) during the early purification steps but not when amyloid is further purified.

DR. BERENSON: Are these akin to type II diabetes?

DR. HOWARD: I think they are a subpopulation of maturity onset type II diabetes.

DR. BERENSON: But with low insulin?

DR. HOWARD: Yes, with low insulin. There have been some studies of islet cell antibodies (ICA) in human type II diabetics. Those individuals with ICA at diagnosis are more inclined to require insulin therapy sooner than those who are ICA-negative. This would indicate to me some deterioration of cells to cause formation of ICA, and very possibly, there is some amyloid. When these people are first diagnosed as overtly diabetic, diet or sulfonylurea therapy will be useful only transiently. They soon will require insulin therapy simply because they don't have enough beta cells present.

DR. GELLER: I just want to comment that this work is done at the Oregon Regional Primate Research Center which some animal rights groups want to close; they picketed the Center two days ago.

DR. HOWARD: We were fortunate because there were no demonstrations in Oregon. There were demonstrations at the Primate Centers in Atlanta, Boston, Davis and Madison, Wisconsin, as I understand, but because Oregon is inaccessible they simply said, "Let's close that Center down."

DR. REAVEN: Would you care to speculate on the high VLDL levels?

DR. HOWARD: I can't answer the question as far as the mechanisms responsible for the increase in triglycerides. Part of our problem is that we are working with such low levels of lipids in the circulation, i.e., low cholesterol and low triglyceride concentrations. It is difficult to even establish significant differences unless we segregate our population. The best information I showed on differences in cholesterol concentrations of diabetics and nondiabetics was limited to male monkeys. If we examine both males and females, we don't see any significant differences. We have also fed monkeys cholesterol and can then differentiate significant lipid concentrations in the groups more adequately.

DR. WISSLER: I have a comment. I have been interested in this model of diabetes for a long time and have had the privilege of seeing much of the material as it has developed. I can't help comparing it to many adult-onset diabetics that we see in which there is extensive hyalinization of pancreatic islets. We frequently do not look for amyloid, and these substances in the human might be a mixed bag in a way.

I wonder, if one did a careful study of a series of 100 adult-onset diabetics, all with hyalinized islets, whether one would find evidence of amyloid in a substantial number of cases? I think it is well worth re-examining adult-onset diabetic human material in relation to this model to see if there is more evidence of an amyloid component there than most of us take the time and trouble to look for.

DR. PARKER: Did you find amyloid in areas other than the islets? Were lymphoid cells seen in the islets? Can you explain the predominant deposition of lipid in the monkey's thoracic aorta in contrast to the human? The

Macaca aortic distribution appears different. Does this have some relationship to the animal's physical features?

DR. HOWARD: Many of the animal models of induced atherosclerosis seem to have higher thoracic than abdominal involvement, for reasons that I could not speak to. As for the first part of your question on the distribution of amyloid, studies in humans and in our monkeys show the deposition of amyloid in the islets is not related to deposits elsewhere. We do find amyloid in the intestines, occasionally in the arteries, spleen or liver, but it has no consistent relationship to amyloid in the islets. It appears to be quite a different phenomenon. Pathologists have made the same observations in human beings; i.e., humans may or may not have islet amyloid regardless of whether there is amyloid present elsewhere in the body. Deposition of amyloid in the islets seems to be a very specific phenomenon.

DR. PARKER: Did you see any lymphocytes?

DR. HOWARD: If you mean insulitis, not often.

DR. WISSLER: This is simply a comment on the topography of the atherosclerosis. We have studied induced or spontaneous aortic atherosclerosis in at least six different primate species now, and they all go through a progression where they are more severe in the thoracic early, and then if they become severe enough they become more severe in the abdominal aorta with time. If you evaluate the severity of the lesions that Dr. Howard showed on a scale of what is possible in primates using atherogenic diets, then the most severe of these would be about 1.5 to 2+ on a scale of 1.0 to 4+. So with time, I am sure that one of these days Dr. Howard is going to autopsy an old diabetic animal from his colony that will have much more disease in the abdominal aorta than in the thoracic aorta. That is not much different than in the human. A human also only develops its great propensity for the abdominal aorta to be more severe with time and age, so it is a part of the usual progression that when the aortic disease gets severe it usually becomes more severe in the abdominal aorta.

Comparative Pathobiology of Major Age-Related Diseases: Current Status and Research Frontiers, pages 307–329

THE EXTRACELLULAR MATRIX IN ATHEROSCLEROSIS

G. S. Berenson, M.D., B. Radhakrishnamurthy*, Ph.D
S. R. Srinivasan*, Ph.D., P. Vijayagopal, Ph.D.,
E. R. Dalferes, Jr., B.S., and C. Sharma, Ph.D.

Departments of Medicine and Biochemistry*,
Louisiana State University Medical Center,
New Orleans, LA 70112

INTRODUCTION AND GENERAL STATEMENT

Manifestations of aging of the cardiovascular system appear to reflect a final common path, likely being governed by numerous host factors. In the instance of large elastic arteries and coronary arteries, pathologic changes become a mixture of development and maturation, aging and atherosclerosis. The arterial wall is a well differentiated tissue structure adapted to be resilient and flexible conduits of circulating elements. As with other tissues that are being subjected to various forms of stress and injury, it must respond with ultimate attempts to preserve the integrity of the arterial wall (Figure 1). Processes that involve hyperplasia, cell growth, possibly transformation of cells and compensatory metabolic alterations respond in an adaptive manner to disease. The matrix components of the arterial wall play an interesting and important role in maintenance of the normal structure and in pathogenesis of atherosclerotic lesions. This presentation will focus primarily on the carbohydrate-protein macromolecules of that intercellular material.

Structural Characteristics of the Arterial Wall and the Developing Atherosclerotic Lesions

The intimal surface of the arterial wall, the aorta and coronary vessels, shows some form of atherosclerotic lesion in cultures with both high and low risk for coronary heart

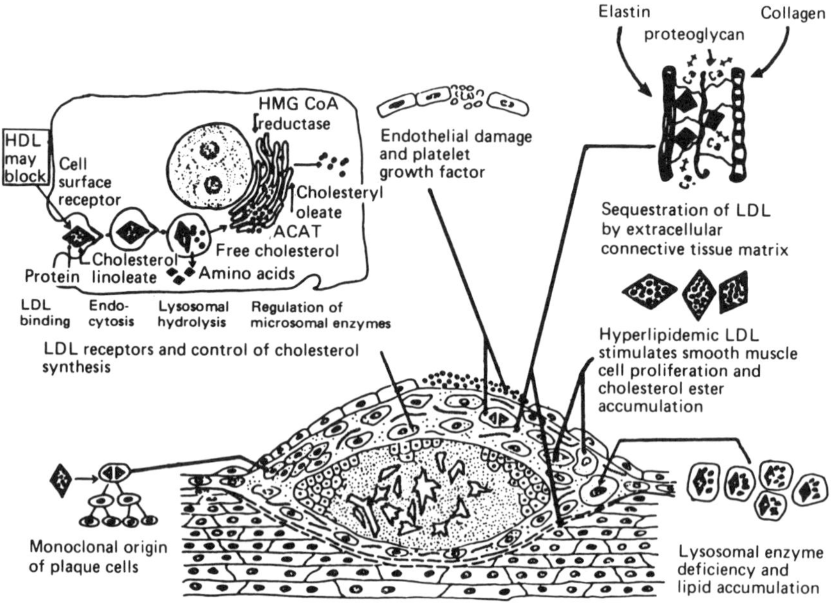

Fig. 1. Diagrammatic representation of mechanisms that are postulated to be involved in the pathogenesis of athero- sclerosis. Sequestration of serum low density lipoproteins (LDL) by extracellular connective tissue components is hypothesized to be one of the early events in the development ment of atherosclerotic lesions. (Reprinted with permission from Academic Press and Radhakrishnamurthy et al 1982a).

disease (McGill 1968). In high risk populations, e.g., United States, atherosclerotic lesions appear at an early age, even infancy, and begin forming obstructive disease by the second to third decade of life. It is then difficult to differentiate changes related to age as compared to atherosclerosis. The initial stages of atherogenesis begin early and pleomorphic lesions begin to develop that suggest episodic arterial reactions to recurrent injury. The very early lesions show minimally detectable variations from the normal with primarily intimal thickening; subsequently, the arterial changes begin to appear in childhood and progress during young adulthood into raised lesions and finally the complicated disease is noted in later life. More severe lesions appear initially in the abdominal aorta, followed by the posterior thoracic region, and finally in the coronary vessels. Fibromuscular intimal thickening occurs in coronary arteries in young people and consists of a thickened intimal layer with increased ground substance, collagen and elastic fibers. These first occur as cushions particularly at sites of arterial branching, and in the abdominal aorta by the end of the first decade cell proliferation is prominent as lesions become associated with focal intracellular lipid deposits. The peculiarity of distributions suggests an element of vascular remodeling resulting from changes in blood flow during development. Further, coronary artery lesions are more extensive in males than in females.

Matrix Components of the Arterial Wall

The extracellular components of the arterial wall consist of fibrous structures, collagen and elastin, and families of carbohydrate-protein macromolecules. The latter are of primary interest to this discussion. The connective tissue elements form an integral part of the cardiovascular structures and obviously undergo changes in response to such stimuli as stress, inflammation, repair, and hormonal activity, and these changes are governed by the local cellular responses to those processes occurring in the arterial wall. Because of the very significant interrelationship of the matrix carbohydrate-protein macromolecules to collagen and elastin, a very brief description of the fibrous structures is given.

Fibrous Components. Extensive reviews are available on both collagen and elastin found in vascular tissue (Bornstein, Sage 1980; Sandberg 1976). Brief consideration must be given to these fibrous components of arterial tissue, since these are major structural materials that occur in unusually high content in the large blood vessels, e.g., aorta. The internal elastic lamina is a landmark in studying vascular disease. Large arteries, such as the aorta, contain a high content of elastic tissue and develop characteristic lamellae with collagen fibers and matrix material interspersed within the elastin structure. In advancing age and with atherosclerosis the lamellar structure and particularly the internal elastic lamina show significant disruption. Associated with this aging and disease process total cellularity of the arterial wall decreases, as indicated by studies of DNA content and decreased turnover of collagen and elastin. While the turnover of collagen fractions is reduced, the total content of insoluble collagen in the vascular wall increases during the aging process. In very early life the physical properties and the composition of connective tissue appear to change, but over the very short span of time from birth to about five years; little change occurs between the ages of 10 and 30 and a further slowing of the progressive changes occurs after the age of 40, as noted by the study of skeletal structures. Changes include increase of fibrodiameter, an increased degree of intrafibrillar crystallinity, thermal shrinkage behavior, chemically-induced swelling, solubility and altered metabolism. Similarly, changes occurring in the elastic tissue include fraying, fragmentation, and changing its staining properties. Cross-linking components including desmosine, isodesmosine, and lysonorleucine appear to increase with maturation.

The nature of microfibrils of elastic fibers indicates the occurrence of two distinct structural elements, fibrillar and amorphous. The microfibrils are distinct from collagen and they surround and interpenetrate the amorphous protein elastin. It is suggested that these aggregates of microfibrils have a role in the morphogenesis of the elastic fiber, and as structural age occurs the amorphous regions appear to become more enveloped by microfibrils. Elastin has a rubber-like property with a lower tensile strength than collagen and by being more extensible, obviously plays an important role in the continual stretching and relaxing associated with hemodynamic forces. Again, extensive reviews on the nature of elastin are available but it is important to mention briefly these major components of connective tissue since they interact so closely with the carbohydrate-protein macromolecules. Kramsch et al (1971) and Urry (1974) have discussed in detail the interaction and binding of elastin to lipids and calcium. The interaction of proteoglycan material with these fibrous elements and calcium being progressively deposited in the vessel wall is considered an important potential mechanism for the development and pathogenesis of atherosclerotic lesions. The involvement of elastin in the atherosclerotic process and in aging appears to be associated with a change in its amino acid composition, i.e., an increase in polar amino acids with atherosclerosis. The cross-linking appears to be lower in elastin isolated from the human aorta and pulmonary tissue from senile subjects with some dilution of cross-links due to associated glycoprotein content. Aging of elastin is defined as a breakdown of the polypeptide chain and an infiltration of glycoprotein material, while in atherosclerosis an infiltration of calcium and lipid also occurs.

Carbohydrate-Protein Macromolecules. The intercellular matrix consists of proteoglycan and glycosaminoglycan (GAG) molecules and glycoprotein materials (Berenson et al 1971; Radhakrishnamurthy et al 1981). A marked interaction occurs between the fibrous components and these carbohydrate-protein molecules. The interaction with different fibers or fibrils takes place, in part, according to the nature and function of cells that produce and maintain these connective tissue components (Figure 2). The arterial wall undergoes changes that can be related to both hemodynamic stress, like hypertension, as well as other influences such as hormonal and metabolic changes. The nature of carbohydrate-protein materials and potential mechanisms that relate to their maintenance of the integrity of the arterial wall in the pathogenesis of atherosclerosis will be considered.

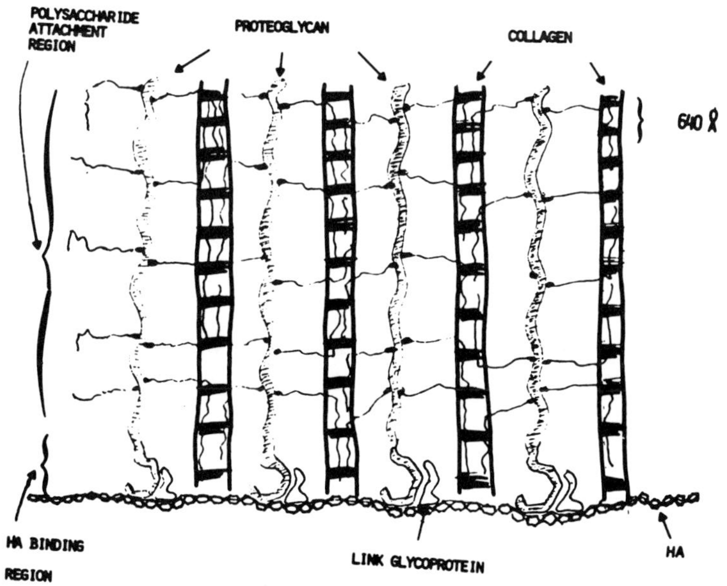

Fig. 2. A schematic representation of mechanisms of proteoglycan aggregation and their interaction with collagen. (Reprinted with permission from Plenum Publishing and Radhakrishnamurthy et al 1981).

GLYCOPROTEINS AND POTENTIAL ROLE IN ATHEROSCLEROSIS

Extracellular matrix glycoproteins are predominantly protein in nature with one or more heterosaccharide chains containing hexosamine, mannose, fucose and sialic acid. Sialic acid is usually linked glycosidically in the terminal position of the oligosaccharide side chains. It is known that many but not all of these carbohydrate chains are -ASN-GlcNAc-containing glycoproteins sharing a common "core" structure. Glycoproteins exist in soluble, easily extractable, or in insoluble material strongly bound to membranes or fibrous structures. Glycoproteins incorporate into fibrils during collagen synthesis and play a role in cementing fibrils into fibers, an interaction that accounts for certain biologic staining properties of fibers.

Several interesting observations on the soluble glycoprotein materials from the arterial wall were described previously in studies from this laboratory. Sialic acid-containing glycoproteins are a very heterogeneous group of materials from aorta, apparently with distinct differences in individuals (Berenson et al 1966) (Figure 3). Individual heterogeneity along with electrophoretic and immunologic identity of material obtained from monozygous twins suggest a genetic order of these compounds. It was shown that these compounds are quite reactive immunologically and their composition varies in different body organs and tissues. Further, a number of enzymatic activities have been noted for these materials and it is now recognized that many enzymes are glycoproteins in structure (Dugan et al 1967). Diabetes mellitus (Srinivasan et al 1970) and myxedema (McFadden, Berenson 1972) alter the tissue composition appreciably.

Other studies from our laboratory of soluble glycoproteins of human aortas related to atherosclerosis show both qualitative and quantitative changes in glycoproteins (Radhakrishnamurthy et al 1977). Fatty streaks have a lower glycoprotein content when compared to fibrous plaques and to control tissue grossly uninvolved. Total hexoses, hexosamines and sialic acid composition are also markedly altered in a similar direction (Schonebeck et al 1962).

Robert (1978) earlier conducted extensive studies on the structural glycoproteins and they also suggest organ and species specificity and immunologic reactivity comparable to that also evident from the soluble materials. The concentra-

Electrophoretic Patterns of Glycoproteins from Individual Human Aortas

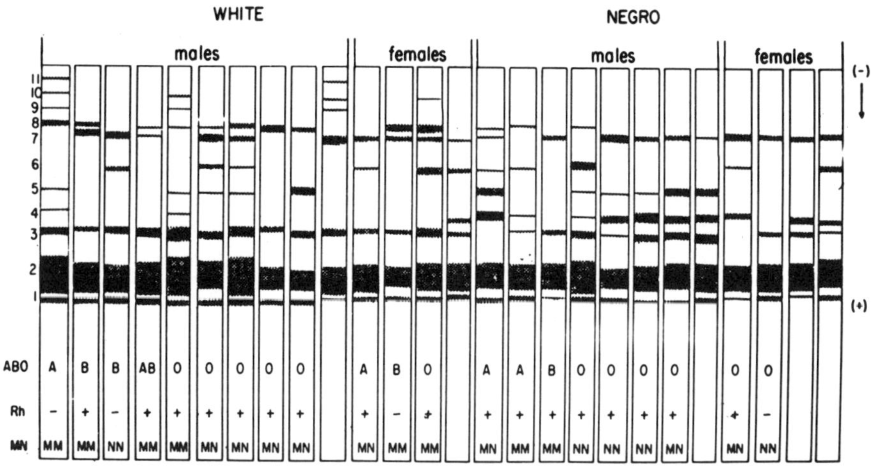

Fig. 3. A composite illustration of electrophoretic patterns of human aorta glycoproteins from 26 individuals. Electrophoresis was performed in polyacrylamide gels using phosphate buffer pH 7.8, μ=0.03, Amido-black stain. An arbitrary numbering system was assigned to the bands corresponding to the mobility. The blood groups of the individuals are shown. (Reprinted with permission from J Atheroscler Res and Berenson et al 1966).

tion of structural glycoproteins is highest in embryonic tissue and decreases with aging while collagen increases. It is suggested that the glycopeptides may have a regulatory function in the spacing and deposition of fibers. Structural glycoproteins appear to be secreted by fibroblasts as extracellular membrane. These materials act as templates upon which fibers of intracelluar matrix are laid down. Electron microscopic studies show the fibrillar nature of aorta structural glycoproteins that apparently serve as a nucleus for the deposition of elastin in addition to collagen.

Very recently, many distinctive structural glycoproteins of arterial wall that form the extracellular matrix have been identified (Poste, Nicolson 1981) (Table 1). Each of these has specific and distinctive interactions with either basement membrane substances or extracellular matrix components. Many glycoproteins are known to be associated with cytoskeletal elements of all cells, especially smooth muscle cells. These cytoskeletal glycoproteins may play an important role in cell activity such as mobility, contraction, spreading and differentiation. The extracellular matrix and cytoskeletal glycoproteins fundamentally play an important role in initiating the process of wound healing. If one visualizes atherosclerosis as a process of injury and repair, it is easy to appreciate the possible role of extracellular arterial wall matrix glycoproteins in the pathogenesis of atherosclerosis.

TABLE 1

EXTRACELLULAR MATRIX GLYCOPROTEINS

Name	Interaction	Cell Type
Fibronectin	Proteoglycans Heparin Hyaluronic acid Collagen (Type I-IV) Fibrin Actin DNA Cell surfaces Bacteria (Staphylococci)	Fibroblasts Smooth muscle Myoblasts Epithelial Endothelial Etc.
Laminin	Proteoglycans Heparin Basement membrane Collagen (Type IV)	Epithelial Smooth muscle
Chondronectin	Proteoglycans Heparin Collagen (Type II)	Chondrocytes
Microfibrillar Proteins	Elastin	Fibroblasts Smooth muscle

Although the association of the processes of aging and atherogenesis is well known, it is difficult to dissociate the effect of one from the other. Moreover, due to lack of efficient methods of isolation and identification of extracellular matrix glycoproteins, quantitation of these glycoproteins in the arterial wall during the process of aging and atherogenesis has been elusive. Further detailed studies are necessary not only in identifying and quantitating individual glycoproteins, but also the process of synthesis during both aging and atherogenesis.

With the idea of quantitating specific extracellular matrix glycoproteins we have recently initiated methods of isolation and identification of laminin and fibronectin. Fibronectin seems to have general distribution being associated with both collagen and elastin fibers. Some fibronectin can be extracted by saline while other enzymic means lead to further solubilization. Laminin can only be extracted by buffered heparin. These results suggest that both fibronectin and laminin are associated with proteoglycans of the human aortic wall; moreover, these results suggest that laminin may well be associated with basement membrane substances while fibronectin could be associated more with other fibrous structures.

PROTEOGLYCANS (GLYCOSAMINOGLYCANS) (GAG)

The proteoglycans consist of GAG components covalently bound to a protein core (Radhakrishnamurthy et al 1981). These monomeric proteoglycans appear often in an aggregating form interacting with hyaluronic acid through a link glycoprotein region (Figure 2). Presumably, proteoglycans are the native form of GAG as they exist with protein in the matrix. Up to the present the clearest structural information is available on GAG. These are hexosamine, uronic acid and sulfate-containing compounds with characteristic repeating units and are associated with a protein core in their native state. One compound, however, hyaluronic acid, has not been shown to be covalently linked to protein. The changes of the GAG with both age and atherosclerotic lesions have been studied and reviewed in detail previously (Berenson et al 1971; Radhakrishnamurthy et al 1982a), although changes are not uniformly stated. Because more current information on the proteoglycan structures in arteries has been obtained, this presentation will consider them primarily.

Most chemistry is known for GAG that are, for the most part, isolated after extensive degradation of tissue. In the aorta there are at least six types of GAG: hyaluronic acid, chondroitin 4-sulfate, chondroitin 6-sulfate, dermatan sulfate, heparan sulfate, and heparin. Variations in sulfate content in some GAG types isolated from different sources have been noted, e.g., over-sulfated chondroitin 6-sulfate from shark cartilage, dermatan sulfate from bovine lung and under-sulfated heparan sulfate from bovine and human aorta tissues. In pig skin and bovine and human aorta, dermatan sulfate and chondroitin 4-sulfate occur as a hybrid. Heparan sulfate is now recognized as an integral part of several cell membranes.

Most of our current knowledge of proteoglycans is derived from the studies of cartilage. With the possible exception of hyaluronic acid, the connective tissue GAG occur in the native state covalently bound to proteins as proteoglycans. Chondroitin sulfates, heparan sulfate and heparin are linked to proteins through an 0-glycosidic bond between D-xylose and the hydroxyl group of serine (Rodén 1980).

A proteoglycan isolated from bovine nasal cartilage contains about 100 chondroitin sulfate chains each with an average molecular weight of 2×10^4 and 30 to 60 keratan sulfate chains each with a molecular weight of 4.8×10^3. The cartilage proteoglycan has a molecular weight of 2.5×10^6 (Hascall, Heinegård 1975).

Arterial Wall Proteoglycans

Recently, attention has been focused on proteoglycans from the arterial wall because of their involvement in the pathogenesis of atherosclerosis. From the studies conducted over the past ten years there is now a general agreement that there are at least two types of proteoglycans in the aorta: 1) chondroitin sulfate-dermatan sulfate proteoglycan (CS-DS-PG) and 2) heparan sulfate proteoglycan (HS-PG). The former is present in aorta in greater amounts and can be extracted from the tissue by dissociative solvents like 4 M guanidine hydrochloride (Radhakrishnamurthy et al 1982a). A proteoglycan isolated from bovine aorta contained 21% protein and 22% uronate. Although not much is known about the protein core, the proteoglycan had chondroitin 6- and 4-sulfates and dermatan sulfate in an 8:3:1 proportion. A hypothetical model of the hybrid proteoglycan is shown in Figure 4. It is not known precisely how different GAG chains are distributed along the length of the protein core. Two different chondroitin sulfate type proteoglycans were isolated from aorta explant culture media extract by Schmidt et al (1982): one rich in

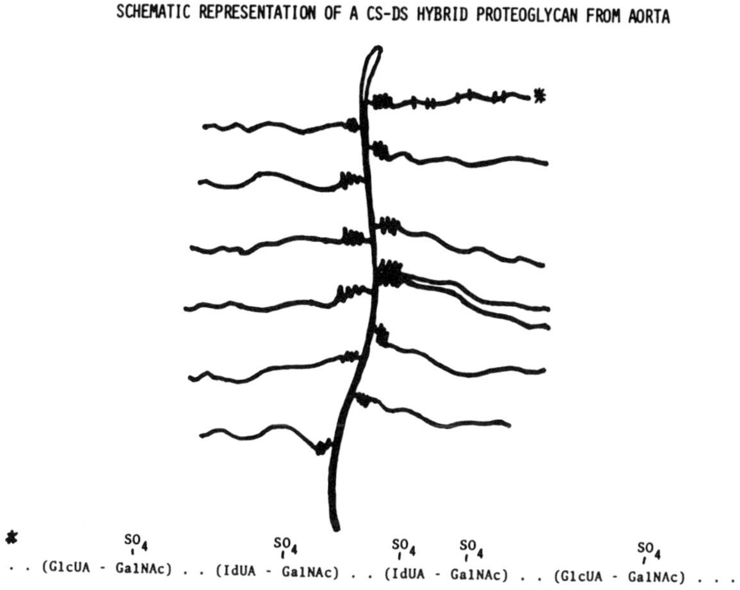

Fig. 4. A model of a chondroitin sulfate-dermatan sulfate hybrid proteoglycan from aorta. GlcUA - glucuronic acid; IdUA - iduronic acid; GalNAc - N-acetyl-D-galactosamine. (Reprinted with permission from S. Karger and Radhakrishnamurthy et al 1982b).

chondroitin 6-sulfate and the other rich in dermatan sulfate. Whether these are fragments of one species of proteoglycan or two individual species is not known.

Unlike the hybrid proteoglycan, HS-PG cannot be extracted easily by dissociative solvents (Radhakrishnamurthy et al 1982a). Only about 10% of the proteoglycan can be extracted by these solvents and the remainder is firmly bound to elastic tissue. Elastase digestion of the tissue provides a method for solubilization of the proteoglycan, but elastase has inherent nonspecific protease activity that can degrade the protein core. Several protease inhibitors need to be added to the extraction medium to inhibit spurious protease activity of the enzyme. Even in the presence of inhibitors, it is possible that some degradation of the core protein can occur, and therefore, one should exercise caution in interpreting the results.

A HS-PG isolated by a sequential extraction of bovine aorta by NaCl, digestion of the tissue with collagenase and then elastase had a molecular weight of 300,000 and protein 19% and uronate 18% (Vijayagopal et al 1983). HS-PG with biologic properties like heparin is an important component of the aorta and is believed to play an important role in the pathogenesis of atherosclerosis.

Aggregation of Proteoglycans

Hascall and Heinegard (1975) showed proteoglycans from bovine nasal cartilage to form large aggregates in the presence of hyaluronic acid and link proteins. Since that time several investigators studied the phenomenon of aggregation of proteoglycans. It was observed that proteoglycans from cartilage aggregate with hyaluronic acid even in the absence of link proteins, although they noted link proteins stabilize the interaction between hyaluronic acid and the proteoglycan. The nature of link proteins is being studied by several investigators.

Unlike proteoglycans from cartilage, aorta proteoglycans do not form large aggregates. Only 10% of CS-DS-PG from bovine aorta was noted by Oegema et al (1979) to form aggregates with exogenous hyaluronic acid. In our laboratory we (Radhakrishnamurthy et al 1982a) isolated two proteoglycan-hyaluronate complexes from bovine aorta by the procedure of Hascall and Heinegard (1975). Complex I sedimented at the bottom 1/3 of the gradient ($\rho_c > 1.7$) and the other (Complex II) sedimented between densities 1.6 and 1.7 g/ml in CsCl density gradient centrifugation. Complex I had protein content of 22% whereas Complex II had about 11%. The only GAG found in the complexes were hyaluronic acid and chondroitin sulfates (plus dermatan sulfate) in a proportion of 13:87 in Complex I and 24:76 in Complex II. Whether link proteins are present in these complexes is not known. Gardell et al (1980) noted the presence of link proteins in their preparation of proteoglycan aggregates from bovine aorta.

These complexes in aorta may be of particular importance in the pathogenesis of atherosclerosis because they act as macromolecular sieves inhibiting the extrusion of large particles like lipoproteins through the arterial wall while they are being sequestered in subendothelial space by highly negatively charged proteoglycans.

Proteoglycan Metabolism

Buddecke and Kresse (1972) observed differences between the turnover rates of chondroitin sulfate and dermatan sulfate in the proteoglycan isolated from the aorta. Proteoglycan material has been isolated with apparently different proportions of chondroitin sulfate and dermatan sulfate. Labelling experiments suggest that the dermatan sulfate portion of the proteoglycan is much more active with a more rapid turnover, and further degradation studies have shown metabolic heterogeneity of the chondroitin sulfate and dermatan sulfate. Their work suggests that dermatan sulfate and chondroitin sulfate clusters develop each with different specific activity with respect to the ester sulfate groups. Fransson and Havsmark (1970) suggest that in a dermatan sulfate isolated from horse aorta iduronic acid-N-acetylgalactosamine 4-sulfate units are located near the linkage regions, followed by glycuronosyl-N-acetylgalactosamine 4-sulfate units with glucuronosyl-N-acetylgalactosamine 6-sulfate units in the center of the chains. Iduronic acid is formed from glucuronic acid in the polymer by a C_5-epimerase. The metabolic heterogeneity might be due to their different locations in the GAG chain or structural differences in uronic acid moieties. With regard to the degradation of the GAG, significant alterations during catabolism of GAG develop even before microscopic abnormalities may be detected. Higher metabolic rates appear in detectable plaques. Endoglycosidases like hyaluronidase and exoglycosidases like ß-glucuronidase and N-acetylhexosaminidases are involved in the degradation of the GAG. These, along with intrinsic proteolytic enzymes, limit precise determinations of the nature of these substances as they occur in tissue and require a considerable number of inhibitors in an effort to obtain the native material.

POTENTIAL MECHANISMS RELATED TO ATHEROSCLEROSIS

A number of specific physiological functions have been attributed to GAG. These include providing structural support to the vessel wall and resistance to infection, regulating fluid and electrolyte balance, influencing blood coagulation, platelet aggregation and calcification, regulating lipid metabolism and transporting lipoproteins across the endothelium (Radhakrishnamurthy et al 1981).

Anticoagulant Activity

Even though many of these functions of GAG are not clearly understood, it has been known for many years that GAG possess anticoagulant activity. Several laboratories (Izuka, Murata 1972) have demonstrated that the anticoagulant properties of GAG are due to dermatan sulfate and heparan sulfate. Since GAG occur in the native state as proteoglycans in the tissue, a better understanding of their physiological functions can be obtained by studying intact proteoglycans. Therefore, we studied the hemostatic properties of a CS-DS-PG and a HS-PG from bovine aorta (Vijayagopal et al 1980, 1983).

The anticoagulant activity was assayed in three clotting systems viz. Stypven time, partial thromboplastin clotting time and thrombin time. The proteoglycans delayed or totally inhibited all three systems, but maximum activity was noted in the thrombin time assay. In all three systems HS-PG exhibited significantly more anticoagulant activity than CS-DS-PG. Both proteoglycans also inhibited thrombin-induced platelet aggregation and at comparable uronic acid levels the HS-PG was a more potent inhibitor of platelet aggregation than the CS-DS-PG. Our studies have shown that the protein core of the proteoglycan molecules is not essential for their hemostatic properties (Vijayagopal et al 1980). These studies suggest that the anticoagulant activities of aorta proteoglycans may be due to the ability of polysaccharides to accelerate the inactivation of serine proteases by antithrombin III. Proteoglycans might do this by increasing the binding affinity of these proteases for antithrombin III as has been suggested for free GAG (Hatton et al 1978). The studies of Buonassisi and Colburn (1982) confirm the anticoagulant activity of arterial HS-PG. These investigators also observed the inhibition of blood coagulation by HS-PG isolated from cultured rabbit aorta endothelial cells.

Recently, Kanaide et al (1982) reported lower anticoagulant activity for chondroitin sulfate isolated from atherosclerotic regions of human aorta as compared to that obtained from normal intima-media regions. According to these authors the lower anticoagulant activity of sclerotic chondroitin sulfate was due to greater accelerating effect on the polymerization of fibrin. Although the importance of arterial proteoglycans in relation to atherosclerosis is now well recognized, little attention has been paid to the study of the alteration in the biological properties of these macromolecules in atherosclerosis.

Lipoprotein-Lipase Binding

Lipoprotein lipase (LPL) is the key enzyme involved in the hydrolysis of plasma chylomicrons and very low density lipoprotein (VLDL)-triglycerides. Several lines of evidence suggest that LPL activity is localized at or near the capillary endothelium. Recently, we (Vijayagopal et al 1980) noted that the CS-DS-PG from bovine aorta when injected into rabbits was about 60% as effective as heparin in causing LPL release.

Proteoglycan-Lipoprotein Interactions

There is now wide agreement that the lipids of atherosclerotic lesions originate from plasma apoB-containing lipoproteins such as low density (LDL), VLDL, and Lp(a) lipoproteins. Modulations in arterial cellular binding and uptake of apoB-containing lipoproteins remain the main focus of attention with respect to lipid accumulation. Histochemical studies have demonstrated a close relationship between arterial GAG, fibrous structures and lipid deposits of atheromatous lesions in both humans and experimental animals. These observations strongly imply that connective tissue macromolecules, especially proteoglycans, are involved in selective retention of certain plasma lipoproteins.

Passage of macromolecules across the arterial wall is greatly affected by subendothelial GAG (proteoglycans). The physicochemical properties of proteoglycans and hyaluronic acid, for example, their capacity for hydrophilic trapping, charge characteristics and interaction with collagen and elastin (Lindahl, Höök 1978) result in a gel-sieve matrix. The permeability and retention of macrocolecules such as lipoproteins which enter the matrix may be modulated by molecular-sieving, steric exclusion and electrostatic interaction. On the other hand, the permeating plasma components, especially LDL in excess amounts, contribute to the microenvironment of cellular and connective tissue elements of vessel wall. Furthermore, an interaction of LDL with arterial GAG should make LDL electronegative. Unlike arterial smooth muscle cells, blood monocytes are known to bind and internalize electronegative LDL by a high affinity process devoid of feedback control. Such a process may result in focal localization of fat-filled foam cells.

Since an increase in lipid content of grossly normal intima with age is greater than the changes of plasma lipids with age, mechanisms other than simple infiltration of plasma lipids into the vessel wall appear to be operative in lipid accumulation. Progressive alterations of connective tissue components likely affect the arterial tissue organization and integrity, which in turn may influence the permeability of macromolecules across the arterial wall. The selective interaction of plasma apoB-containing lipoproteins with proteoglycans and transfer of lipids from LDL to elastin and collagen favor enrichment of normal arterial wall with lipids gradually during life. While all of these changes may be the normal adaptive processes of the arterial wall, focal response to chronic hemodynamic stress and even slightly elevated levels of plasma LDL over time may initiate lesion formation.

In Vitro Interactions with Lipoproteins

The ability of GAG to form both soluble and insoluble complexes with plasma LDL is well known (Srinivasan et al 1975). For selective precipitation of apoB-containing lipoproteins from serum, the nature and concentration of cations appear to be important. We (Srinivasan et al 1975) studied the complexing ability of different plasma lipoproteins in the presence of Ca^{++}, Mg^{++} and Mn^{++} using a heparin-substituted Sepharose gel. The heparin-LDL interaction was quantitative only within a narrow range of metal ion concentration (0.02 to 0.04 M); the relative stability of the complexes depended on the type of cation ($Mn^{++} > Mg^{++} > Ca^{++}$). While similar results were observed with VLDL, virtually no interaction was noted between HDL and heparinated gel in the presence of Ca^{++} or Mg^{++}. Unlike Mn^{++}, the presence of Ca^{++} did not promote an interaction between heparin and apoE (arginine-rich) containing HDL subfractions.

The chemical characteristics of isolated GAG seem to influence significantly the formation of complexes with serum lipoproteins. The ability of different GAG to form insoluble complexes in the presence of Ca^{++} was found to be in the following order: heparin > heparan sulfate > chondroitin 6-sulfate > chondroitin 4-sulfate > dermatan sulfate. The above order of affinity for interaction appears to be different in the absence of Ca^{++}. Further N-desulfation of heparin eliminated complexing of this GAG which has the greatest ability to form insoluble complexes. It has been demonstrated that certain plasma GAG cause conformational changes on lipoproteins by increasing the viscosity and swelling of hydrophilic region.

Hitherto, the *in vitro* lipoprotein-GAG interaction studies were mainly focused on sulfated GAG instead of native proteoglycans. We recently demonstrated that the CS-DS-PG from bovine aorta can be potent and selective as heparin in terms of complex formation (Vijayagopal et al 1981) (Figure 5). On the other hand, the complex forming ability of HS-PG from

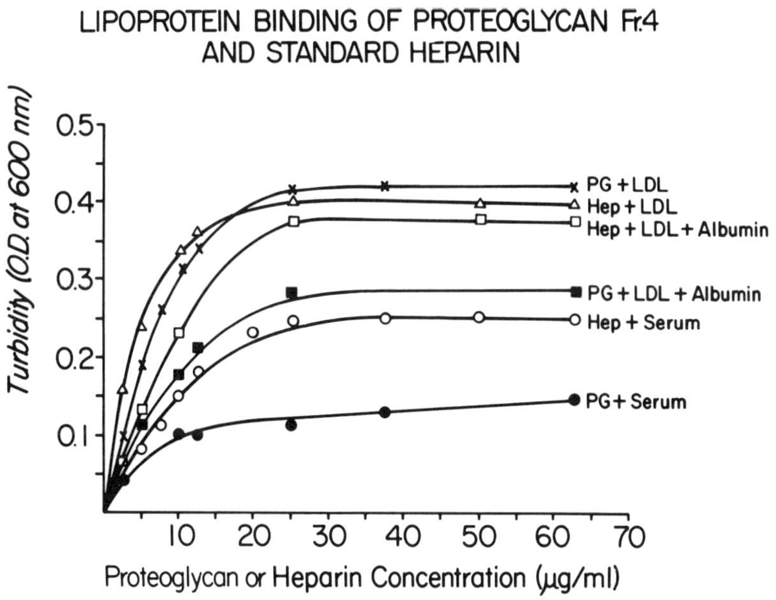

Fig. 5. Lipoprotein binding of a proteoglycan (PG) from bovine aorta and standard heparin. Serum or serum low density lipoprotein (LDL) was incubated with varying amounts of PG or heparin with or without albumin in the presence of $CaCl_2$. Degree of insoluble complex formation was measured in terms of turbidity produced. (Reprinted with permission from Lab Invest and Vijayagopal et al 1980).

bovine aorta is far less when compared to the CS-DS-PG. These differences may be functionally important because heparan sulfate proteoglycans, which are synthesized predominantly by the endothelial cells, might increase the cell surface negative charge (antithrombogenic) without binding LDL.

The fact that the removal of the protein core or the GAG chains of proteoglycan prevented interaction with LDL indicates that the native state of carbohydrate-protein macromolecules confers optimum charge density for specific interaction with apoB-containing lipoproteins. Recently, Camejo et al (1980) reported isolation of proteoglycan(s) from human arterial extracts that rendered serum LDL insoluble; this "lipoprotein-complexing factor" represented a heterogeneous population of "quasi-spherical particles" composed of protein, GAG (heparin, dermatan sulfate and chondroitin 6-sulfate) and lipids.

The nature of interaction between apoB-containing lipoproteins and GAG at physiologic pH is interesting because both the macromolecular species are anionic at this pH. The reaction mechanism between LDL and GAG can be conceived of as an electrostatic binding occurring in the following manner: 1) in the absence of divalent metal ions, the polyanionic groups of GAG primarily interact with the basic amino groups of LDL protein (apoB) to form less stable soluble complexes; 2) independent of this, the addition of divalent cations can bridge the anionic groups of GAG and LDL phospholipids (GAG---Ca^{++}---LDL and GAG---Ca^{++}---GAG), thereby promoting aggregation and insolubility of the complexes. The binding of Ca^{++} with arterial GAG in association with connective tissue components is likely to alter the charge characteristics of the extracellular matrix and trigger rapid accumulation of plasma apoB-containing lipoproteins.

In Vivo Interactions

Although indirect evidence based on electrophoretic and thermoanalytic methods for the association of lipoproteins and proteoglycans in atherosclerotic lesions was proposed, the actual isolation of intact LDL-GAG complexes from human normal intima and atherosclerotic lesions in our laboratory provided evidence for an *in vivo* interaction and complexing (Radhakrishnamurthy et al 1982a). They contain both LDL and VLDL with the former being predominant. Our studies that show the presence of Ca^{++} in significant quantities and the morphologic evidence that these complexes have a highly aggregated nature indicate an interaction similar to that observed *in vitro*. The observations have been confirmed by several other laboratories in human and rabbit (Mawhinney et al 1978) atherosclerotic lesions.

Extracellular lipoprotein pools in arterial wall are associated with GAG and the different fibrous structures to varying degrees. However, whether the binding of lipoproteins to arterial wall structures is promoted independently or cooperatively by GAG, collagen and/or elastin remains unknown. Recently, we have demonstrated in a rabbit model that sustained hypercholesterolemia causes atherosclerosis associated simultaneously with an increase in LDL uptake by aorta, alterations in GAG metabolism, and formation of LDL complexes of GAG in association with collagen and elastin (Srinivasan et al 1982). The specific activities of GAG in the complexes obtained by different extraction procedures differed markedly (elastase > collagenase > saline), emphasizing the presence of different pools of complexes.

The occurrence of GAG in complexes from human atherosclerotic lesions varies depending upon the extraction procedure and isolation techniques. While saline-extracted lipoprotein-GAG complexes contained chondroitin 6-sulfate and hyaluronic acid as the major and minor GAG, respectively, the collagenase-solubilized complexes contained these GAG in reverse proportions. Interestingly, heparin, the most potent complexing agent, was detected in trace amounts only in saline-solubilized complexes of fibrous plaque lesions. Furthermore, the association of hyaluronic acid with an apparent molecular weight of 400,000 and 75,000 as the only GAG in the elastase-solubilized lipoprotein fraction is an unexpected finding that needs to be clarified.

Thus there is both *in vitro* and *in vivo* evidence highly in favor of a role for proteoglycans in selective retention of certain plasma lipoproteins. Further studies are needed to elucidate the dynamic nature and complexity of the physicochemical changes occurring in the extracellular matrix that may affect the lipoprotein flux and retention.

SUMMARY

From the above discussion, potential mechanisms in the role of carbohydrate-protein macromolecules in maintenance of the integrity of the matrix of arterial wall and their role in aging and atherosclerosis is suggested. Prominent is their role in anticoagulant activity and in platelet aggregation. The interaction of proteoglycans and glycoprotein material with the fibrous structures of the aorta and with the serum lipoproteins shows important roles for the connective tissue macromolecules in the pathogenesis of atherosclerosis. It is apparent that the carbohydrate-protein macromolecules of the arterial wall matrix have a number of biologic functions important to both maintenance in health and pathogenesis of disease.

REFERENCES

Berenson GS, Radhakrishnamurthy B, Dalferes ER Jr, Srinivasan SR (1971). Carbohydrate-protein macromolecules and atherosclerosis. Hum Pathol 2:57.

Berenson GS, Radhakrishnamurthy B, Fishkin AF, Dessauer H, Arquembourg P (1966). Individuality of glycoproteins in human aorta. J Atheroscler Res 6:214.

Bornstein P, Sage H (1980). Structurally distinct collagen types. Annu Rev Biochem 190:393.

Buddecke E, Kresse H (1972). Metabolic heterogeneity of arterial tissue glycosaminoglycans and proteoglycans. In Vogel HG (ed): "Connective Tissue and Aging," Vol I, Amsterdam, The Netherlands: Excerpta Medica, p 14.

Buonassisi V, Colburn P (1982). Biological significance of heparan sulfate proteoglycans. Ann NY Acad Sci 401:76.

Camejo G, Lalaruna F, Lopez F, Starosta R (1980). Characterization and properties of a lipoprotein-complexing proteoglycan from human aorta. Atherosclerosis 35:307.

Dugan FA, Radhakrishnamurthy B, Berenson GS (1967). Enzymes of glycoprotein preparations from connective tissue. Enzymologia 33:215.

Fransson L-A, Havsmark B (1970). Structure of dermatan sulfate. VII. The copolymeric structure of dermatan sulfate from horse aorta. J Biol Chem 245:4770.

Gardell S, Baker J, Caterson B, Heinegard D, Roden L (1980). Link protein and a hyaluronic acid-binding region as components of aorta proteoglycan. Biochem Biophys Res Commun 95:1823.

Hascall VC, Heinegard D (1975). The structure of proteoglycans. In Slavkin HC, Greulich RC (eds): "Extracellular Matrix Influences on Gene Expressions," New York: Academic Press, p 267.

Hatton MWC, Berry LR, Regoeczi E (1978). Inhibition of thrombin by antithrombin III in the presence of certain glycosaminoglycans found in the mammalian aorta. Thromb Res 13:655.

Izuka K, Murata K (1972). Inhibitory effects of human aortic and venous acid glycosaminoglycans and thrombus formation. Atherosclerosis 16:3217.

Kanaide H, Urarishi T, Nakashima Y, Nakamura M (1982). The anticoagulant effect of chondroitin sulfates isolated from normal and atherosclerotic regions of human aortas. Br J Exp Pathol 63:82.

Kramsch DM, Franzblau C, Hollander W (1971). The protein and lipid composition of arterial elastin and its relationship to lipid accumulation in the atherosclerotic plaque. J Clin Invest 50:1666.

Lindahl U, Höök M (1978). Glycosaminoglycans and their binding to biological macromolecules. Annu Rev Biochem 47:385.

Mawhinney TP, Augustyn JM, Fritz KE (1978). Glycosaminoglycan-lipoprotein complexes from aortas of hypercholesterolemic rabbits. Atherosclerosis 31:155.

McGill HC Jr (1968). "The Geographic Pathology of Atherosclerosis." Baltimore: Williams and Wilkins.

McFadden PM, Berenson GS (1972). Basement membrane changes in myocardial and skeletal muscle capillaries in myxedema. Circulation 45:808.

Oegema TR Jr, Hascall VC, Eisenstein R (1979). Isolation of bovine aorta proteoglycan extracted with guanidine hydrochloride in the presence of protease inhibitors. J Biol Chem 254:1312.

Poste G, Nicolson GL (eds) (1981). "Cytoskeletal Elements and Plasma Membrane Organization." Amsterdam, The Netherlands: North-Holland Publishing.

Radhakrishnamurthy B, Berenson GS, Dalferes ER Jr (1977). Complex carbohydrates of arterial wall connective tissue. In Schettler G, Gotto Y, Hata Y, Klose G (eds): "Atherosclerosis IV," New York: Springer-Verlag, p 353.

Radhakrishnamurthy B, Srinivasan SR, Berenson GS (1982a). Glycosaminoglycans in atherosclerosis. In Horowitz MI (ed): "The Glycoconjugates," Vol IV, New York: Academic Press, p 265.

Radhakrishnamurthy B, Srinivasan SR, Dalferes ER Jr, Pargaonkar

PS, Berenson GS (1981). Arterial wall carbohydrate-protein macromolecules. In Schwartz CJ, Werthessen NT, Wolf S (eds): "Structure and Function of the Circulation," Vol 3, New York: Plenum, p 157.

Radhakrishnamurthy B, Srinivasan SR, Vijayagopal P, Dalferes ER Jr, Berenson GS (1982b). Mesenchymal injury and proteoglycans of arterial wall in atherosclerosis. In Varma RS, Varma R (eds): "Glycosaminoglycans and Proteoglycans in Physiological and Pathological Processes of Body Systems," Basel, Switzerland: S. Karger, p 231.

Robert L (1978). Structural glycoproteins of connective tissue. In Robert AM, Robert L (eds): "Biochemistry of Normal and Pathological Connective Tissue," Colloque du CNRS, No 287, Vol 2, Paris: CNRS, p 189.

Rodén L (1980). Structure and metabolism of connective tissue proteoglycans. In Lennarz L (ed): "The Biochemistry of Glycoproteins and Proteoglycans," New York: Plenum, p 267.

Sandberg LB (1976). Elastin structure in health and disease. Int Rev Connect Tissue Res 7:159.

Schmidt A, Prager M, Selmke P, Buddecke (1982). Isolation and properties of proteoglycans from bovine aorta. Eur J Biochem 125:95.

Schonebeck L, Werber U, Voigt KD (1962). Protein-bound carbohydrate containing constituents of serum and vessel wall in atherosclerosis. J Atheroscler Res 2:332.

Srinivasan SR, Berenson GS, Radhakrishnamurthy B (1970). Glycoprotein changes in diabetic kidneys. Diabetes 19:171.

Srinivasan SR, Radhakrishnamurthy B, Berenson GS, (1975). Studies on the interaction of heparin with serum lipoproteins in the presence of Ca^{2+}, Mg^{2+} and Mn^{2+}. Arch Biochem Biophys 170:334.

Srinivasan SR, Yost C, Bhandaru RR, Radhakrishnamurthy B, Berenson GS (1982). Lipoprotein-glycosaminoglycan interactions in aortas of rabbits fed atherogenic diets containing different fats. Atherosclerosis 43:289.

Urry DW (1974). On the molecular basis for vascular calcification. Perspect Biol Med 18:68.

Vijayagopal P, Radhakrishnamurthy B, Srinivasan SR, Berenson GS (1980). Studies of biologic properties of proteoglycans from bovine aorta. Lab Invest 42:190.

Vijayagopal P, Srinivasan SR, Radhakrishnamurthy B, Berenson GS (1981). Interaction of serum lipoproteins and a proteoglycan from bovine aorta. J Biol Chem 256:8234.

Vijayagopal P, Srinivasan SR, Radhakrishnamurthy B, Berenson GS (1983). Hemostatic properties and serum lipoprotein binding of heparan sulfate proteoglycan from bovine aorta.

Biochim Biophys Acta (in press).

DISCUSSION

DR. REGELSON: Could you say something about proteoglycan control of smooth muscle proliferation?

DR. BERENSON: I don't know. There presumably could be a feedback from proteoglycan on smooth muscle, but it may be the other way around, i.e., that smooth muscle proliferation is associated with synthesis of the proteoglycans. Several of us have been trying to explore the effect of proteoglycan on internalization of lipoproteins which enhances growth of cells, but we haven't been able to show that proteoglycans clearly alter the LDL or other lipoproteins being internalized.

DR. REGELSON: I am thinking more specifically of work from Harvard with regard to the platelet growth factor causing smooth muscle hyperplasia being a heparinase.

DR. BERENSON: That is an enzyme, not a proteoglycan.

DR. REGELSON: The enzyme would affect the proteoglycans, i.e., affecting the heparin content of the smooth muscle of the vascular wall resulting in proliferation.

DR. BERENSON: I can't comment. Certainly heparan sulfate and heparin are both digested by the heparinase enzymes. Are you referring to Rosenberg's study?

DR. REGELSON: Yes.

DR. POTTENGER: Is the inhibitory effect of the glycosaminoglycans thought to be due to their ability to clear lipid from the bloodstream?

DR. BERENSON: Yes, I think that that may be a major effect. Also they could compete with the heparan sulfate on the endothelial surface complexing with lipoproteins or even transport across the arterial wall by complexing them in serum.

III. THE AGING BRAIN

Comparative Pathobiology of Major Age-Related Diseases: Current Status and Research Frontiers, pages 333–355

NERVE CELL AND SYNAPTIC DECLINE IN BRAIN AGING: IMPLICATIONS FOR ANIMAL MODELS AND FOR A HYPOTHESIS OF ALZHEIMER'S DISEASE

P. W. Landfield, Ph.D., T. A. Pitler, and M. D. Applegate

Department of Physiology and Pharmacology, Bowman Gray School of Medicine, Wake Forest University, Winston-Salem, NC 27103

INTRODUCTION

In a symposium on comparative pathobiology it seems relevant to consider how animal models, particularly rodent models, of brain aging may relate to human brain aging and to a major age-correlated form of neuropathology, Alzheimer's disease. Consequently, this paper addresses two questions that are central to an assessment of rodent models for research on normal brain aging and on Alzheimer's disease. These are: 1) how analogous are mechanisms and patterns of brain aging in rodents to those in other mammals, including humans? and 2) what is the nature of the relationship, if any, between normal brain aging and senile dementia of the Alzheimer's type (SDAT)?

These are key issues since the extent to which studies of normal brain aging mechanisms in rodents can be generalized to other mammalian species will be an important factor in determining the extent to which many current neuroscience techniques can be used to study basic mechanisms of normal and pathological brain aging. That is, many of our more sophisticated technical procedures require fresh tissue and/or surgical approaches, for which rodents are often the most practical experimental animals. Moreover, rodents by far constitute the most abundant source of aged animals of defined health, genetic, and age status. Nevertheless, while rodents possess many practical advantages as experimental animals, it is also clearly valuable to study model species in which the basic neurobiological mechanisms and principles of brain aging can be generalized to those in other vertebrate species. Therefore, it appears essential that we begin to systematically evaluate the likelihood that mechanisms of rodent brain aging are at some level analogous to brain aging mechanisms in other species. Although the relevance of rodents as models for general aging mechanisms has been treated in some depth in several earlier volumes (Gibson et al 1978; National Academy of Sciences 1981; Burek, Hollander 1980), this issue has been only minimally considered with specific regard to brain aging (National Academy of Sciences 1981). However, it is certainly conceivable that brain aging mechanisms are regulated independently of non-neural aging processes.

With respect to non-neural aging mechanisms, it appears that nearly all vertebrate species exhibit analogous phases of development, sexual maturity, reproductive senescence, physiological decline, and the onset of extensive pathology, during approximately similar fractions of the life span (Finch 1976). This suggests that generalized aging processes are fundamentally similar across vertebrates, and therefore, that aging is deeply entrenched in vertebrate biology. In turn, this implies that common etiological mechanisms may well underlie such common patterns of progressive senescence, rather than that separate and convergent mechanisms of aging have evolved in different mammalian orders (Landfield 1981, 1982). The apparent similarity of mechanisms of non-neural aging in many vertebrate species suggests that neural mechanisms may also be similar across species; however, such *a priori* arguments must of course be supported by empirical observations on the similarities and differences in brain aging patterns across species.

In this context, it is already clear that there are species differences in overt patterns of age-related brain change. Neuritic (senile) plaques are not generally found in aged rats, although they occur in humans, nonhuman primates, and dogs. Moreover, significant amounts of neurofibrillary tangles are only found in aging human brain (Wisniewski, Terry 1973). However, it appears useful to distinguish between detailed patterns of overt brain aging and broader categories of brain change in assessing brain aging analogies across species. That is, it seems likely that even if underlying mechanisms are precisely the same across species, the overt expressions of this process will differ, since these are presumably the result of interactions between the common underlying aging process and species-specific adaptations and pathological processes. Therefore, it appears more valuable to evaluate the degree of generality of brain aging processes based on broad categories of neural aging changes rather than upon the detailed patterns of expression.

For these reasons, then, this paper briefly surveys and compares data on several major correlates of brain aging, including neuronal loss, synaptic decline, and glial changes, for rats and other mammals.

In addition, a hypothesis on the relationship of SDAT to normal brain aging is proposed here. Although this problem has received considerable attention, it remains highly controversial. As noted, however, it is a key issue in determining whether spontaneously aging experimental animals are likely to be of value in the study of SDAT; this hypothesis therefore attempts to contribute to a framework for considering SDAT within the context of brain aging studies.

BRAIN AGING CHANGES IN MAMMALIAN SPECIES

Neuronal Density and Aging

Nerve cell loss is among the most widely cited correlates of human brain aging, but there have been a number of conflicting reports about whether the phenomenon is consistently found in normal aging. The initial quantitative studies of neocortex in which neuronal loss was found (Brody 1955) were followed by several studies that observed no age-related nerve cell loss in human subcortical nuclei (Konigsmark, Murphy 1972; Brody, Vijayashankar 1977), or in neocortex of aged rats (Brizzee et al 1968). More recent studies, however, have confirmed and clarified Brody's data on normal aging of the human brain. It now seems evident from numerous reports (Corsellis 1976; Tomlinson, Henderson 1976; Brizzee et al 1980; Terry at al 1981) that nerve cell loss does occur with normal aging in human and monkey cortical structures (including hippocampus and cerebellar cortex), but it is not generally found in subcortical nuclei. The pigmented nuclei (locus ceruleus, substantia nigra) are among the only human subcortical nuclei in which cell loss has been reported (Brody 1976; Mann, Yates 1979).

Nevertheless, while the issue of nerve cell loss in humans has been substantially clarified, the question of cell loss in rodent brain remains controversial. As noted, initial studies by Brizzee and colleagues (1968) did not find neuronal loss in the neocortex of aged rats. However, the aged group of rats was relatively young in that study, and methods of cell selection and quantification are also major factors in such analyses. Subsequently, in a study with older rats, Brizzee and Ordy (1979) did find age-related neuronal decreases in the neocortex of one strain of rats.

In several studies from our laboratory, we have found a clear decrease in neuronal density in the hippocampus (Landfield et al 1977, 1981a,b) and possibly the neocortex (Landfield et al 1977) of aged Fischer rats. Brizzee and Ordy (1979) have also seen an age-related decrease in hippocampal neuronal density in rats. Conversely, several recent experiments have not found evidence of age-dependent neuronal loss in other brain regions of rats, including dentate gyrus (Geinisman et al 1977), olfactory cortex (Hinds, McNelly 1980), or locus ceruleus (Goldman, Coleman 1981).

Measures of numerical cell density in a cortical structure can of course be influenced by subtle differences in the regions sampled, by alterations in cortical volume, and by changes in cell size. These considerations may be particularly relevant to the findings on hippocampal cell density, since there is evidence that hippocampal depth continues to increase with aging in rats (Diamond et al 1975; Lindsey et al 1979). Thus, the clear-cut decreases in hippocampal pyramidal cell density that we have observed in aging rats (Figure 1), both qualitatively and quantitatively (Landfield et al 1977, 1981a,b), could in part be due to increased hippocampal volume rather than to cell loss.

On the other hand, in recent studies in which we simultaneously counted neurons and measured hippocampal depth, we did not find consistent evidence that altered structural volume can account for age-related changes in neuronal density. Moreover, it seems unlikely that the age-related decline in neuronal density in the neocortex of rats (Brizzee, Ordy 1979) can be accounted for by increases in cortical volume, since neocortical depth appears to be reduced in aged rats (Diamond et al 1975). Nevertheless, until a complete analysis is performed, based on sections systematically taken throughout the entire length of the hippocampus, it will not be possible to rule out changes in structural volume, or to conclude with total confidence that neuronal loss occurs in hippocampus of aged rats. It seems of interest, however, that one of the few studies in aging rats in which sections were taken throughout an entire brain stucture (the medial nucleus of the trapezoid

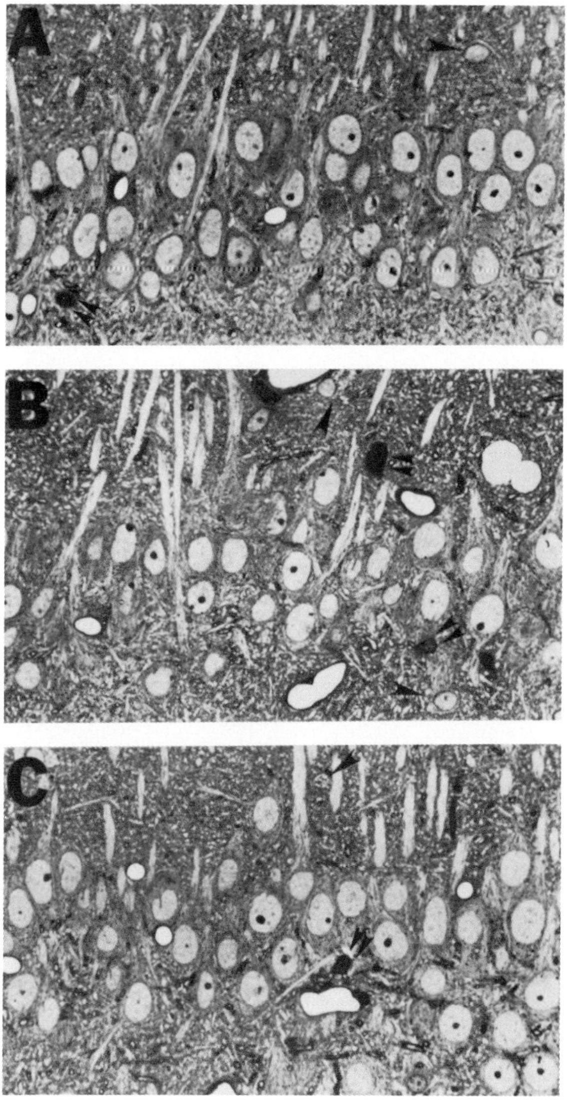

Fig. 1. (legend on next page)

Fig. 1. Examples of CA1 pyramidal cells in the somal layer in semithin sections from young rats (A), aged controls (B), and aged rats adrenalectomized 9 months earlier (C). Long-term adrenalectomy protects against the age-related decrease in neuronal density, and some aspects of increased glial reactivity. All sections are cut perpendicular to the somal layer, from the CA1 region just dorsal to the tip of the dorsal limb or the dentate gyrus granule cells. Neuronal nuclei and major glial species can be recognized - astrocytes with lucent cytoplasm (arrowheads) and the darker microglia and oligodendrocytes, with chromatin clumps in the nucleus (double arrowheads). From Landfield et al 1981a. Copyright 1981 by the AAAS.

---

body) found an age-related decrease in total neurons in that structure (Casey, Feldman 1982).

In summary then, the age-related increase in hippocampal volume does not seem large enough to account for decreased neuronal density during aging in rats, but this possibility has not yet been definitively ruled out. However, it seems unlikely that reported cell loss during aging in a subcortical auditory relay nucleus, and in neocortex, can be readily accounted for by structural volume changes. Conversely, there is evidence that neuronal loss does not occur with aging in a number of brain regions of the rat. At present, therefore, there appears to be evidence of neuronal loss with aging in some, but not all, regions of the rat brain; this pattern seems relatively analogous to that found in human aging studies.

Synaptic Density and Aging

The data regarding synaptic loss in the brains of aged animals are no more clear-cut than are the data on neuronal loss. Again, however, considerations of structural volume, comparable sampling fields, and corrections for unit size and shape, are of obvious relevance to the interpretation of findings.

The question of synaptic deterioration is of major importance in the assessment of rodent models, since ultrastructural studies have shown that degenerating axon terminals are the primary component of neuritic (senile) plaques (Terry, Wisniewski 1972; Wisniewski et al 1973; Terry, this symposium), and such plaques are one of the hallmarks of morphological aging changes in the brains of aged humans, monkeys and dogs, and humans with Alzheimer's disease (Wisniewski, Terry 1973). Using a Golgi method, Scheibel and Scheibel (1975) reported massive dendritic degeneration in cortical neurons from humans with SDAT. Golgi studies in animals have also generally found that dendrites appear to lose small branches and spines, and are reduced in extent, as a function of aging (Feldman 1976; Vaughan 1977; Mervis 1978). More recent Golgi analyses of human material, however, have suggested that neuronal dendrites may continue to grow with aging, although this growth process may cease in SDAT (Buell, Coleman 1979). Dendritic growth also appears to occur in normal adult brain in several species (Morest 1971), and we recently found that mean axon terminal volume may be larger in aging rats (Landfield et al 1982). These studies, then, emphasize that there may be different aspects of age-related dendritic or axonal change.

Electron microscopic studies are required to directly address the issues of synaptic density or deteroriation and, as noted, ultrastructural studies (Terry, Wisniewski 1972; Wisniewski et al 1973) have clearly pointed to deteriorating axon terminals as a key factor in neuritic plaque development.

However, quantitative E.M. studies in rodents have found evidence both for and against synaptic loss with aging. Feldman (1976) initially reported E.M. evidence of synaptic declines in the neocortex of aging rats. Subsequently, extensive studies by Geinisman et al (1977, 1978a) found quantitative ultrastructural evidence of a reduction in synaptic density in the dentate gyrus of aging rats. This finding was confirmed by one study (Hoff et al 1982), but not by another (Cotman, Scheff 1979).

In addition, a more recent analysis of the dentate gyrus, in which tissue volume and unit size were taken into account, found no evidence of synaptic loss or spine volume changes in the dentate gyrus of aged rats (Curcio, Hinds 1983). However, an electrophysiological analysis of the dentate gyrus in aging rats found that the extracellular excitatory postsynaptic potential (EPSP), which is an extracellular summation of EPSPs from individual cells, was reduced in aged rats (Barnes 1979). This result would be predicted if reduced synaptic density were present, although the animals in this electrophysiological study were quite aged.

In two recent and relatively extensive quantitative E.M. studies, we have also found consistent age-related reductions in synaptic density, in a well-defined region of the stratum radiatum of field CA1 in hippocampus of rats (MD Applegate, PW Landfield, unpublished observations; Landfield et al 1982). This region of the hippocampus is a site of dense termination of Schaffer collaterals and commissural afferents (Swanson et al 1978), in which the great majority of terminals are axospinous (Figure 2).

In addition, we found that the input-output curve for the extracellular field EPSP as a function of stimulation intensity in these same terminal fields is decreased with age (PW Landfield et al, unpublished observations). This electrophysiological observation is directly comparable to our morphological findings on decreased synaptic density, since the animals studied electrophysiologically and morphologically were of similar ages and of the same strain.

Other reports suggest that there may be a decline of synaptic density in the cerebellar cortex of aged rats (Glick, Bondareff 1979; Bertoni-Freddari, Giuli 1980), but not in the olfactory bulb (Hinds, McNelly 1980).

However, it should be emphasized that there are age-related functional alterations in synapses, as well as possible alterations in numerical density. For example, we have reported that, while many aspects of neurophysiology are relatively normal in hippocampus of aged rats, there is an age-related impairment in the frequency potentiation of monosynaptic responses during repetitive electrical stimulation (Landfield, Lynch 1977; Landfield et al 1978b). More recently, a similar phenomenon was found in synapses of neuromuscular junction of aged rats (Smith 1979). Recent intracellular studies in this laboratory using the hippocampal slice suggest that the age deficit in responsiveness to repetitive stimulation is presynaptic (Landfield et al 1983; Pitler, Landfield 1983).

In summary, it may be noted that E.M. studies of neuritic plaques strongly indicate that synaptic degeneration, at least in cortical structures, is a major correlate of primate brain aging in general, and is greatly increased in SDAT.

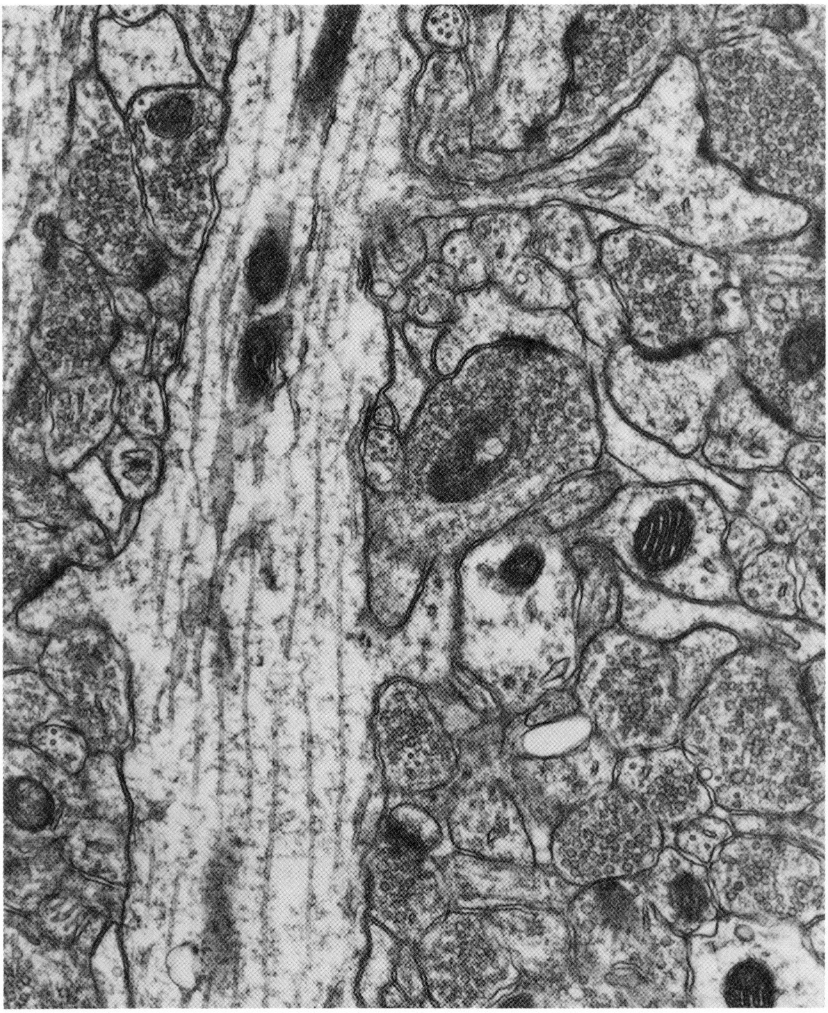

Fig. 2. Electron micrograph from the apical dendrites (stratum radiatum) of CA1 pyramidal cells in rat hippocampus. High density of synapses and a predominance of axospinous synaptic contacts over dendritic shaft contacts can be seen.

In rodents, neuritic plaques are not found, but in some brain regions there are consistent reports of a decline in synaptic density or in dendritic ramification. Because of the small amount of tissue sampled in the E.M. studies, however, particular care must be taken to ensure sampling from comparable regions, and controls for tissue volume and unit size must be included. At present, the data suggest that synaptic loss in some regions is a correlate of aging in rodents as well as in humans. However, there are a sufficient number of methodological problems involved to require caution and to hold open the possibility that some of these observed declines are due to increased tissue volume or reduced synaptic size, rather than to actual loss.

Glial Changes in the Aging Brain

In contrast to the studies on neuronal or synaptic density, there appears to be a relative degree of agreement on the glial changes that accompany brain aging in rodents. Moreover, the patterns of glial change seen in rodents are very similar to those seen in aged primates.

Early E.M. studies of neuritic plaques first noted that plaques were often surrounded by reactive cells, and that astrocytic processes were frequently seen in association with the plaques (Terry, Wisniewski 1972). However, until relatively recently there had been few studies that directly focused on glial changes during brain aging.

Brizzee et al (1968) initially reported an increase in glial cell density in the neocortex of aged rats, but it was unclear from the conventional light microscopic methods employed which classes of glial cells were responsible for the increase. Using quantitative and qualitative electron microscopy, Vaughan and Peters (1974) found that the numerical increase in glia was largely accounted for by increased microglia. Subsequently, we found evidence in semithin sections of a similar but less substantial microglial (or possibly dark oligodendroglial) increase in the hippocampus of aged rats (Landfield et al 1981b). Vaughan and Peters (1974) also described a variety of inclusions found in glial cells in aged rat brain in considerable detail, and interpreted some of those seen in the microglia to be remnants of degenerated synapses.

In addition to the microglial proliferation and glial inclusions noted above, we found, using a gold sublimate staining method, that astrocytes undergo major hypertrophy of the soma and processes in the hippocampus of normally aging rats (Landfield et al 1977), and that these changes have already begun by midlife (Lindsey et al 1979). Figure 3 shows the appearance of this hypertrophy. Although earlier studies had not found alterations in astrocytes in aging rats (Hasan, Glees 1973), the observation that astrocytes are hypertrophied in aging has now been confirmed for rats at the ultrastructural level (Landfield et al 1978a; Geinisman et al 1978b; MD Applegate, PW Landfield, unpublished observations), and in the hippocampus of aging monkeys (Brizzee et al 1980).

Metallic stains have also revealed that extensive astroglial hypertrophy is present in the brains of humans with SDAT (Schechter et al 1982), and the presence of astrocyte processes in plaques, which are found in the normal human elderly, suggests that some degree of glial reactivity also accompanies normal human aging.

Human and Animal Normal Brain Aging: Conclusions

There seems to be little doubt that decreased neuronal and synaptic density occurs in some regions of aged rat brain, but the evidence that this decrease is not due to tissue volume or unit size alterations does not yet seem conclusive, except in a very few studies.

Nonetheless, age-related glial changes appear extremely similar across species; this suggests that glial cells are reacting to an underlying pathological process in all species, or, alternatively, to an ongoing growth process, since dendritic growth apparently continues in the brains of adult animals (Morest 1971) and humans (Buell, Coleman 1979).

Despite some differences from the human pattern, then, there is little doubt that the brains of rodents change with age and that the synapse is a critical site of such change in both rodents and primates. Further, it seems likely that at least some of the reported density declines reflect neuronal or synaptic loss in rodent brain.

Thus, it appears that in rodents, as in humans, brain neurons undergo significant changes with aging, and these appear to be deleterious, to involve synaptic alterations, and to induce glial reactivity. Nerve cell loss appears to accompany these changes in some but not all brain regions in

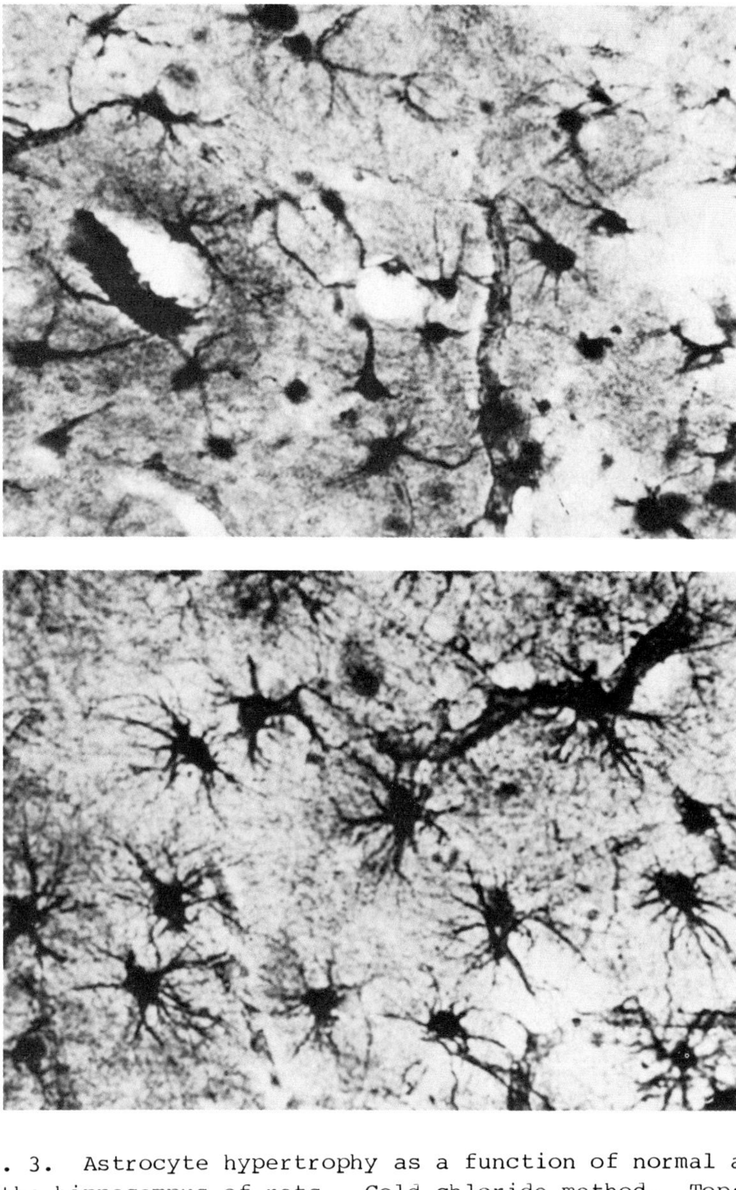

Fig. 3. Astrocyte hypertrophy as a function of normal aging in the hippocampus of rats. Gold chloride method. Top: Astrocytes from perforant path terminal fields of a young, mature rat. Bottom: Hypertrophied astrocytes from the same region of a healthy aged rat. Astrocyte changes can be seen as early as mid-life in rats.

rodents and humans. Since nerve cell loss is likely to be a late stage of deterioration, and therefore presumably dependent on interactions with numerous species-specific processes, it is perhaps not surprising that the topographical pattern of this loss may be different across species.

It appears, therefore, that there are considerable similarities between the processes of brain aging in rodents and humans, although there are also some clear differences in the detailed patterns of expression; moreover, some questions remain on the nature of the changes seen in rat brain. However, in conjunction with the evidence noted earlier that progressive patterns of non-neural senescence are generally similar across most vertebrate species (Finch 1976), the apparent similarity of some measures of brain aging suggests that the underlying mechanisms of brain aging are also shared by most mammalian species, including rats and humans. Thus, it seems likely that studies in aging rats, to the extent that they address fundamental mechanisms, will prove relevant to our understanding of the basic processes of normal mammalian brain aging in general.

A HYPOTHESIS ON THE RELATIONS OF NORMAL BRAIN AGING TO ALZHEIMER'S DISEASE

If the conclusion noted above (e.g., that studies of normal brain aging in one species are likely to be relevant to normal brain aging in other mammalian, or possibly all vertebrate, species) is correct, then the question of whether studies of aging animals may be relevant to Alzheimer's disease essentially reduces to the question of whether there is any overlap between Alzheimer's disease and normal brain aging in humans. At present, this is an unresolved and controversial issue. According to some views, SDAT is a neuropathological condition completely unrelated to brain aging, while other investigators suggest that SDAT is the extreme end of the continuum of normal brain aging changes. In the latter view, SDAT is seen as a state in which the accumulation of normal brain aging changes has reached a threshold of clinical dysfunction.

The arguments for considering SDAT to be an extreme form of normal brain aging have been extensively reviewed elsewhere (Wisniewski, Terry 1973; Tomlinson, Henderson 1976; Terry 1978). The major argument in favor of this view is that apparently all of the qualitative patterns of neuropathology found in SDAT are also seen (to considerably lesser extent) in the clinically normal elderly. By the ninth decade of life essentially all of the elderly exhibit some of the neuropathological changes associated with SDAT (Matsuyama, Nakamura 1978). Further, the brain topographical distribution of this pathology is the same in normal brain aging and in SDAT. Neuritic ("senile") plaques, which accompany SDAT, are also found in aged dogs and monkeys (Terry, Wisniewski 1972), species which are not generally thought to suffer from SDAT. A second argument in favor of considering SDAT to be somehow associated with normal aging is that the frequency of the disease increases rapidly above age 65. Estimates of the incidence of mild and severe SDAT combined range from 10-20% of the population above 65 years (Katzman et al 1978).

On the other hand, the primary argument against the view that SDAT is a continuation of normal aging is that the majority of the elderly are not affected by SDAT. In fact, once a substantially advanced age is reached, the incidence of SDAT appears to decline somewhat. Another argument against this view is that the neuropathology associated with SDAT is far too extensive to represent the simple accumulation of normal changes. Moreover, there is a clear evidence of genetic susceptibility to SDAT and there is increasing evidence that environmental factors (e.g., aluminum, viruses) may in some way be linked to SDAT-like neuropathology (Perl, Brody 1980; Wisniewski 1978).

In this section, a hypothesis is proposed which appears able to at least reconcile these main lines of evidence. Advancing a hypothesis on this problem, even at our early stage of knowledge, may be useful if it serves to more sharply define some of the unresolved issues and key questions on the relations between SDAT and normal aging.

A primary tenet of the hypothesis suggested here is that SDAT results from the interaction of some non-age-related etiological factor, either genetic or environmental, with the "machinery" of the normal brain aging process. As aging progresses, the machinery of brain aging becomes more susceptible to this etiological factor, and the result of the interaction is a "telescoping" of the normal brain aging process into a greatly reduced period. Thus, SDAT is not viewed as a continuation of normal aging, but rather as a distinct state in which the rate of brain aging is greatly accelerated.

Conversely, SDAT is not viewed as a process that is fully independent of normal aging, since its expression in some manner depends on an increase in brain aging processes.

This view can apparently account for the qualitative similarities between pathological patterns of brain aging and SDAT, for the great disparity in the quantitative expression of these pattern manifestations, and for the observation that most of the elderly are never affected by severe SDAT.

However, if SDAT does represent a telescoping of normal brain aging, then it appears that the potential for a remarkable degree of age-related neuropathology is present in the human brain. In turn, this potential for pathological change suggests that some inhibitory mechanism normally operates to hold the development of neuropathology in check. In this view, therefore, normal brain aging involves the gradual weakening of a pathology-inhibiting, or cellular "defense," mechanism. At some point this pathology-retarding mechanism may bcome sufficiently susceptible, and simultaneously be exposed to an interaction with deleterious genetic or environmental factors, so that the mechanism is rapidly rather than gradually disrupted, resulting in "runaway" brain aging (i.e., in SDAT).

Wisniewski and Terry (1973) have drawn attention to an analogy between SDAT and cancer, in that the probability of both is substantially increased by aging, but not all of the elderly are affected by either. In addition, there is another characteristic of cancer that seems to share something in common with SDAT; that is, cancer bears many qualitative similarities to a normal biological process (e.g., cell proliferation), but is by definition a quantitatively extreme example of the cell division process. Considerable evidence suggests that many cancers result from damage to genes that normally repress the expression of oncogenic potential; such damage can result from either genetic fragility or from environmental factors (Yunis 1983). Since SDAT is also a quantitatively extreme state that qualitatively resembles what can be viewed as a normal biological process (brain aging), and since SDAT has been suggested to result from either genetic or environmental factors, the analogy with cancer seems reasonably close. However, there is at least one notable conceptual distinction between cancer and SDAT, which is that cancer appears to be an uncontrolled form of development and growth (e.g., cell proliferation), while SDAT resembles an uncontrolled form of aging and decline (e.g., cell or synaptic death).

This is of course not the first hypothesis to suggest that SDAT represents an acceleration of normal brain aging. For example, Appel (1981) recently proposed the interesting view, which is elaborated further in this symposium, that neuronal decline occurs during normal aging due to the gradual loss of peptide trophic factors, and that this loss is substantially accelerated in SDAT and other neuropathological conditions by intrinsic neuronal properties. However, since neural trophic influences, either chemical or electrical, could well be important in the maintenance of pathology-retarding mechanisms, these hypotheses of SDAT as accelerated brain aging are clearly not mutually exclusive.

Thus, if the viewpoints and the evidence on which they are based, suggesting that SDAT and normal human brain aging are qualitatively similar, are correct, it may be feasible to use animal models to examine aspects of SDAT-like neuropathology which overlap with components of normal brain aging. Recent experiments have in fact used aged monkeys to examine the nature and origins of neuritic plaques (Struble et al 1982; Coyle et al 1983; Price, this symposium).

STUDIES ON THE MODIFICATION OF BRAIN AGING IN RATS

The conclusions reached in earlier sections on the relevance of rodent models of brain aging are of course tentative, since the data are not yet definitive. However, if correct, there may be significant implications of recent studies indicating that the rate of brain aging in rats may be subject to experimental modification.

During the past several years, our laboratory has been pursuing studies on the brain effects of long-term (8-9 months) experimental alterations of physiological processes in aging rats. These long-term studies have been aimed at testing specific hypotheses on etiological mechanisms of brain aging (Landfield 1978; Landfield et al 1981a), and we view the ability to alter the rate of brain aging by an appropriate treatment to be an essential test of such hypotheses. In these experiments we found that the patterns and rate of brain aging in rats can apparently be altered by several experimental treatments (e.g., Figure 1C). Among the factors that appear effective in this regard are glucocorticoid alterations (Landfield 1978; Landfield et al 1979, 1981a; Figure 1C), a neurally-active peptide analog of an adrenocorticotropin fragment (ORG 2766), and low doses of the well-established neural stimulant, pentylenetetrazol (PTZ) (Landfield et al 1981a). The data suggest that endogenous steroids, and possibly peptides, as well as neural activity, may normally regulate brain aging. The effect of the neural stimulant PTZ raises the possibility that there may be trophic effects of neural activity _per se_ which counteract brain aging (Landfield et al 1981a). This observation may be the electrical counterpart to the evidence that loss of chemical trophic substances could play a role in neuropathology (Appel 1981; this symposium).

The results obtained in our long-term paradigms provide evidence that brain aging in rats is not an immutable or inexorable process. Clearly, if similar mechanisms of brain aging operate across mammalian species, then these and other data raise the possibility that human brain aging may also be labile, and consequently, subject to modification by chronic treatments.

In addition, if SDAT does eventually prove to be a form of accelerated brain aging (though possibly initiated by interactions of brain aging with non-age-related etiological factors), then methods that are capable of modifying the course of normal brain aging may also be able to modify accelerated brain aging (SDAT). Finally, it may be noted that if normal brain aging can be slowed, then the period of susceptibility to SDAT might also be substantially postponed.

REFERENCES

Appel SH (1981. A unifying hypothesis for the cause of amyotrophic lateral sclerosis, parkinsonism and Alzheimer's disease. Ann Neurol 10:499.

Barnes CA (1979). Memory deficits associated with senescence: A neurophysiological and behavioral study in the rat. J Comp Physiol Psychol 93:74.

Bertoni-Freddari C, Giuli C (1980). A quantitative morphometric study of synapses of rat cerebellar glomeruli during aging. Mech Ageing Dev 12:127.

Brizzee KR, Ordy JM (1979). Age pigments, cell loss and hippocampal function. Mech Ageing Dev 9:143.

Brizzee KR, Ordy JM, Bartus RT (1980). Localization of cellular changes within multimodal sensory regions in aged monkey brain: Possible implications for age-related cognitive loss. Neurobiol Aging 1:45.

Brizzee KR, Sherwood N, Timiras PS (1968). A comparison of cell populations at various depths in cerebral cortex of young adult and aged Long-Evans rats. J Gerontol 23:289.

Brody H (1955). Organization of the cerebral cortex. III. A study of aging in the human cerebral cortex. J Comp Neurol 102:511.

Brody H (1976). An examination of cerebral cortex and brain stem aging. In Terry RD, Gershon S (eds): "Neurobiology of Aging," New York: Raven Press, p 171.

Brody H, Vijayashankar N (1977). Anatomical changes in the nervous system. In Finch CE, Hayflick L (eds): "Handbook of the Biology of Aging," New York: Van Nostrand Reinhold, p 241.

Buell SJ, Coleman PD (1979). Dendritic growth in aged human brain and failure of growth in senile dementia. Science 206:854.

Burek JD, Hollander CF (1980). Experimental gerontology. In Baker HJ, Lindsey JR, Weisbroth SH (eds): "The Laboratory Rat," Vol II, New York: Academic Press, p 149.

Casey MA, Feldman ML (1982). Aging in the rat medial nucleus of the trapezoid body. I. Light microscopy. Neurobiol Aging 3:187.

Corsellis JAN (1976). Some observations on the Purkinje cell population and on brain volume in human aging. In Terry RD, Gershon S (eds): "Neurobiology of Aging," New York: Raven Press, p 205.

Cotman CW, Scheff SW (1979). Compensatory synapse growth in aged animals after neuronal death. Mech Ageing Dev 9:103.

Coyle JT, Price DL, DeLong MR (1983). Alzheimer's disease: A disorder of cortical cholinergic innervation. Science 219:1184.

Curcio CA, Hinds JW (1983). Stability of synaptic density and spine volume in dentate gyrus of aged rats. Neurobiol Aging 4:77.

Diamond MC, Johnson RE, Ingham C (1975). The development, adult and aging patterns of the cerebral cortex, hippocampus and diencephalon. Behav Biol 14:163.

Feldman ML (1976). Aging changes in the morphology of cortical dendrites. In Terry R, Gershon S (eds): "Neurobiology of Aging," New York: Raven Press, p 211.

Finch CE (1976). The regulation of physiological changes during mammalian aging. Q Rev Biol 51:49.

Geinisman Y, Bondareff W, Dodge JT (1977). Partial deafferentation of neurons in the dentate gyrus of the senescent rat. Brain Res 134:541.

Geinisman Y, Bondareff W, Dodge JT (1978a). Dendritic atrophy in the dentate gyrus of the senescent rat. Am J Anat 152:321.

Geinisman Y, Bondareff W, Dodge JT (1978b). Hypertrophy of astroglial processes in the dentate gyrus of the senescent rat. Am J Anat 153:537.

Gibson DC, Adelman RC, Finch CE (1978). "Development of the Rodent as a Model System of Aging." Book II. (DHEW Publication No. 79-161), Bethesda, Maryland: National Institutes of Health.

Glick R, Bondareff W (1979). Loss of synapses in the cerebellar cortex of the senescent rat. J Gerontol 34:818.

Goldman G, Coleman PD (1981). Neuron numbers in locus coeruleus do not change with age in Fishcher 344 rat. Neurobiol Aging 2:33.

Hasan M, Glees P (1973). Ultrastructural changes in hippocampal neurons, synapses and neuroglia. Exp Gerontol 8:75.

Hinds JW, McNelly NA (1980). Correlation of aging changes in the olfactory epithelium and olfactory bulb of the rat. Soc Neurosci Abstr 6:739.

Hoff SF, Scheff SW, Bernardo LS, Cotman CW (1982). Lesion-induced synaptogenesis in the dentate gyrus of aged rats. I. Loss and reacquisition of normal synaptic density. J Comp Neurol 205:246.

Katzman R, Terry RD, Bick KL (1978). "Alzheimer's Disease: Senile Dementia and Related Disorders." New York: Raven Press.

Konigsmark BW, Murphy EA (1972). Volume of the ventral cochlear nucleus in man: Its relationship to neuronal population and age. J Neuropathol Exp Neurol 31:304.

Landfield PW (1978). An endocrine hypothesis of brain aging and studies on brain-endocrine correlations and monosynaptic neurophysiology during aging. In Finch CE, Potter D, Kenny A (eds): "Parkinson's Disease--II: Aging and Neuroendocrine Relationships," New York: Plenum Press, p 179.

Landfield PW (1981). Adrenocortical hypotheses of brain and somatic aging. In Schimke RT (ed): "Biological Mechanisms of Aging," (NIH Publication No. 81-2194), Bethesda, Maryland: National Institutes of Health, p 658.

Landfield PW (1982). Measurement of brain aging: Conceptual issues and neurobiological indices. In Adelman R, Roth G (eds): "Endocrine and Neuroendocrine Mechanisms of Aging," Boca Raton, Florida: CRC Press, p 183.

Landfield PW, Applegate MD, Pitler TA (1982). Increased synaptic density in hippocampus of aging rats chronically treated with a neural stimulant. Soc Neurosci Abstr 8:439.

Landfield PW, Baskin RK, Pitler TA (1981a). Brain aging correlates: Retardation by hormonal-pharmacological treatments. Science 214:581.

Landfield PW, Braun LD, Pitler TA, Lindsey JD, Lynch G (1981b). Hippocampal aging in rats: A morphometric study of multiple variables in semithin sections. Neurobiol Aging 2:265.

Landfield PW, Lindsey J, Braun L, Wurtz C, Maxwell M, Lynch G (1978a). Quantitative E.M. and semithin studies on synaptic vesicles and degeneration, astrocyte reactivity, microglia, lipofuscin and displaced nucleoli in hippocampal neurons of rat during aging. Proc Gerontol Soc 31:92.

Landfield PW, Lynch G (1977). Impaired monosynaptic potentiation in _in vivo_ hippocampal slices from aged, memory-deficient rats. J Gerontol 32:523.

Landfield PW, McGaugh JL, Lynch G (1978b). Impaired synaptic potentiation processes in the hippocampus of aged, memory-deficient rats. Brain Res 150:85.

Landfield PW, Pitler TA, Applegate MD, Robinson JH (1983). Intracellular studies of the age-related deficit in hippocampal frequency potentiation: Apparent calcium saturation in synapses of aged rats. Soc Neurosci Abstr 9.

Landfield PW, Rose G, Sandles L, Wohlstadter T, Lynch G (1977). Patterns of astroglial hypertrophy and neuronal degeneration in the hippocampus of aged, memory-deficient rats. J Gerontol 32:3.

Landfield PW, Wurtz C, Lindsey JD, Lynch G (1979). Long-term adrenalectomy reduces some morphological correlates of brain aging. Soc Neurosci Abstr 5:20.

Lindsey JD, Landfield PW, Lynch G (1979). Early onset and topographical distribution of hypertrophied astrocytes in hippocampus of aging rats. A quantitative study. J Gerontol 34:661.

Mann DMA, Yates PO (1979). The effect of ageing in the pigmented nerve cells of the human locus coeruleus and substantia nigra. Acta Neuropathol 47:93.

Matsuyama H, Nakamura S (1978). Senile changes in the brain in the Japanese: Incidence of Alzheimer's neurofibrillary change and senile plaques. In Katzman R, Terry RD, Bick KL (eds): "Alzheimer's Disease: Senile Dementia and Related Disorders," New York: Raven Press, p 287.

Mervis R (1978). Structural alterations in neurons of aged canine neocortex: A Golgi study. Exp Neurol 62:417.

Morest DK (1971). Dendrodendritic synapses of cells that have axons: The fine structure of the Golgi Type II cell in the medial geniculate body of the cat. Z Anat Entwickl-Gesch 133:216.

National Academy of Sciences (1981). "Mammalian Models for Research on Aging." Washington, DC: National Academy Press.

Perl DP, Brody AR (1980). Alzheimer's disease: X-ray spectrometric evidence of aluminum accumulation in neurofibrillary tangle-bearing neurons. Science 208:297.

Pitler TA, Landfield PW (1983). Intracellular studies of hippocampal frequency potentiation: Evidence for a presynaptic, residual Ca^{2+} mechanism. Soc Neurosci Abstr 9.

Schechter R, Yen S-H, Terry RD (1982). Fibrous astrocytes in senile dementia of the Alzheimer's type. J Neuropathol Exp Neurol 53:413.

Scheibel ME, Scheibel AB (1975). Structural changes in the aging brain. In Brody H, Harman D, Ordy JM (eds): "Clinical, Morphologic, and Neurochemical Aspects in the Aging Central Nervous System," [Aging, Vol 1], New York: Raven Press, p 11.

Smith DO (1979). Reduced capabilities of synaptic transmission in aged rats. Exp Neurol 66:650.

Struble RG, Cork LC, Whitehouse PJ, Price DL (1982). Cholinergic innervation in neuritic plaques. Science 216:413.

Swanson LW, Wyss JM, Cowan WM (1978). An autoradiographic study of the organization of intrahippocampal association pathways in the rat. J Comp Neurol 181:681.

Terry RD (1978). Aging, senile dementia and Alzheimer's disease. In Katzman R, Terry RD, Bick KL (eds): "Alzheimer's Disease: Senile Dementia and Related Disorders," New York: Raven Press, p 11.

Terry RD, Peck A, DeTeresa R, Schechter R, Horoupian DS (1981). Some morphometric aspects of the brain in senile dementia of the Alzheimer's type. Ann Neurol 10:184.

Terry RD, Wisniewski HM (1972). Ultrastructure of senile dementia and of experimental analogs. In Gaitz CM (ed): "Aging and the Brain," New York: Plenum Press, p 89.

Tomlinson BE, Henderson G (1976). Some quantitative cerebral findings in normal and demented old people. In Terry RD, Gershon S (eds): "Neurobiology of Aging," New York: Raven Press, p 183.

Vaughan DW (1977). Age-related deterioration of pyramidal cell basal dendrites in rat auditory cortex. J Comp Neurol 171:501.

Vaughn DW, Peters A (1974). Neuroglial cells in the cerebral cortex of rats from young adulthood to old age: An electron microscope study. J Neurocytol 3:405.

Wisniewski HM (1978). Possible viral etiology of neurofibrillary changes and neuritic plaques. In Katzman R, Terry RD, Bick KL (eds): "Alzheimer's Disease: Senile Dementia and Related Disorders," New York: Raven Press, p 555.
Wisniewski HM, Ghetti B, Terry RD (1973). Neuritic (senile) plaques and filamentous changes in rhesus monkeys. J Neuropathol Exp Neurol 32:566.
Wisniewski HM, Terry RD (1973). Morphology of the aging brain, human and animal. In Ford DM (ed): "Progress in Brain Research," Vol 40, Amsterdam: Elsevier/North Holland, p 167.
Yunis JJ (1983). The chromosomal basis of human neoplasia. Science 221:227.

DISCUSSION

DR. GLEISER: What do you call an aging rat and what do you call an aged rat?

DR. LANDFIELD: I guess an aging rat is one that is on the way to becoming aged.

DR. GLEISER: At what point in time is a rat considered aged?

DR. LANDFIELD: A rat is generally viewed as aged at about 25 months old, but anywhere from perhaps 22 months to 30 months can be considered aged, depending upon whether one wishes to look at very extreme aging, which makes statistical analysis easier, or whether one wishes to examine the onset of these changes, which may provide clues to etiology.

DR. PARKER: Did you weigh the rat brain in your studies?

DR. LANDFIELD: Unfortunately, we have not done the volumetric analyses that we need to do to resolve some of these questions. If we had known that brain growth with aging might be a problem, we would have studied this as we went along. However, a conclusive answer will very likely be available within a few years, either from us or another laboratory.

DR. APPEL: I am not clear on what synapse or group of synapses you are referring to specifically within the hippocampus.

DR. LANDFIELD: Our research has focused on the Schaffer collaterals arising from CA 3 pyramidal cells, which probably use glutamate as a transmitter. These fibers terminate in the middle regions of the apical dendrites of CA 1 pyramids.

DR. APPEL: Your profiles showed a decrease in synaptic density, a decrease in vesicle density and an increase in synaptic terminal area which by analogy with the periphery would suggest that the major brunt of the deficit is presynaptic as opposed to postsynaptic. Would you comment on that?

DR. LANDFIELD: I didn't show our data on functional changes, but we are also performing extensive electrophysiological studies of these same synapses which suggest that there are functional changes in synaptic physiology apart from changes in number. These changes appear to be presynaptic. With regard to structure, the decrease in synaptic density implies a decrease in spines as well as a decrease in terminals. There does appear to be an increase in mean presynaptic terminal area with aging. For technical reasons, however, we do not yet have good data on spine area. Regarding vesicle density, I do not put much emphasis on data collected under these sacrifice conditions. Vesicle density is extremely labile, depending on how the animals are killed, how they are fixed, how aroused they are, and so on and we need additional information on this problem. In summary, while we have data from several lines of research that point to a presynaptic locus as being of particular importance, our findings do not yet rule out the possibility that major postsynaptic changes may also occur.

Comparative Pathobiology of Major Age-Related Diseases: Current Status and Research Frontiers, pages 357–371

ALZHEIMER'S DISEASE

Robert D. Terry, M.D.

Professor and Chairman, Department of Neuropathology, Albert Einstein College of Medicine, The Bronx, NY 10461

One of the most frightening aspects of old age is the very real possibility of becoming senile. Senile dementia (SD) is clearly an age-related disorder, rare in the 50's and 60's, but increasingly common through the 70's and 80's such that nearly 25% of people in their ninth decade of life will manifest it significantly (Gruenberg 1960-1961). One Scandinavian group (CG Gottfries, personal communication) has found that the prevalence continues to rise into the tenth decade, reaching about 45%, but another (Hagnell et al 1981) has noted a fall-off in that age group, probably as a survivor phenomenon. Just as we find few ninety-year-old diabetics, so it is with senile dementia; most of those who will get it have already done so, and have died. There are close to a quarter million deaths per year related to SD in the United States. It is said that about 60% of nursing home beds in this country are occupied by patients with SD. The current cost of nursing home care is close to 25 billion dollars a year, and therefore the annual cost of institutional senile dementia must be about 15 billion.

The disorder is devastating to the patient, and all too often ruinous to his family. It is characterized by loss of memory, initiative, judgment, ability to calculate, to orient oneself in space and time, and to find appropriate words. It usually progresses quite steadily over a period of years, ultimately reducing the patient to a vegetative state before he is carried off by an intercurrent infection, a vascular episode, or some other incidental disease. One might postulate a causal relationship between the most common dementing process and the final non-neurologic disorder: the hypothalamus is involved in the former, thus altering immune function (Cross et al 1980), stress resistance and nutrition.

Senile dementia is a class of disorders including especially senile dementia of the Alzheimer type (SDAT), which accounts for 50 to 60% of cases and is essentially identical to the classical pre-senile form; multi-infarct dementia due to cerebrovascular disease, accounting for 20 to 25%; and a large group of infectious, metabolic, and neoplastic diseases each of which can occasionally cause dementia (Tomlinson 1977). SDAT is by far the most important member of the class, and it is with this subject that we are concerned.

Individuals in at least two nonhuman species seem to become senile, and this may be on a basis similar to that of Alzheimer's disease. Aged dogs (Wisniewski et al 1970), at least of some breeds, often display loss of memory, disorientation in time, and a decreasing retention of their former training. Old monkeys (Wisniewski et al 1973) display an arcus senilis, and thin papery skin with gray hair. They retreat to the back of the cage, and are much less vivacious than earlier. Psychologic deficits have been measured (Bartus et al 1982). Their pathologic similarities to Alzheimer's disease are discussed below.

Aside from these monkeys and dogs, this writer is unaware of any other spontaneous models of senile dementia at all similar to Alzheimer's among domestic or laboratory animals. Old specimens in the wild state must be very rare since they would fall to predators. Only to a very limited extent can one induce in laboratory animals some of the organic abnormalities characteristic of SDAT.

It is the purpose of this presentation to demonstrate the structural and morphometric aspects, to touch on the biochemical alterations in Alzheimer's disease, and to discuss briefly some of those aspects of the aged or experimentally altered animal brain which resemble particular aspects of Alzheimer's disease.

In the course of normal aging the human brain undoubtedly shrinks to a certain extent. Measurements based simply on large autopsy series have not been very satisfactory for several reasons: there is a wide range of normal weight; many patients entering the series might not have been clinically normal; there is known to have been an increase in normal brain weight during the past century (Corsellis 1978). The best way to assay brain size is somewhat awkward, involving measurement of the volume of the cranial cavity for comparison with the volume of the brain. It has been found that in youth the brain occupies 92% of the cavity (Davis, Wright 1977), whereas in normal aging this decreases to about 84%. There is an additional 8% loss in the presence of SDAT (Hubbard, Anderson 1981). If one simply compares the average brain weight of a group of SDAT patients between ages 70 and 90 with similarly aged normal counterparts, there is about a 10% difference (Terry et al 1981).

This weight loss has a counterpart noted on sectioning the brain, where in normal aging there is a variable, mild dilatation of the ventricles, shrinkage of white matter, and narrowing of cortex. All these changes are somewhat exaggerated in SDAT, but none provides a diagnostic feature with statistically significant difference. The gray-to-white ratio is approximately the same in SDAT as in the age-matched normals (AMN) (Miller et al 1980). Shrinkage of the aged animal brain has not been thoroughly examined.

Age-related loss of neurons from the CNS is not uniform throughout the brain. Several cranial nerve nuclei (Van Buskirk 1945; Konigsmark, Murphy 1972; Vijayashankar, Brody 1973) and the inferior olivary nucleus (Monagle, Brody 1974) of the medulla maintain normal populations throughout life span. On the other hand, the locus ceruleus (Vijayashankar, Brody 1979), the major source of norepinephrine; the substantia nigra (McGeer et al 1977), the source of dopamine; the spinal cord (Tomlinson, Irving 1977), the cerebellar cortex (Corsellis 1976), the putamen (Bugiani et al 1978), and the cerebral cortex (Brody 1955; Henderson et al 1980) all lose neurons. Brody's hand tallies of the cerebral neocortex indicate a loss of as much as 54% from the superior temporal gyrus in the course of normal aging. Other parts of the neocortex and the paleocortex also undergo this decremental process but to a somewhat lesser extent. Brody emphasized the particular loss of small neurons, although our own data (RD Terry, R DeTeresa, unpublished observations) and that of Henderson et al (1980) are not in agreement on this point since we found large neurons to be more vulnerable. These are the neurons which are greater than 90 microns square in cross section, as we see them in paraffin sections. In SDAT there is an additional loss which, in the mid-frontal, superior temporal, and inferior parietal area ranges from 35% to 45%, almost exclusively among the large neurons (Terry et al 1981). This work compared cases of SDAT aged 70-90 with age-matched normals. It is not known whether susceptible cells are from a uniform group in terms of transmitter or receptor, but the cell loss, significant among large neurons at a p value less than 0.001, is additive to that of normal aging.

There are no significant differences between the average counts of small neurons (cells 40 - 90 μ^2) or of glial cells (5 - 40 μ^2) in these two groups (Terry et al 1981). However, the composition of the cortical glial population is altered in SDAT. It has been found that there are about four times as many fibrous astrocytes in the neocortex in SDAT as in the AMN controls (Schechter et al 1981). Since the total number of glia has not changed, we must assume that there has been a transformation from the normal protoplasmic type to the fibrous type of astrocyte. The loss of neurons and the fibrous astrocytosis result in a disruption and disorganization of the cortex, as well as a simple decrement.

Two transmitter-specific areas of the brain suffer particular cell loss in SDAT. The basal nucleus of Meynert in the substantia innominata undergoes very severe loss of its cholinergic, cortical projecting neurons (Whitehouse et al 1981). This will be discussed in greater detail by Dr. Price. Also affected is the noradrenergic locus ceruleus which in many, if not all, cases of advanced Alzheimer's disease, demonstrates a significant loss of pigmented neurons (Bondareff et al 1981; Perry et al 1981). The cortex in SDAT reflects losses from these two areas in that it is severely deficient in choline acetyltransferase (ChAT) (Davies, Maloney 1976; Perry et al 1977; White et al 1977) and often in norepinephrine (Mann et al 1980; Cross et al 1981). Based on therapeutic trials (Drachman, Leavitt 1974; Thal et al 1983), we have reason to believe that the cholinergic deficiency is the more significant one, especially since the number of cortical muscarinic receptor sites is normal (Davies, Maloney 1976). At this time, there is no general agreement about the effects of normal aging on the concentration of choline acetyltransferase or of cholinergic receptors in the human or rodent (Bartus et al 1982).

In any case, it must be kept in mind that the cause of the pharmacologic deficiency in SDAT and the penultimate cause of the disease is loss of neurons in particular parts of the brain. The reasons for neuronal death as a part of normal aging are probably different from those in SDAT, but in either situation the cause or causes might well come from one or more of the following seven general classes:

1. A genetic program of pre-determined cell death. Alzheimer's disease, in a small percentage of cases, is indeed familial, being expressed as a simple Mendelian dominant (Cook et al 1979). Most cases, however, are sporadic although a sizeable portion of these have at least one first-order relative involved with a similar disease.

2. Failure of a maintenance or trophic factor analogous to nerve growth factor. While this has been hypothesized for Alzheimer's disease (Appel 1981), we have no evidence for it. Furthermore, this reasoning simply puts the question back one step as to which cells are failing to produce the maintenance factor.

3. Autoimmunity. An anti-brain serum factor has been demonstrated to increase with age and with the presence of Alzheimer's disease (Nandy 1977), but its cytotoxicity and specificity are still uncertain at this time. Furthermore, tissue inflammation is lacking and serum changes are inconsistent.

4. An endogenous toxin such as lysolecithin or an analogue of a neurotransmitter such as 6-HT might be formed by an error of metabolism. Again, this has not been demonstrated.

5. An exogenous toxic factor, such as aluminum, has been suggested. Some investigators have demonstrated an increase in aluminum in SDAT brain tissue (Crapper et al 1973; Perl, Brody 1980), while others have found it to be present in normal concentrations in these cases (Markesbery et al 1981). The difference may depend upon the environmental concentration of the metal.

6. An unconventional "slow" virus. Transmission studies on nonhuman primates were originally reported to be positive in two of six familial cases, but not in any sporadic cases (Gibbs, Gajdusek 1978). The report of the positive transmission has, however, been retracted (Goudsmit et al 1980). At this time there is no direct evidence of a transmissible factor responsible for SDAT.

7. Abnormally increased peroxidation of cell membranes. This should cause increased lipofuscin, which is not the case in SDAT (Mann, Sinclair 1978).

There are two major histologic lesions which have been

used since Alzheimer's time to make the anatomical diagnosis of Alzheimer's disease. The first is the neurofibrillary tangle, which involves the perikarya of large and medium sized neurons in the cerebral cortex, innominata, amygdaloid, hypothalamus, and mesencephalic and pontine tegmentum. In patients older than 75, one finds many cases without neocortical tangles (Constantinidis 1978; Terry et al 1982). The second lesion is the neuritic or senile plaque, found in the neuropil of the same locations, but relatively uncommon in the basal nucleus. A few plaques are found in most aged normals.

The tangle is made up of argentophilic, congophilic fibers coursing through the neuronal cytoplasm. At electron microscopic magnifications, each fiber is seen to be made up of a pair of helically wound 100 A filaments, crossing over each other at about 800 A intervals (Kidd 1963; Wisniewski et al 1976). The presence of side arms on these structures has been debated since they are not usually apparent with the standard fixation methods. These paired helical filaments (PHF) are very insoluble, and this insolubility in beta-mercaptoethanol, SDS, etc., accounts for the electrophoretic patterns of SDAT tissue being identical to those of normal controls (Selkoe et al 1982). Selkoe has suggested that the reason for the insolubility is that they are covalently linked by means of a glutamyl-lysine moiety induced by transglutaminase. Now, however, isolates of PHF are being attacked vigorously with more powerful solvents in order to study the products of their partial and total dissolution. Some antisera made against normal brain tissue and against normal neurofilament proteins react with at least some tangles (Gambetti et al 1980; Yen et al 1981; Anderton et al 1982). This may indicate a partial identity or that many shared sites are blocked in PHF, or that the tangles contain a consistent contaminant.

Aluminum salts and metallic aluminum placed in the subarachnoid space of several animal species cause the multiplication of normal neurofilaments in certain neuronal cell bodies (Klatzo et al 1965; Terry, Pena 1965). These have the superficial appearance of neurofibrillary tangles, but are in fact made up of biochemically and immunocytochemically normal filaments (Liem et al 1978). Several mitotic inhibitors, the best known of which is colchicine, produce similar results, best seen in cultured nervous tissue (Wisniewski et al 1968).

A very few clusters of PHF have been reported in the aged monkey (Wisniewski et al 1973), but these have a period about half that found in the human. The giant neurons of the whip spider's extremities have also been found to contain twisted filaments each about 60 A thick and with a half period of about 180 A (Foelix, Hauser 1979). It can be said, therefore, that there is not a very satisfactory animal model of Alzheimer's neurofibrillary tangle.

The neuritic plaque, as stained by any one of a number of silver impregnations or with thioflavine S, is made up of a central core of amyloid surrounded by a halo of filaments and granules. Electron microscopy confirms the filamentous amyloid core, and shows that the surrounding structures are primarily pre-synaptic unmyelinated terminals, which are enlarged because of their content of PHF, lamellar lysosomes, and degenerating mitochondria (Terry et al 1964). A few post-synaptic boutons may be involved (Terry, Wisniewski 1970). The synaptic gap and membranes are usually normal, even where the bouton is markedly affected (Gonatas et al 1967). Some of these pre-synaptic boutons are presumed to come from cells of the innominata, since they stain for acetylcholinesterase (Perry et al 1980; Struble et al 1982). Golgi preparations have shown that nearby neurons also participate in the composition of the plaque, sending short dystrophic dendrites into it (Probst et al 1983). The amyloid in the center of the plaque has been identified as containing many different products including immunoglobulins (Ishii et al 1975), pre-albumin (Shirahama et al 1982), and APUD-amyloid (Powers, Spicer 1978).

Plaques are found in the neocortex of aged dogs (Wisniewski et al 1970) and monkeys (Wisniewski et al 1973), but they are not common in these species. In the nonhuman brains, the plaques contain amyloid and abnormal boutons, with degenerating mitochondria and lamellar lysosomes. In short, the plaques here are identical to those in the human except that they lack the PHF.

Of perhaps greater interest is the fact that plaques can be induced in susceptible strains of mice inoculated intracerebrally with extracts of certain genetic strains of scrapie (Bruce, Fraser 1975; Wisniewski et al 1975). Again these plaques are identical to those of the human but for the absence of PHF. This experimental model provides at this time the only link between SDAT and a possible transmissible etiology.

In conclusion, one can point out that while Alzheimer's disease has clinical, genetic, structural, and biochemical aspects, the animal models resemble it only very partially. While these models have, therefore, some utility, the major source of experimental material remains as human tissue gained through autopsy.

REFERENCES

Anderton BH, Breinburg D, Downes MJ, Green PJ, Tomlinson BE, Ulrich J, Wood JN, Kahn J (1982). Monoclonal antibodies show that neurofibrillary tangles and neurofilaments share antigenic determinants. Nature 298:84.

Appel SH (1981). A unifying hypothesis for the cause of amyotrophic lateral sclerosis, Parkinsonism, and Alzheimer's disease. Ann Neurol 10:499.

Bartus RT, Dean RL III, Beer B, Lippa AS (1982). The cholinergic hypothesis of geriatric memory dysfunction. Science 217:408.

Bondareff W, Mountjoy CQ, Roth M (1981). Selective loss of neurones of origin of adrenergic projection to cerebral cortex (nucleus locus coeruleus) in senile dementia. Lancet I:783.

Brody H (1955). Organization of the cerebral cortex. III. A study of aging in the human cerebral cortex. J Comp Neurol 102:511.

Bruce ME, Fraser H (1975). Amyloid plaques in the brains of mice infected with scrapie: Morphological variation and staining properties. Neuropathol Appl Neurobiol 1:189.

Bugiani O, Salvarani S, Perdelli F, Mancardi GL, Leonardi A (1978). Nerve cell loss with aging in the putamen. Eur Neurol 17:286.

Constantinidis J (1978). Is Alzheimer's disease a major form of senile dementia? Clinical, anatomical, and genetic data. In Katzman R, Terry RD, Bick KL (eds): "Alzheimer's Disease: Senile Dementia and Related Disorders," [Aging, Vol 7], New York: Raven Press, p 15.

Cook RH, Ward BE, Austin JH (1979). Studies in aging of the brain: IV. Familial Alzheimer's disease: Relation to transmissible dementia, aneuploidy, and microtubular defects. Neurology 29:1402.

Corsellis JAN (1976). Some observations on the Purkinje cell population and on brain volume in human aging. In

Terry RD, Gershon S (eds): "Neurobiology of Aging," [Aging, Vol 3], New York: Raven Press, p 205.

Corsellis JAN (1978). Discussion. In Katzman R, Terry RD, Bick KL (eds): "Alzheimer's Disease: Senile Dementia and Related Disorders," [Aging, Vol 7], New York: Raven Press, p 397.

Crapper DR, Krishnan SS, Dalton AJ (1973). Brain aluminum distribution in Alzheimer's disease and experimental neurofibrillary degeneration. Science 180:511.

Cross AJ, Crow TJ, Perry EK, Perry RH, Blessed G, Tomlinson BE (1981). Reduced dopamine-beta-hydroxylase activity in Alzheimer's disease. Br Med J 282:93.

Cross RJ, Markesbery WR, Brooks WH, Roszman TL (1980). Hypothalamic-immune interactions. I. The acute effect of anterior hypothalamic lesions on the immune response. Brain Res 196:79.

Davies P, Maloney AJR (1976). Selective loss of central cholinergic neurons in Alzheimer's disease. Lancet II:1403.

Davis PJM, Wright EA (1977). A new method for measuring cranial cavity volume and its application to the assessment of cerebral atrophy at autopsy. Neuropathol Appl Neurobiol 3:341.

Drachman DA, Leavitt J (1974). Human memory and the cholinergic system. Arch Neurol 30:113.

Foelix RF, Hauser M (1979). Helically twisted filaments in giant neurons of a whip spider. Eur J Cell Biol 19:303.

Gambetti P, Velasco ME, Dahl D, Bignami A, Roessmann U, Sindely SD (1980). Alzheimer neurofibrillary tangles: An immunohistochemical study. In Amaducci L, Davison AN, Antuono P (eds): "Aging of the Brain and Dementia," [Aging, Vol 13], New York: Raven Press, p 55.

Gibbs CJ Jr, Gajdusek DC (1978). Subacute spongiform virus encephalopathies: The transmissible virus dementias. In Katzman R, Terry RD, Bick KL (eds): "Alzheimer's Disease: Senile Dementia and Related Disorders," [Aging, Vol 7], New York: Raven Press, p 559.

Gonatas NK, Anderson A, Evangelista I (1967). The contribution of altered synapses in the senile plaque: An electron microscopic study in Alzheimer's dementia. J Neuropathol Exp Neurol 26:25.

Goudsmit J, Morrow CH, Asher DM, Yanagihara RT, Masters CL, Gibbs CJ Jr, Gajdusek DC (1980). Evidence for and against the transmissibility of Alzheimer's disease. Neurology 30:945.

Gruenberg EM (1960-1961). A mental health survey of older

people. III. Psychiatr Q Suppl 34-35:34.

Hagnell O, Lanke J, Rorsman B, Ojesjo L (1981). Does the incidence of age psychosis decrease? Neuropsychobiology 7:201.

Henderson G, Tomlinson BE, Gibson PH (1980). Cell counts in human cerebral cortex in normal adults throughout life using an image analysing computer. J Neurol Sci 46:113.

Hubbard BM, Anderson JM (1981). A quantitative study of cerebral atrophy in old age and senile dementia. J Neurol Sci 50:135.

Ishii T, Haga S, Shimizu F (1975). Identification of components of immunoglobulins in senile plaques by means of fluorescent antibody techniques. Acta Neuropathol 32:157.

Kidd M (1963). Paired helical filaments in electron microscopy in Alzheimer's disease. Nature 197:192.

Klatzo I, Wisniewski H, Streicher E (1965). Experimental production of neurofibrillary degeneration. I. Light microscopic observations. J Neuropathol Exp Neurol 24:187.

Konigsmark BW, Murphy EA (1972). Volume of ventral cochlear nucleus in man: Its relationship to neuronal population and age. J Neuropathol Exp Neurol 31:304.

Liem RKH, Yen S-H, Salomon GD, Shelanski ML (1978). Intermediate filaments in nervous tissues. J Cell Biol 79:637.

Mann DMA, Lincoln J, Yates PO, Stamp JE, Toper S (1980). Changes in the monoamine containing neurones of the human CNS in senile dementia. Br J Psychiatry 136:533.

Mann DMA, Sinclair KGA (1978). The quantitative assessment of lipofuscin pigment, cytoplasmic RNA and nucleolar volume in senile dementia. Neuropathol Appl Neurobiol 4:129.

Markesbery WR, Ehmann WD, Hossain TIM, Alauddin M, Goodin DT (1981). Brain trace element levels in Alzheimer's disease by instrumental neutron activation analysis. J Neuropathol Exp Neurol 40:359.

McGeer PL, McGeer EG, Suzuki JS (1977). Aging and extrapyramidal function. Arch Neurol 34:33.

Miller AKH, Alston RL, Corsellis JAN (1980). Variation with age in the volumes of grey and white matter in the cerebral hemispheres of man: Measurements with an image analyser. Neuropathol Appl Neurobiol 6:119.

Monagle RD, Brody H (1974). The effects of age upon the main nucleus of the inferior olive in the human. J Comp Neurol 155:61.

Nandy K (1977). Immune reactions in aging brain and senile dementia. In Nandy K, Sherwin I (eds): "The Aging Brain and Senile Dementia," New York: Plenum Press, p 181.

Perl DP, Brody AR (1980). Alzheimer's disease: X-ray spectrometric evidence of aluminum accumulation in neurofibrillary tangle-bearing neurons. Science 208:207.

Perry EK, Perry RH, Blessed G, Tomlinson BE (1977). Necropsy evidence of central cholinergic deficits in senile dementia. Lancet I:189.

Perry EK, Tomlinson BE, Blessed G, Perry RH, Cross AJ, Crow TJ (1981). Neuropathological and biochemical observations on the noradrenergic system in Alzheimer's disease. J Neurol Sci 51:279.

Perry RH, Blessed G, Perry EK, Tomlinson BE (1980). Histochemical observations on cholinesterase activities in the brains of elderly normal and demented (Alzheimer type) patients. Age Ageing 9:9.

Powers JM, Spicer SS (1978). Histochemical similarity of senile plaque amyloid to apudamyloid. Virchows Arch (Pathol Anat) 376:107.

Probst A, Basler V, Bron B, Ulrich J (1983). Neuritic plaques in senile dementia of Alzheimer type: A Golgi analysis in the hippocampal region. Brain Res (in press).

Schechter R, Yen S-HC, Terry RD (1981). Fibrous astrocytes in senile dementia of the Alzheimer type. J Neuropathol Exp Neurol 40:95.

Selkoe DJ, Ihara Y, Salazar FJ (1982). Alzheimer's disease: Insolubility of partially purified paired helical filaments in sodium dodecyl sulfate and urea. Science 215:1243.

Shirahama T, Skinner M, Westermark P, Rubinow A, Cohen AS, Brun A, Kemper TL (1982). Senile cerebral amyloid. Prealbumin as a common constituent in the neuritic plaque, in the neurofibrillary tangle, and in the microangiopathic lesion. Am J Pathol 107:41.

Struble RG, Cork LC, Whitehouse PJ, Price DL (1982). Cholinergic innervation in neuritic plaques. Science 216:413.

Terry RD, Davies P, DeTeresa R, Katzman R (1982). Are both plaques and tangles required to make it Alzheimer's disease? J Neuropathol Exp Neurol 41:364.

Terry RD, Gonatas NK, Weiss M (1964). The ultrastructure of the cerebral cortex in Alzheimer's disease. Trans Am Neurol Assoc 89:12.

Terry RD, Peck A, DeTeresa R, Schechter R, Horoupian DS (1981). Some morphometric aspects of the brain in senile dementia of the Alzheimer type. Ann Neurol 10:184.

Terry RD, Pena C (1965). Experimental production of neurofibrillary degeneration. 2. Electron microscopy, phosphatase histochemistry and electron probe analysis. J Neuropathol Exp Neurol 24:200.

Terry RD, Wisniewski HM (1970). The ultrastructure of the neurofibrillary tangle and the senile plaque. In Wolstenholme GEW, O'Connor M (eds): "CIBA Foundation Symposium on Alzheimer's Disease and Related Conditions," London: Churchill, p 145.

Thal LJ, Fuld PA, Masur DM, Sharpless ND (1983). Oral physostigmine and lecithin improve memory in Alzheimer's disease. Ann Neurol 13:491.

Tomlinson BE (1977). The pathology of dementia. In Wells CE (ed): "Dementia," 2nd edition, [Contemporary Neurology Series, Vol 15], Philadelphia: F. A. Davis Company, p 113.

Tomlinson BE, Irving D (1977). The numbers of limb motor neurons in the human lumbosacral cord throughout life. J Neurol Sci 34:213.

Van Buskirk C (1945). The seventh nerve complex. J Comp Neurol 82:303.

Vijayashankar N, Brody H (1973). The neuronal population of the nuclei of the trochlear nerve and the locus coeruleus in the human. Anat Rec 172:421.

Vijayashankar N, Brody H (1979). A quantitative study of the pigmented neurons in the nuclei locus coeruleus and subcoeruleus in man as related to aging. J Neuropathol Exp Neurol 38:490.

White P, Goodhardt MJ, Keet JP, Hiley CR, Carasco LH, Williams IEI, Bowen DM (1977). Neocortical cholinergic neurons in elderly people. Lancet I:668.

Whitehouse PJ, Price DL, Clark AW, Coyle JT, DeLong MR (1981). Alzheimer's disease: Evidence for selective loss of cholinergic neurons in the nucleus basalis. Ann Neurol 10:122.

Wisniewski HM, Bruce ME, Fraser H (1975). Infectious etiology of neuritic (senile) plaques in mice. Science 190:1108.

Wisniewski HM, Ghetti B, Terry RD (1973). Neuritic (senile) plaques and filamentous changes in aged rhesus monkeys. J Neuropathol Exp Neurol 32:566.

Wisniewski HM, Johnson AB, Raine CS, Kay WJ, Terry RD (1970). Senile plaques and cerebral amyloidosis in aged dogs. A histochemical and ultrastructural study. Lab Invest 23:287.

Wisniewski HM, Narang HK, Terry RD (1976). Neurofibrillary tangles of paired helical filaments. J Neurol Sci 27:173.

Wisniewski HM, Shelanski ML, Terry RD (1968). Effects of mitotic spindle inhibitors on neurotubules and neurofilaments in anterior horn cells. J Cell Biol 38:224.

Yen S-HC, Gaskin F, Terry RD (1981). Immunocytochemical studies of neurofibrillary tangles. Am J Pathol 104:77.

DISCUSSION

DR. MORGAN: I noticed that you said muscarinic receptor binding was normal in senile dementia patients you studied as compared to age-matched controls, yet there is a 30 to 40% cell loss where those receptors would presumably be. Do you think that these have actually supersensitized to the loss of acetylcholine innervation?

DR. TERRY: There is, as far as I know, no real evidence that supersensitization occurs in the central cholinergic system.

DR. MORGAN: No, there is. Perhaps not in humans, but diisopropylfluorophosphate will supersensitize or, no, desensitize.

DR. TERRY: That is different. We have not yet found what transmitter the lost cortical cells use or what receptors they would have had.

DR. TURTURRO: Is the general loss in the neocortex a focal loss or just spread throughout the entire cortex? Are there any characteristics that can be associated with some physiological parameters?

DR. TERRY: Are you referring to normal or abnormal aging?

DR. TURTURRO: I am referring to normal aging.

DR. TERRY: In normal aging, according to Brody, the lost cells are mostly small and therefore come from the small cell layers. Our own work and that of Henderson would indicate that large cells are more vulnerable.

DR. TURTURRO: Are they distributed all over the brain?

DR. TERRY: They are fairly well distributed in terms of the laminae of the cortex and in all three areas that I have examined so far.

DR. LANDFIELD: In terms of the animal model issue, it is interesting that the astrocytes shown in your slides closely resemble reactive astrocytes found in the aged rat hippocampus.

DR. TERRY: One must count them in order to demonstrate that they really are increased in number.

DR. LANDFIELD: We have not found an increase in number of astrocytes in aged rats, only an increase in their size or degree of hypertrophy, and consequently an increase in the number of astrocyte processes.

DR. TERRY: We have found an increased number in SDAT.

DR. SCARPELLI: Has there been any support for the notion that intermediate filaments might be altered in Alzheimer's?

DR. TERRY: When I was speaking about the antigens shared between PHF and normal neurofibrous proteins, I was referring to the neurofilament which is a class of intermediate filament. There may be some shared antigenic sites, but it is still not clear.

DR. SCARPELLI: Do these insoluble fibrils withstand rigorous treatment such as eight molar guanidine?

DR. TERRY: That is right.

DR. APPEL: Recently some investigators reported alterations in locus ceruleus as a prominent part of changes in Alzheimer's. Have you had a chance in your studies to look at this and to confirm this or not?

DR. TERRY: I have the impression from gross dissections, of which I have done several hundred in Alzheimer's and relatively fewer normal controls, which are really quite rare, that there is a significant majority of SDAT cases with pallor in the region of the locus ceruleus. Cells have been counted in that area by two groups, one in Newcastle and the other in Cambridge. They found that in about 50% of the cases there is a decreased number of neurons. Norepinephrine has been found to be decreased in the cortex but not necessarily in the same cases. This would indicate to me that there is probably sprouting of neurons in some cases and less in others, and the sprouting supplies sufficient norepinephrine to bring the level back to normal. But there is, indeed, a loss of norepinephrine and cells in the ceruleus.

DR. PARKER: Do you feel that it is necessary to have cerebral atrophy demonstrated by either CAT Scan or autopsy to make a diagnosis of Alzheimer's disease?

DR. TERRY: Absolutely and unequivocally, no. I have seen 1,350-gram brains with very severe microscopic changes, and I have seen 1,050-gram brains without any changes at all. The diagnosis is a clinical-pathologic one based on the finding of microscopic lesions in a patient with dementia. I must also say that a large number of patients over 80, or even over 75, have only plaques in the neocortex without tangles, and there are many pathologists who do not include those cases in Alzheimer's disease. I do, and according to Dr. Harry Zimmerman, Alzheimer did too.

DR. MAURER: I am not familiar with any immunological studies done with Alzheimer patients, but I am certainly interested in them. I was wondering whether sera from patients with Alzheimer's have been used to see whether any of them can block the immunohistochemical studies to which you referred? More specifically, might there be antigen-antibody complexes rather than just antibody or soluble antigen in the serum?

DR. TERRY: Kal Nandy, who apparently is not at this meeting, has done more of that type of work than anybody else I know. Numbers of us have thought about those data, and we are just not very comfortable with them. May I leave it at that, that the conclusions are inconsistent and that cytotoxicity has not been demonstrated in terms of complexes. Dr. Wisniewski believes that plaque amyloid is, in fact, a complex which has somehow passed through a permeable blood-brain barrier. There is, however, not adequate evidence of an increased permeability of the blood-brain barrier in either normal or abnormal aging, and in fact, there is evidence against it. I don't know how such things would get out into the brain.

There are some reactions between aging serum and neurons and glia in sections of brain, but the significance of these has never been convincing.

Comparative Pathobiology of Major Age-Related Diseases: Current Status and Research Frontiers, pages 373–384

NEUROCHEMICAL STUDIES OF ALZHEIMER-TYPE NEUROFIBRILLARY DEGENERATION AND A RELATED EXPERIMENTAL MODEL

Kenneth S. Kosik, M.D., Yasuo Ihara, M.D., Carmela Abraham, Chaudri G. Rasool, Ph.D., Alan McCluskey, and Dennis J. Selkoe, M.D.

Departments of Neurology and Neuropathology, Harvard Medical School, Boston, MA 02115, and Ralph Lowell Laboratories, Mailman Research Center, McLean Hospital, Belmont, MA 02178

INTRODUCTION

The classic morphological hallmarks of presenile and senile dementia of the Alzheimer type (Alzheimer's disease, AD) are neurofibrillary tangles (NFT) and neuritic (senile) plaques. While high densities and widespread distribution of these lesions in human brain tissue lead to a diagnosis of AD, neither of these lesions is specific for the disease. The majority of normal aged individuals develop some NFT and neuritic plaques, although in much smaller numbers and in a topographically restricted distribution compared to AD. Neurofibrillary tangles are non-membrane-bound cytoplasmic collections of filaments found in neurons of the hippocampus, amygdala, cerebral cortex, and certain deep gray nuclear structures. Electron microscopic studies from numerous laboratories have concluded that NFT consist of masses of helically wound pairs of filaments. These structures are referred to as paired helical filaments (PHF) and have a maximum width of about 20 nm and a periodicity of approximately 80 nm (Kidd 1963, Terry et al 1964; Wisniewski et al 1976). They are found not only in neuronal perikarya (as NFT) but also in the abnormal neurites (including axonal terminals) forming the peripheral rim of the senile plaque (Gonatas et al 1967). Because the individual filaments of the PHF are approximately 10 nm, it has been suggested that they are related to a class of cytoskeletal elements referred to as intermediate filaments. Such filaments vary greatly in their molecular composition, principally as a function of the cell type in which they are found. The intermediate filaments of neurons are referred to as neurofilaments.

Recently, reports have appeared that bundles of straight (non-helical) filaments of approximately 15 nm width may also be found in Alzheimer cortex and may possibly coexist within perikarya containing PHF (Shiboyama, Kitoh 1978; Yagishita et al 1981; Metuzals et al 1981; Rudelli et al 1982). Collections of 15 nm straight filaments predominate in another age-related human neuronal degeneration, progressive supranuclear palsy (Tellez-Nagel, Wisniewski 1973; Bugiana et al 1979). Such straight filaments are slightly wider than the normal 10 nm neurofilaments of the neuron (Metuzals et al 1981).

The number of neuritic plaques and NFT in Alzheimer cortex appears to correlate semi-quantitatively with the degree of intellectual impairment during life (Tomlinson et al 1970; Ball 1976; Farmer et al 1976; Ball 1977). The number of tangles present in hippocampus may also be related to the extent of neuronal loss in this tissue (Ball 1976). The decrease of choline acetyltransferase activity in Alzheimer cortex has been found to correlate statistically with the number of neuritic plaques (Perry et al 1978). The marked depletion of cholinergic perikarya recently discovered in the nucleus basalis of Meynert and the septal nuclei in Alzheimer brains is associated with the presence of NFT in some of the remaining neurons in these nuclei (Whitehouse et al 1982; Nakano, Hirano 1982).

These various correlations underscore the importance of identifying the molecular nature of the PHF and the mechanisms responsible for their progressive accumulation. We have therefore focused specifically upon three areas: (1) biochemical and immunological characterization of PHF; (2) the development of model systems in which perturbations of intermediate filament organization and metabolism can be studied; and (3) the role that pathological alteration of the neuronal cytoskeleton may play in the accelerated death of certain neuronal populations during normal aging and in AD. Data will be presented here which address the first two areas of research.

MOLECULAR STUDIES OF ALZHEIMER PAIRED HELICAL FILAMENTS

Recent investigations in our laboratory were undertaken with the goal of ascertaining the chemical identity of the PHF by attempting to extract these unusual organelles from postmortem brain and separate and characterize their presumed protein subunits. Initially, fractions enriched in PHF or in tangle-bearing neuronal perikarya were obtained by conventional cellular fractionation methods and extraction with the non-ionic detergent Triton X-100. Although electron microscopy demonstrated that these initial crude fractions derived from AD cortex were enriched in PHF, the polypeptide composition of such fractions was identical to control (PHF-free) brain fractions when examined by both one- and two-dimensional gel electrophoresis with silver or Coomassie staining (Selkoe et al 1982b). This unexpected and anomalous finding of lack of protein differences led us to postulate that PHF might be insoluble in sodium dodecyl sulfate (SDS), urea, and other solvents used to solubilize proteins before gel electrophoresis. Such insolubility would prevent PHF proteins from entering the acrylamide gel matrix and thus preclude their visualization. This hypothesis was confirmed by pelleting the insoluble residue from a PHF-enriched fraction which had been heated to 100°C for 5 min in a gel sample buffer containing 2% SDS and 5% ß-mercaptoethanol (ßME), a disulfide reducing agent. The pellet, when examined by electron microscopy, contained abundant PHF which retained their structural integrity. Even after isolation under these harsh denaturing conditions, PHF had a maximum width of 18-21 nm and an interperiod distance of 75-80 nm, dimensions highly similar to those reported for *in situ* PHF from freshly biopsied Alzheimer cortex (Selkoe et al 1982b).

While the marked insolubility of PHF demonstrated in these studies made biochemical analysis difficult, it did permit the development of strategies to purify the PHF to a greater extent than previously believed possible. The PHF purification procedure we have now developed relies on extensive extraction of AD cortex in SDS/ßME at room temperature followed by differential centrifugation and sucrose density gradient centrifugation. By electron microscopy, these preparations contain abundant isolated NFT as well as skeins of PHF. Such preparations, although highly enriched in PHF, are not homogeneously pure. The major SDS-insoluble contaminants remaining are: (1) electron dense granular masses that resemble lipofuscin, (2) small electron dense particles, (3) fragments of basement membrane-like material, and (4) some amyloid cores from senile plaques (most of which are separated out at an early step in the purification).

In order to depolymerize and analyze the PHF chemically, numerous additional harsh denaturants and solvents have been tried. None of the reagents tried to date has resulted in quantitatively detectable solubilization of PHF (Table 1). The lack of significant solubilization has been concluded on the basis of these criteria: (1) gel electrophoretic analysis of the supernatant after attempted solubilization

Table 1

Apparent Insolubility of Paired Helical Filaments

Reagents used to assess PHF solubility:

sodium dodecyl sulfate (5%, 100°C)
ß-mercaptoethanol (2%, 100°C)
urea (9.5 M)
guanidine HCl (6 M, 100°C)
potassium thiocyanate (10 M, 100°C)
lithium bromide (5 M, overnight)
trifluoroacetic acid (20%, 2 hr)
monochloracetic acid (1%)
chloral hydrate (100%)
phenol/acetic acid/water (2:1:1)
chloroform/methanol (2:1)
0.2 N hydrochloric acid
0.2 N sodium hydroxide

Enzymatic hydrolysis (48 hr, 37°C; with or without SDS) used to assess PHF solubility:

proteinase K
Streptomyces griseus protease ("pronase E")
elastase
papain
thermolysin
chymotrypsin
trypsin
pepsin

in the reagents listed reveals no significant soluble protein bands; (2) light microscopy demonstrates intact Congo red-birefringent tangles; (3) electron microscopic analysis of the pellet after exposure to some of these reagents demonstrates intact PHF. An example of the effects on PHF of a strong chaotropic solvent that would be expected to alter noncovalent forces (hydrophobic, hydrogen bonds, etc.) in the fiber is provided by lithium bromide treatment. Three M concentrations of LiBr do not significantly affect the structure of PHF and NFT. At 5 M, a marked decrease in Congo red-detectable NFT occurs, but EM demonstrates recovery of intact PHF in the pellet. After 7 M LiBr, PHF can no longer be seen by EM; they are apparently replaced by an amorphous, but still particulate material that has a vaguely fibrous appearance but no structural features of PHF. Gel electrophoresis of such 7 M LiBr-treated samples still demonstrates significant amounts of insoluble, Coomassie-positive material excluded at the top of the gel and no soluble protein bands appear in the running gel, although some very low molecular weight material which is Coomassie-positive is seen at the dye front. Similar results are noted after treatment of PHF with saturated guanidine thiocyanate. Currently, attempts are being made to digest the PHF proteolytically by sequential application of various proteases as well as by treatment with salts such as lithium bromide followed by protease treatment.

From these experiments, which have demonstrated the resistance of PHF to strong solvents and enzymatic hydrolysis, we have drawn certain conclusions regarding the molecular interactions that maintain the structural integrity of PHF. The chemical inertness of these filaments suggests a polymeric structure maintained in part by nondisulfide covalent cross-links. Since solvents known to be effective in breaking hydrogen bonds and other noncovalent interactions in proteins are ineffective in depolymerizing the PHF into soluble subunits, it is unlikely that such noncovalent forces are solely responsible for maintaining the rigid, helically wound configuration of PHF. The resistance to strong solvents and enzymatic hydrolysis suggests that the macromolecule is cross-linked; such a process could lead to the sites for enzymatic digestion on PHF being inaccessible to proteases.

Since neurofilaments, perhaps in some altered form, remain the leading candidate for the subunit proteins of

PHF, studies were undertaken to determine if neurofilaments *in vitro* can serve as a substrate for the cross-linking enzyme, transglutaminase (Selkoe et al 1982a). This enzyme was selected because it is a well-characterized enzyme known to covalently cross-link mammalian intracellular and extra-cellular proteins by forming ε-(γ-glutamyl)lysine isopeptide bonds. Examples of ε-(γ-glutamyl)lysine-cross-linked polymers include proteins in the erythrocyte membrane (Dutton, Singer 1975; Lorand et al 1976), proteins in human lens tissue during senile cataract formation (Lorand et al 1981), and proteins in the cornified envelope of terminally differentiated keratinocytes in human epidermis (Rice, Green 1979). In our experiments, human brain neurofilament fractions incubated in the presence of transglutaminase, Ca^{2+}, and the fluorescent amine, dansylcadaverine, formed a fluorescent, nondisulfide-bonded, SDS-insoluble polymer. The insoluble, fluorescent material can be visualized at the top of gels because it fails to enter the acrylamide matrix. The formation of these cross-linked polymers is associated with a decrease in the amount of soluble, neurofilament polypeptides in the preparations. Cystamine, an inhibitor of transglutaminase, prevents such *in vitro* neurofilament cross-linking. Electron micrographs of the cross-linked material show an extensive, complex network of connecting filaments which can be immunostained with various neuro-filament antisera. Glial fibrillary acidic protein and myelin basic protein, which are present in the crude, brain filament fractions utilized, can also serve as substrates for transglutaminase *in vitro* and are likely to contribute to the meshwork of cross-linked, interconnecting fibrous structures seen by electron microscopy in our preparations. Although AD-type PHF are not formed under the specific *in vitro* conditions employed, the data suggest one possible mechanism for the covalent cross-linking of neurofilaments into insoluble polymers during human neuronal aging (Selkoe et al 1982a).

Since solubilization and protein chemical analysis of PHF have not yet been achieved, we have developed immuno-chemical probes to purify and study PHF. PHF purified in the presence of SDS were used to raise a polyvalent anti-serum in rabbits. This antiserum, at dilutions up to 1:5000, stains a large number of NFT in AD cortex and some of the neurites in the rims of senile plaques. The antiserum also stains many abnormal neuritic profiles scattered diffusely throughout AD cortical neuropil. It does not specifically immunolabel any structures in normal aged human brain except the occasional NFT seen in such tissue. The NFT staining pattern in AD cortical sections using this new antiserum was compared to that obtained with certain anti-neurofilament antibodies previously reported to stain _in situ_ NFT. For this purpose, well-characterized monoclonal antibodies which specifically recognize the 160 kilodalton and 200 kilodalton neurofilament proteins, respectively, were used (Anderton et al 1982). Double immunofluorescent staining using the rabbit anti-PHF antibodies with fluorescein-conjugated secondary antibodies and the mouse anti-neurofilament antibodies with rhodamine-conjugated secondary antibodies revealed that many NFT-bearing neurons appear to stain with both antisera. In many cells, the same fibrous structure (i.e., NFT) was stained with both antibodies. However, when NFT are isolated from cortex, the respective antigens recognized by each immune reagent are separated. Specifically, isolated NFT, regardless of the method of isolation (i.e., gentle or harsh extraction conditions), no longer immunostain with the anti-neurofilament monoclonal antibodies, but retain their reactivity with the anti-PHF antiserum. That the anti-PHF antiserum does not recognize determinants in normal neurofilaments is further substantiated by the failure of this antiserum to stain any of the neurofilament triplet polypeptides in immunoblotted gels. Interpretation of these different reactivity patterns of _in situ_ and extracted NFT with the two antibodies awaits further experimental clarification. However, a closely associated complex of neurofilament-reactive antigens and PHF may be present in tangle-bearing perikarya _in situ_; the neurofilament antigen, which is apparently soluble, may be lost from this complex when the tangles are extracted, while the insoluble PHF remain in the extracted tangle and are still recognized by our anti-PHF antibodies. The apparent high degree of specificity of our antiserum for PHF makes it a suitable ligand for immunoaffinity purification of PHF to homogeneity, a step that is critical to the further protein chemical analysis of these unusual pathological organelles. Experiments directed at this goal are now underway in our laboratory.

STUDIES OF ALUMINUM-INDUCED NEUROFIBRILLARY DEGENERATION IN AN ANIMAL MODEL

In our efforts to study the pathobiology of neurofibrillary degeneration, we have modified existing animal models of aluminum intoxication in which massive collections of neurofilaments accumulate in neuronal perikarya (Kosik et al 1983). Our modification, in which aluminum salts are microinjected directly into the lumbar spinal cord of rabbits, engenders a denser involvement of neuronal perikarya with filamentous lesions than the more classical intracisternal route of aluminum administration. Of particular importance in the studies described below is the extensive involvement of anterior horn cells achieved in this model. Because in diseases with Alzheimer-type neurofibrillary degeneration a specific relationship to loss of cholinergic activity has been postulated, we sought to determine whether a relationship between filamentous accumulation in cholinergic neurons and lack of cholinergic activity was present in aluminum intoxication. In our studies, choline acetyltransferase (ChAT) activity in aluminum-treated rabbits was decreased from one-third to one-half of control values over the entire length of the sciatic nerve in all aluminum-treated rabbits studied. This marked biochemical alteration associated with the development of filamentous accumulations in the anterior horn cells was not accompanied by any morphometric evidence of axonal degeneration at four weeks following the aluminum injections. There was no significant loss of myelinated axons in sciatic nerve despite the fact that the cell bodies for these axons contained massive collections of neurofilaments. Although the static levels of ChAT activity were markedly diminished, the rate of accumulation of ChAT activity proximal to a sciatic nerve ligature was increased in aluminum intoxication. Thus, it appeared that the decrease in the static levels of ChAT activity in the axon was being compensated for in part by an increased rate of distal delivery of the enzyme. Support for this hypothesis derived from calculations which determined the total amount of ChAT activity accumulating proximal to a sciatic nerve ligature in a 24-hr period. These calculations revealed no difference between control and aluminum-treated animals. Thus, cholinergic neurons containing aluminum-induced neurofibrillary tangles appear able to maintain distal delivery of the synthetic enzyme over the time-course studied despite the fact that their perikarya contain an abnormal accumulation of neurofilaments.

REFERENCES

Anderton BH, Breinburg D, Downes MJ, Green PJ, Tomlinson BE, Ulrich J, Wood JN, Kahn J (1982). Monoclonal antibodies show that neurofibrillary tangles and neurofilaments share antigenic determinants. Nature 298:84.

Ball MJ (1976). Neurofibrillary tangles and the pathogenesis of dementia: A quantitative time study. Neuropathol Appl Neurobiol 2:394.

Ball MJ (1977). Neuronal loss, neurofibrillary tangles and granulovacuolar degeneration in the hippocampus with aging and dementia: A quantitative study. Acta Neuropathol (Berl) 37:111.

Bugiana L, Marcardi GL, Brusa A, Ederli E (1979). The fine structure of subcortical tangles in progressive supranuclear palsy. Acta Neuropathol (Berl) 45:147.

Dutton A, Singer SJ (1975). Crosslinking and labeling of membrane proteins by transglutaminase-catalyzed reactions. Proc Natl Acad Sci USA 72:2568.

Farmer PM, Peck A, Terry RD (1976). Correlations among numbers of neuritic plaques, neurofibrillary tangles, and the severity of senile dementia. J Neuropathol Exp Neurol 35:367.

Gonatas NK, Anderson W, Evangelista I (1967). The contribution of altered synapses in the senile plaque: An electron microscopic study in Alzheimer's dementia. J Neuropathol Exp Neurol 26:25.

Kidd M (1963). Paired helical filaments in electron microscopy of Alzheimer's disease. Nature 197:192.

Kosik KS, Bradley WG, Good PF, Rasool CG, Selkoe DJ (1983). Cholinergic function in lumbar aluminum myelopathy. J Neuropathol Exp Neurol (in press).

Lorand L, Hsu LKH, Siefring GE, Rafferty NS (1981). Lens transglutaminase and cataract formation. Proc Natl Acad Sci USA 78:1356.

Lorand L, Weissmann LB, Epel DL, Brunner-Lorand J (1976). Role of the intrinsic transglutaminase in the Ca^{2+}-mediated crosslinking of erythrocyte proteins. Proc Natl Acad Sci USA 73:4479.

Metuzals J, Monpetit V, Clapin DF (1981). Organization of the neurofilamentous network. Cell Tissue Res 214:455.

Nakano I, Hirano A (1982). Loss of large neurons of the medial septal nucleus in an autopsy of Alzheimer's disease. J Neuropathol Exp Neurol 41:341.

Perry EK, Tomlinson BE, Blessed G, Bergmann K, Gibson PH, Perry RH (1978). Correlation of cholinergic abnormalities

with senile plaques and mental test scores in senile dementia. Br Med J 2:1457.
Rice RH, Green H (1979). Presence in human epidermal cells of a soluble protein precursor of the cross-linked envelope: Activation of the cross-linking of calcium ions. Cell 18:681.
Rudelli R, Strom JO, Welch PT, Ambler MW (1982). Post-traumatic premature Alzheimer's disease: Neuropathologic findings and pathogenetic considerations. Arch Neurol 39:570.
Selkoe DJ, Abraham C, Ihara Y (1982a). Brain transglutaminase: *In vitro* crosslinking of human neurofilament proteins into insoluble polymers. Proc Natl Acad Sci USA 79:6070.
Selkoe DJ, Ihara Y, Salazar FJ (1982b). Alzheimer's disease: Insolubility of partially purified paired helical filaments in sodium dodecyl sulfate and urea. Science 215:1243.
Shiboyama H, Kitoh J (1978). Electron microscopic structure of the Alzheimer's neurofibrillary changes in case of atypical senile dementia. Acta Neuropathol (Berl) 41:229.
Tellez-Nagel I, Wisniewski HM (1973). Ultrastructure of neurofibrillary tangles in Steele-Richardson-Olszewski syndrome. Acta Neurol 29:324.
Terry RD, Gonatas NF, Weiss M (1964). Ultrastructural studies in Alzheimer's presenile dementia. Am J Pathol 44:269.
Tomlinson BE, Blessed G, Roth M (1970). Observations of the brains of demented old people. J Neurol Sci 11:205.
Whitehouse PJ, Price DL, Struble RG, Clark AW, Coyle JT, DeLong MR (1982). Alzheimer's disease and senile dementia: Loss of neurons in the basal forebrain. Science 215:1237.
Wisniewski HM, Narong HK, Terry RD (1976). Neurofibrillary tangles of paired helical filaments. J Neurol Sci 27:173.
Yagishita S, Itoh Y, Nan W, Amano N (1981). Reappraisal of the fine structure of Alzheimer's neurofibrillary tangles. Acta Neuropathol (Berl) 54:239.

DISCUSSION

DR. TURTURRO: Given the possible cross-link nature of the protein that you are having trouble isolating, have you tried digestion with collagenase?

DR. KOSIK: Yes, collagenase was tried because one of the things that we think might be a contaminant in the preparations is collagen. We thought we could clean it up with collagenase, which it did do, but it didn't affect the paired helical filaments (PHF).

DR. MORGAN: Along that same line, you mentioned the fact that you tried transglutaminase on neurofibrillary or neurofilament proteins. That enzyme forms a specific type of linkage between amino acids. Can that linkage be dissolved? Lazlo Lorand worked with that enzyme linkage. Have you tried his procedure on the neurofibrillary tangles?

DR. KOSIK: In Dr. Lorand's procedure the linkage itself is not actually digested. The bonds around the glutamine-lysine are digested so that one is left with the two cross-linked amino acids alone which can then be detected.

I'd like to emphasize that at this stage we have no evidence that there is a gamma glutamyl epsilon lysine cross-link in PHF. However, we are attempting to digest the PHF by sequential proteolytic digestion to detect a cross-link in collaboration with Dr. Lorand.

DR. MORGAN: What good evidence is there that it is even a protein? Have you digested it?

DR. KOSIK: While it is possible that PHF contain non-protein components, they do contain protein. Neurofibrillary tangles on a slide stain with Coomassie blue which stains proteins. Preparations highly enriched in PHF contain amino acids which are detected after complete hydrolysis in strong acid.

DR. REGELSON: As I remember, when Laki first described transglutaminase with Factor 13 fibrin cross-linkage, serotonin had a striking enhancing effect on the cross-linkage. Is there any evidence that serotonin affects your transglutaminase model?

DR. KOSIK: I don't know. We haven't looked at that.

DR. APPEL: In your first experiments with the antibodies, even though the PHF antibodies do not react in the Western blot technique, can you preincubate with your PHF antibodies to block the effect of the monoclonal antibodies against neurofilaments in any of your systems to see whether the PHF antibodies might recognize the same antigenic site as the monoclonal antibodies?

DR. KOSIK: We definitely plan to do that. We haven't tried that.

DR. APPEL: You showed us some effects in the anterior horn cells. Is there evidence that there actually is aluminum in the anterior horn cells, or is this a trans-synaptic effect that you are documenting?

DR. KOSIK: We have not measured aluminum in the neurofibrillary-containing anterior horn cells, and I think that is an important thing to do; but other investigators who have used an aluminum model have performed a similar analysis. I believe that aluminum is increased in neurons after the treatment with aluminum. Dr. Terry may be able to answer this better than I can.

DR. TERRY: Donald Crapper did that.

DR. POTTENGER: Have you tried cyanogen bromide?

DR. KOSIK: Yes we have; similar to seven molar lithium bromide, cyanogen bromide destroys their ultrastructural integrity, but they still do not enter a gel system.

Comparative Pathobiology of Major Age-Related Diseases: Current Status and Research Frontiers, pages 385–399

THE BASAL FOREBRAIN CHOLINERGIC SYSTEM AND ALZHEIMER'S DISEASE

Donald L. Price, M.D., Peter J. Whitehouse, M.D., Ph.D., Mahlon R. DeLong, M.D., Cheryl A. Kitt, Ph.D., John C. Hedreen, M.D., Susan J. Mitchell, Ph.D., Robert G. Struble, Ph.D., Donald L. Price, Jr., and Linda C. Cork, D.V.M., Ph.D.

Departments of Pathology, Neurology, and Neuroscience, School of Medicine, The Johns Hopkins University, Baltimore, MD 21205

INTRODUCTION

Neurobiological investigations in several species have demonstrated a basal forebrain cholinergic (Ch) system which innervates the amygdala, hippocampus, and neocortex (Divac 1975; Kievit, Kuypers 1975; Pearson et al 1983; Tigges et al 1982; Mesulam et al 1983). In primates, this magnocellular cholinergic cell population, termed the Ch1-4 complex (Mesulam et al 1983), consists of neurons in the medial septum (Ch1), diagonal band of Broca (dbB) (Ch2), and nucleus basalis of Meynert (nbM) (Ch4). Although definite statements concerning the functions of this system are premature, behavioral and physiological investigations suggest that the Ch system may play roles in arousal and in learning and memory behaviors (DeLong 1971; Drachman, Leavitt 1974; Weingartner et al 1979; Davis et al 1979; Rolls et al 1979; Drachman et al 1980; Bartus et al 1982). Moreover, recent evidence suggests that dysfunction/death of the Ch1-4 complex may be, in part, responsible for the reductions in cholinergic markers occurring in Alzheimer's disease (AD) and its late-life variant, senile dementia of the Alzheimer's type (SDAT) (Whitehouse et al 1981, 1982; Price et al 1982a,b, 1983; Coyle et al 1983).

The present review addresses several questions. What is the neurochemical evidence for cholinergic abnormalities in AD/SDAT? What is the anatomy/neurochemistry of the Ch system projecting to forebrain? What is the evidence for changes in the Ch1-4 system in AD/SDAT? What are the possible functional roles of the Ch1-4 system? Finally, we describe a hypothetical model linking Ch1-4 neurons, neuritic plaques, and reductions in cholinergic markers and describe preliminary studies addressing several predictions of this model.

NEUROTRANSMITTER SYSTEM ABNORMALITIES IN ALZHEIMER'S DISEASE/SENILE DEMENTIA OF THE ALZHEIMER'S TYPE

Reductions in cholinergic markers appear to be one of the earliest and most consistent transmitter-specific abnormalities detected in the cerebrum of patients with AD/SDAT (Pope et al 1964; Bowen et al 1976, 1982; Davies, Maloney 1976; Perry et al 1977, 1980; Reisine et al 1978; Rossor et al 1980, 1982b; Wilcock et al 1982; Sims et al 1983). In the neocortex, the activities of choline acetyltransferase (ChAT) and acetylcholinesterase (AChE) are reduced; high-affinity uptake of choline is decreased; and the synthesis of acetylcholine from $[^{14}C]$glucose is diminished (Bowen et al 1982; Sims et al 1983). Certainly, the Ch system is not the only neuronal population affected in AD. Evidence exists for loss of neurons in the neocortex (Shefer 1972; Colon 1973; Terry et al 1981), hippocampus (Ball 1978), amygdala (Herzog, Kemper 1980), and locus ceruleus (Tomlinson et al 1981; Bondareff et al 1982; Perry et al 1981), but it is not clear how these morphological changes correlate with noncholinergic neurotransmitter abnormalities documented in AD/SDAT (Davies, Terry 1981; Davies et al 1980, 1982; Cross et al 1981; Perry et al 1981; Rossor et al 1982a).

ORGANIZATION OF THE Ch1-4 SYSTEM

Ch1-4 neurons are the major source of cholinergic innervation of the amygdala, hippocampus, and neocortex (Mesulam et al 1983). There appear to be few, if any, cholinergic neurons intrinsic to the primate neocortex (Mesulam et al 1983; JC Hedreen, SJ Bacon, LC Cork, CA Kitt, PM Salvaterra, DL Price, unpublished observations). The nbM is the largest part of the Ch system and has been subdivided into five subgroups (Mesulam et al 1983) which have different overlapping topographical projections to neocortex: the anterior Ch4 projects to prefrontal neocortex; the more caudal Ch4 innervates more posterior areas of neocortex; the medial group of neurons projects to medial neocortex; the lateral group innervates the convexities; the caudolateral Ch4 projects to the temporal lobe; and neurons in the posterior part of Ch4 project to visual neocortex (Tigges et al 1982; Mesulam et al 1983; Pearson et al 1983). Efferents of the Ch1 and Ch2 groups terminate in the hippocampus (Daitz, Powell 1954; Segal, Landis 1974; Swanson, Cowan 1979). The majority of the cholinergic innervation of neocortex appears to be mediated through muscarinic receptors.

Inputs from lateral septal neurons, as well as a wide variety of ascending afferents from the hypothalamus and brainstem, innervate Ch1 and rostral Ch2 neurons (Segal, Landis 1974; Swanson, Cowan 1979). Caudal Ch2 and Ch4 neurons receive afferents from the peripeduncular nucleus of the midbrain, hypothalamus, amygdala, and a variety of brainstem nuclei (Jones et al 1976; Krettek, Price 1978; Saper, Loewy 1980; Price, Amaral 1981; Veazey et al 1982; CA Kitt, JC Hedreen, DL Price, unpublished observations).

INVOLVEMENT OF THE Ch1-4 SYSTEM IN ALZHEIMER'S DISEASE

To test the hypothesis that the Ch1-4 system was, in part, responsible for the cholinergic deficits in neocortex, we set out to examine this neuronal population in the brains of patients with AD. Our first patient was a 74-year-old man who had onset of disease at the age of 60 and who died after a 14-year history of progressive loss of memory, impairment of judgment, and deterioration of other cognitive functions. His father, paternal aunt, and uncle suffered similar illnesses. At autopsy, the brain showed neurofibrillary tangles and neuritic plaques typical of AD. Sections through the basal forebrain disclosed a profound loss of nerve cells within the nbM (Whitehouse et al 1981). Subsequent analysis of the brains of five putative sporadic cases of AD disclosed consistent loss of large neurons in Ch2 and Ch4 (Whitehouse et al 1982). The majority of our initially reported cases had AD; loss of neurons and reductions in cholinergic markers appeared to be more severe in this group. Our experience (Whitehouse et al 1983) and that of others (Tagliavini, Pilleri 1983) suggest that, in patients with SDAT as a group, both the loss of Ch1-4 neurons and changes in cortical ChAT activity are less striking (Bowen et al 1979; Davies 1979; Rossor et al 1982b).

POSSIBLE FUNCTION OF THE Ch1-4 SYSTEM

Cholinergic systems have been implicated in a variety of physiological activities, including arousal and memory and learning behaviors. Indirect evidence suggests that the behavioral arousal and electroencephalographic desynchronization following stimulation of the reticular formation are mediated by cholinergic systems (Szerb 1967; Jasper, Tessier 1971; Lo Conte et al 1982). It is conceivable that the Ch1-4 complex may be an important link in this activating system. Parts of the Ch system have been implicated in memory processes. Blockade of central muscarinic receptors with scopolamine in young adults is associated with memory and other cognitive deficits similar to those found in aged subjects, and age-related changes in cholinergic activity may be associated with the memory deficits of aging (Deutsch 1971; Drachman, Leavitt 1974; Drachman et al 1980; Bartus et al 1982). In addition, some studies suggest that this system plays a role in learning paradigms, e.g., in the acquisition of conditioned reflexes (Woody et al 1978). Finally, physiological studies of primate Ch4 neurons during behavior have shown that these nerve cells exhibit a characteristic tonic firing pattern as well as phasic changes in discharge in relation to different sensory stimuli and directional movements, and following reward delivery (DeLong 1971; Rolls et al 1979; Mitchell et al 1982). These studies suggest both tonic and phasic roles for Ch4 neurons. The tonic activity may relate to the possible role of the Ch system in electroencephalographic and behavioral arousal, while the phasic modulation of neuronal discharge may be related to the aspects of learning, memory, or attention.

MODEL OF DYSFUNCTION/DEATH OF Ch NEURONS

Whatever the etiology of AD, this disorder appears to preponderantly affect certain neuronal populations, including the Ch1-4 system; it is this pathology which appears to be associated with cholinergic deficits. Moreover, it appears that there may be links between dementia, changes in cholinergic markers, the presence of neuritic plaques, and the Ch1-4 system in AD patients. With this as a background, we have formulated a model linking these various processes (Price et al 1982a,b, 1983). For the purposes of the model, the pathological process affects cholinergic neurons in the basal forebrain, although this does not imply that the cholinergic circuits are the only transmitter-specific pathways affected in this disease. The substrate of this pathology could be local changes in terminal fields or a failure of synthesis or delivery of essential materials from the perikarya in the Ch1-4 complex. The result is a decrease in presynaptic cholinergic cortical markers in amygdala, hippocampus, and neocortex. With time, axonal arborizations undergo structural arrangements, e.g., distal axons and nerve terminals enlarge and accumulate organelles. The histopathological counterpart of this structural rearrangement is the immature plaque, comprised of argentophilic neurites (filled with filaments). As plaques mature, they show increased neurites and an extracellular core of amyloid. At late stages in the evolution of individual plaques, the number of argentophilic neurites may be decreased, and the site of the plaque is marked by an amyloid core. In this model, some of the neurites in plaques would be derived from the Ch1-4 system, and the evolution of plaques would be accompanied by gradual loss of the activities of AChE and ChAT in the neocortex, a hypothesis consistent with observations that the presence of plaques correlates with the reduction in cholinergic markers (Perry et al 1978). In this model, it is suggested that Ch neurons do not suddenly die but may survive in a dysfunctional state for long periods.

What is the evidence for this suggestion? First, biopsy studies have shown that changes in cortical cholinergic markers occur early in the disease (Bowen et al 1982). Second, Perry et al (1982) have reported a 75-90% reduction in ChAT activity in the temporal neocortex and substantia innominata with only a 33% loss of neurons in the nbM. These observations are consistent with the hypothesis that Ch neurons are viable but dysfunctional; perhaps they cannot synthesize or deliver essential constituents to their distal arborizations (Price et al 1983). Finally, neurons in the Ch1-4 complex, like neurons in the amygdala, hippocampus, and neocortex, exhibit cytoskeletal pathology involving the perikarya (neurofibrillary tangles) and possibly distal axon terminals (neurites and neuritic plaques). This change must develop over time. These observations support our hypothetical model and have encouraged us to test predictions of this model.

Predictions of Model

Preliminary evidence pertinent to the predictions of this model are described below.

Ablation of the nbM and dbB in primates should result in loss of cholinergic markers in the neocortex. Recently, we have injected ibotenic acid, an excitotoxin which selectively destroys nerve cell bodies but spares fibers of passage, into the substantia innominata of nonhuman primates. This lesion causes a reduction in AChE and ChAT activities in the neocortex ipsilateral to the lesions (Struble et al 1982b).

The distribution of plaques should bear some relationship to the topography of cholinergic innervation. Plaques are most common in the amygdala, hippocampus, and neocortex (Jamada, Mehraein 1968); these areas have a high concentration of cholinergic markers. On the basis of our preliminary tracing studies (Kitt et al 1982), we know that these regions receive innervation from the Ch1-4 system. Certain parts of the primate amygdala, particularly the basolateral amydgala, receive acetylcholine-rich inputs from the nbM, and some cases of AD/SDAT have high plaque densities in the amygdala, particularly in the basolateral nucleus.

As plaques evolve from immature to end stage, there should be a change in cholinergic markers. Aged monkeys show both behavioral abnormalities and neuritic plaques similar to those occurring in aged humans (Davis 1978; Wisniewski, Terry 1973). Recently, we have begun to map the type, density, and distribution of plaques in the neocortex of aged primates (Struble et al 1982a; RG Struble, LC Cork, DL Price, unpublished observations). Immature (neurite-rich) plaques usually begin to appear in the neocortex of monkeys after 20 years of age, and they are particularly apparent in the prefrontal and anterior temporal regions. With time, plaque densities increase and the number of mature and end-stage plaques increases. In the oldest monkeys (31 years old), plaque densities are similar to those occurring in aged nondemented humans.

If some neurites in plaques are derived from cholinergic neurons in the basal forebrain, they should stain for AChE, a marker present in (although not completely specific for) cholinergic axons. During the evolution of plaques, as some neurites disappear, AChE activity should decline and be diminished in end-stage plaques. Our initial studies in monkeys are consistent with this hypothesis (Struble et al

1982a). Immature plaques showed neurites and were rich in AChE activity. As plaques matured, there was some reduction in the number of neurites and activity of AChE, and the amount of amyloid increased. End-stage plaques showed fewer neurites and a marked reduction in AChE activity but were rich in amyloid. Some of these abnormal axon terminals in neuritic plaques may be derived from the Ch system, but it seems likely that a significant number of neurites may be derived from other sources, e.g., from AChE-containing, noncholinergic neurons located in subcortical sites (ventral tegmental area, raphe nuclei, locus ceruleus, and hypothalamus) or from non-AChE-containing, noncholinergic neurons intrinsic or extrinsic to neocortex (Price et al 1982a,b, 1983). Using the aged nonhuman primate model, the transmitter specificity of neurites in plaques can be assessed by immunocytochemical methods to visualize transmitter-specific probes (antibodies directed against transmitters or their synthesizing enzymes), while the sources (neuronal perikarya) of abnormal axons can be traced by connectivity studies utilizing the anterograde transport of [^{3}H]amino acids injected into various regions (Ch1-4, raphe, locus ceruleus, etc.) projecting to neocortex.

Plaque densities in aged monkeys are similar to those in relatively intact aged humans (Tomlinson et al 1968). There is some controversy about changes in cholinergic markers in human brain as a function of age (Perry et al 1977, 1980; Davies 1979; Bowen et al 1982); it is unlikely that monkeys with plaque densities of mild-to-moderate degree will show major reductions in ChAT activity.

CONCLUSION

Available evidence indicates that the Ch1-4 system plays important roles in normal cognitive functions, memory, and arousal and that this system may be mildly dysfunctional in old age and severely impaired in AD/SDAT. Integrated behavioral, neuropsychological, physiological, neuropathological, and neurochemical investigations of normal, aged, and demented individuals should clarify the roles of this system in health and disease.

ACKNOWLEDGEMENTS

This work was supported by grants from the U.S. Public

Health Service NIH NS 07179, NS 15721, and AG 03359 and fellowships from The Commonwealth Fund, The Sloan Foundation, and the McKnight Foundation. Dr. Cork is supported by a Research Career Development Award, NIH NS 00488.

REFERENCES

Ball MJ (1978). Topographic distribution of neurofibrillary tangles and granulovacuolar degeneration in hippocampal cortex of aging and demented patients. A quantitative study. Acta Neuropathol (Berl) 42:73.

Bartus RT, Dean RL III, Beer B, Lippa AS (1982). The cholinergic hypothesis of geriatric memory dysfunction. Science 217:408.

Bondareff W, Mountjoy CQ, Roth M (1982). Loss of neurons of origin of the adrenergic projection to cerebral cortex (nucleus locus ceruleus) in senile dementia. Neurology 32:164.

Bowen DM, Benton JS, Spillane JA, Smith CCT, Allen SJ (1982). Choline acetyltransferase activity and histopathology of frontal neocortex from biopsies of demented patients. J Neurol Sci 57:191.

Bowen DM, Smith CB, White P, Davison AN (1976). Neurotransmitter-related enzymes and indices of hypoxia in senile dementia and other abiotrophies. Brain 99:459.

Bowen DM, Spillane JA, Curzon G, Meier-Ruge W, White P, Goodhardt MJ, Iwangoff P, Davison AN (1979). Accelerated ageing or selective neuronal loss as an important cause of dementia? Lancet I:11.

Colon EJ (1973). The cerebral cortex in presenile dementia. A quantitative analysis. Acta Neuropathol (Berl) 23:281.

Coyle JT, Price DL, DeLong MR (1983). Alzheimer's disease: A disorder of cortical cholinergic innervation. Science 219:1184.

Cross AJ, Crow TJ, Perry EK, Perry RH, Blessed G, Tomlinson BE (1981). Reduced dopamine-ß-hydroxylase activity in Alzheimer's disease. Br Med J 282:93.

Daitz HM, Powell TPS (1954). Studies of the connexions of the fornix system. J Neurol Neurosurg Psychiatry 17:75.

Davies P (1979). Neurotransmitter-related enzymes in senile dementia of the Alzheimer type. Brain Res 171:319.

Davies P, Katz DA, Crystal HA (1982). Choline acetyltransferase, somatostatin, and substance P in selected cases of Alzheimer's disease. In Corkin S, Davis KL, Growdon JH, Usdin E, Wurtman RJ (eds): "Alzheimer's Disease: A

Report of Progress in Research," [Aging, Vol 19], New York: Raven Press, p 9.
Davies P, Katzman R, Terry RD (1980). Reduced somatostatin-like immunoreactivity in cerebral cortex from cases of Alzheimer disease and Alzheimer senile dementia. Nature 288:279.
Davies P, Maloney AJF (1976). Selective loss of central cholinergic neurons in Alzheimer's disease. Lancet II:1403.
Davies P, Terry RD (1981). Cortical somatostatin-like immunoreactivity in cases of Alzheimer's disease and senile dementia of the Alzheimer type. Neurobiol Aging 2:9.
Davis KL, Mohs RC, Tinklenberg JR, Pfefferbaum A, Hollister LE, Kopell BS (1979). Physostigmine: Improvement of long-term memory processes in normal humans. Science 201:272.
Davis RT (1978). Old monkey behavior. Exp Gerontol 13:237.
DeLong MR (1971). Activity of pallidal neurons during movement. J Neurophysiol 34:414.
Deutsch JA (1971). The cholinergic synapse and the site of memory. Science 174:788.
Divac I (1975). Magnocellular nuclei of the basal forebrain project to neocortex, brain stem, and olfactory bulb. Review of some functional correlates. Brain Res 93:385.
Drachman DA, Leavitt JL (1974). Human memory and the cholinergic system. A relationship to aging? Arch Neurol 30:113.
Drachman DA, Noffsinger D, Sahakian BJ, Kurdziel S, Fleming P (1980). Aging, memory, and the cholinergic system: A study of dichotic listening. Neurobiol Aging 1:39.
Herzog AG, Kemper TL (1980). Amygdaloid changes in aging and dementia. Arch Neurol 37:625.
Jamada M, Mehraein P (1968). Vertielungmuster der senilen Veranderungen im Gehirn. Die Beteiligung des limbischen Systems bei hirnatrophischen Prozessen des Seniums und bei Morbus Alzheimer. Arch Psychiatr Nervenkr 211:308.
Jasper HH, Tessier J (1971). Acetylcholine liberation from cerebral cortex during paradoxical (REM) sleep. Science 172:601.
Jones EG, Burton H, Saper CB, Swanson LW (1976). Midbrain, diencephalic and cortical relationships of the basal nucleus of Meynert and associated structures in primates. J Comp Neurol 167:385.
Kievit J, Kuypers HGJM (1975). Basal forebrain and hypothalamic connections to frontal and parietal cortex in the rhesus monkey. Science 187:660.
Kitt CA, Price DL, DeLong MR, Struble RG, Mitchell SJ, Hedreen JC (1982). The nucleus basalis of Meynert: Projections to the cortex, amygdala, and hippocampus. Neurosci Abstr 8:212.

Krettek JE, Price JL (1978). Amygdaloid projections to subcortical structures within the basal forebrain and brainstem in the rat and cat. J Comp Neurol 178:225.

Lo Conte G, Casamenti F, Bigl V, Milaneschi E, Pepeu G (1982). Effect of magnocellular forebrain nuclei lesions on acetylcholine output from the cerebral cortex, electrocorticogram and behaviour. Arch Ital Biol 120:176.

Mesulam M-M, Mufson EJ, Levey AI, Wainer BH (1983). Cholinergic innervation of cortex by the basal forebrain: Cytochemistry and cortical connections of the septal area, diagonal band nuclei, nucleus basalis (substantia innominata), and hypothalamus in the rhesus monkey. J Comp Neurol 214:170.

Mitchell SJ, Richardson RT, Baker RH, DeLong MR (1982). Electrophysiological and functional characteristics of neurons in the nucleus basalis of Meynert in macaque monkeys. Neurosci Abstr 8:212.

Pearson RCA, Gatter KC, Brodal P, Powell TPS (1983). The projection of the basal nucleus of Meynert upon the neocortex in the monkey. Brain Res 259:132.

Perry EK, Perry RH, Blessed G, Tomlinson BE (1977). Necropsy evidence of central cholinergic deficits in senile dementia. Lancet I:189.

Perry EK, Perry RH, Blessed G, Tomlinson BE (1978). Changes in brain cholinesterases in senile dementia of Alzheimer type. Neuropathol Appl Neurobiol 4:273.

Perry EK, Tomlinson BE, Blessed G, Perry RH, Cross AJ, Crow TJ (1981). Neuropathological and biochemical observations on the noradrenergic system in Alzheimer's disease. J Neurol Sci 51:279.

Perry RH, Blessed G, Perry EK, Tomlinson BE (1980). Histochemical observations on the cholinesterase activities in the brains of elderly normal and demented (Alzheimer-type) patients. Age Ageing 9:9.

Perry RH, Candy JM, Perry EK, Irving D, Blessed G, Fairbairn AF, Tomlinson BE (1982). Extensive loss of choline acetyltransferase activity is not reflected by neuronal loss in the nucleus of Meynert in Alzheimer's disease. Neurosci Lett 33:311.

Pope A, Hess HH, Lewin E (1964). Microchemical pathology of the cerebral cortex in pre-senile dementias. Trans Am Neurol Assoc 89:15.

Price DL, Whitehouse PJ, Struble RG, Clark AW, Coyle JT, DeLong MR, Hedreen JC (1982a). Basal forebrain cholinergic systems in Alzheimer's disease and related dementias. Neurosci Comment 1:84.

Price DL, Whitehouse PJ, Struble RG, Coyle JT, Clark AW, DeLong MR, Cork LC, Hedreen JC (1982b). Alzheimer's disease and Down's syndrome. Ann NY Acad Sci 396:145.

Price DL, Whitehouse PJ, Struble RG, Price DL Jr, Cork LC, Hedreen JC, Kitt CA (1983). Basal forebrain cholinergic neurons and neuritic plaques in primate brain. In Katzman R (ed): "Biological Aspects of Alzheimer's Disease," [Banbury Report, Vol 15], Cold Spring Harbor, New York: Cold Spring Harbor Laboratory, p 65.

Price JL, Amaral DG (1981). An autoradiographic study of the projections of the central nucleus of the monkey amygdala. J Neurosci 1:1242.

Reisine TD, Yamamura HI, Bird ED, Spokes E, Enna SJ (1978). Pre- and postsynaptic neurochemical alterations in Alzheimer's disease. Brain Res 159:477.

Rolls ET, Sanghera MK, Roper-Hall A (1979). The latency of activation of neurones in the lateral hypothalamus and substantia innominata during feeding in the monkey. Brain Res 164:121.

Rossor MN, Emson PC, Iverson LL, Mountjoy CQ, Roth M, Fahrenkrug J, Rehfeld JF (1982a). Neuropeptides and neurotransmitters in cerebral cortex in Alzheimer's disease. In Corkin S, Davis KL, Growdon JH, Usdin E, Wurtman RJ (eds): "Alzheimer's Disease: A Report of Progress in Research," [Aging, Vol 19], New York: Raven Press, p 15.

Rossor MN, Emson PC, Mountjoy CQ, Roth M, Iversen LL (1980). Reduced amounts of immunoreactive somatostatin in the temporal cortex in senile dementia of Alzheimer type. Neurosci Lett 20:373.

Rossor MN, Garrett NJ, Johnson AL, Mountjoy CQ, Roth M, Iversen LL (1982b). A post-mortem study of the cholinergic and GABA systems in senile dementia. Brain 105:313.

Saper CB, Loewy AD (1980). Efferent connections of the parabrachial nucleus in the rat. Brain Res 197:291.

Segal M, Landis S (1974). Afferents to hippocampus of the rat studied with the method of retrograde transport of horseradish peroxidase. Brain Res 78:1.

Shefer VF (1972). Absolute number of neurons and thickness of the cerebral cortex during aging, senile and vascular dementia, and Pick's and Alzheimer's diseases. Zh Nevropatol Psikhiatr 72:1024.

Sims NR, Bowen DM, Allen SJ, Smith CCT, Neary D, Thomas DJ, Davison AN (1983). Presynaptic cholinergic dysfunction in patients with dementia. J Neurochem 40:503.

Struble RG, Cork LC, Whitehouse PJ, Price DL (1982a). Cholinergic innervation in neuritic plaques. Science 216:413.

Struble RG, McKinney M, Sanberg PR, Kitt CA, DeLong MR, Coyle JT, Price DL (1982b). Ibotenic acid lesions of the primate nucleus basalis of Meynert result in decreased cortical choline acetyltransferase. Neurosci Abstr 8:211.

Swanson LW, Cowan WM (1979). The connections of the septal region in the rat. J Comp Neurol 186:621.

Szerb JC (1967). Cortical acetylcholine release and electro-encephalographic arousal. J Physiol 192:329.

Tagliavini F, Pilleri G (1983). Neuronal counts in basal nucleus of Meynert in Alzheimer disease and in simple senile dementia. Lancet I:469.

Terry RD, Peck A, DeTeresa R, Schechter R, Horoupian DS (1981). Some morphometric aspects of the brain in senile dementia of the Alzheimer type. Ann Neurol 10:184.

Tigges J, Tigges M, Cross NA, McBride RL, Letbetter WD, Anschel A (1982). Subcortical structures projecting to visual cortical areas in squirrel monkey. J Comp Neurol 209:29.

Tomlinson BE, Blessed G, Roth M (1968). Observations on the brains of non-demented old people. J Neurol Sci 7:331.

Tomlinson BE, Irving D, Blessed G (1981). Cell loss in the locus coeruleus in senile dementia of Alzheimer type. J Neurol Sci 49:419.

Veazey RB, Amaral DG, Cowan WM (1982). The morphology and connections of the posterior hypothalamus in the cynomolgus monkey (Macaca fascicularis). II. Efferent connections. J Comp Neurol 207:135.

Weingartner H, Sitaram N, Gillin JC (1979). The role of the cholinergic nervous system in memory consolidation. Bull Psychonomic Soc 13:9.

Whitehouse PJ, Hedreen JC, White CL III, Clark AW, Price DL (1983). Neuronal loss in the basal forebrain cholinergic system is more marked in Alzheimer disease than senile dementia of the Alzheimer type. Abstr Ann Neurol (in press).

Whitehouse PJ, Price DL, Clark AW, Coyle JT, DeLong MR, (1981). Alzheimer disease: Evidence for selective loss of cholinergic neurons in the nucleus basalis. Ann Neurol 10:122.

Whitehouse PJ, Price DL, Struble RG, Clark AW, Coyle JT, DeLong MR (1982). Alzheimer's disease and senile dementia: Loss of neurons in the basal forebrain. Science 215:1237.

Wilcock GK, Esiri MM, Bowen DM, Smith CCT (1982). Alzheimer's disease. Correlation of cortical choline acetyltransferase activity with the severity of dementia and histological abnormalities. J Neurol Sci 57:407.

Wisniewski HM, Terry RD (1973). Morphology of the aging

brain, human and animal. Prog Brain Res 40:167.
Woody CD, Swartz BE, Gruen E (1978). Effects of acetylcholine and cyclic GMP on input resistance of cortical neurons in awake cats. Brain Res 158:373.

DISCUSSION

DR. KOSIK: Do you think the loss in basalis is cell body death or a dying back?

DR. PRICE: My present view is that the cholinergic cell bodies survive for quite a long time and that dysfunction is expressed in the distal fields. It is not known whether the postulated changes in these axons represent a dying-back process similar to that occurring in several other models of disease in the peripheral nervous system. In late stages of Alzheimer's disease, like our index case, nerve cells are severely reduced (90-95%) in the basal forebrain cholinergic system. Our first case showed severe end-stage pathology presumably because of the early onset, long course, and positive family history. In contrast, individuals with late onset disease have less striking reductions of cholinergic neurons. There is precedent, particularly in studies of the lower motor neuron system, for neurons being dysfunctional for long periods before they die. Aluminum myelopathy, IDPN intoxication, and hereditary canine spinal muscular atrophy are three models in which experimental evidence suggests that axonal transport of specific polypeptides may be abnormal for sustained periods before cell death occurs. I think some similar processes may be occurring in cholinergic neurons and certain other at-risk populations in Alzheimer's disease.

DR. REGELSON: This is very exciting because it implies trophic effects from a brain nucleus affecting a pathologic system which is very similar to what Hoffer, Olson, Wyatt and others have done in relation to substantia nigral abnormalities in Parkinson's disease where embryonic transplantation may be correcting the pathology, at least the behavioral pathology of the animal.

Vernon Mark has organized a meeting in June of this year with the American Paralysis Association, and they will discuss the ethical and technical issues of embryonic--neuro-embryonic transplantation. It is obviously a major ethical problem, but I wonder whether anybody, picking up on what you have observed, is seeking to isolate the CH1 through 4 region and using embryonic cells, putting them into the adult model to see whether or not a trophic effect could restore function. (Note: Carl Cotran has done this in rats with hippocampal repair following surgical injury and embryonic transplantation.)

DR. PRICE: When the hippocampi of rats are destroyed, these animals show impaired performance on behavioral tasks. There are recent reports in which cholinergic neurons from the medial septum have been grafted into the hippocampi of rats. When these septal grafts were put into the hippocampus, the performance of the animals improved. It is not known if this approach will be feasible in other species. Using excitotoxin, we have destroyed nerve cells in the basal forebrain cholinergic system in monkeys with the idea that these animals may provide a model of forebrain cholinergic deficiency which could be manipulated with pharmacological agents, like physostigmine and arecholine, and perhaps for studies of the efficacy of grafts or trophic factors.

DR. MORGAN: What do you think of Ray Bartus' work with presumably non-demented monkeys that shows an improvement in memory with his agonist for the cholinergic system?

DR. PRICE: My view is that Dr. Bartus has been a pioneer in this field. He and Dr. Roger Davis were among the first investigators to call attention to the fact that old monkeys develop cognitive deficits similar to those occurring in humans. Future investigations should be multidisciplinary and focus on aged nonhuman primates with correlations linking behavioral responses, neuropathology, and neurochemistry. I believe that old monkeys provide an excellent model, not of Alzheimer's disease, but for analysis of the neuropathological and neurochemical substrates of behavioral deficits occurring in aged individuals. We have begun studies of the nonhuman primate model because one can do behavioral testing of these animals, carry out a variety of invasive studies, including anterograde transport tracing methods (to look at sources of neurites in plaques), and then do detailed neuropathological studies, including transmitter-specific immunocytochemical and [^{3}H]ligand receptor autoradiography, in conjunction with neurochemical analysis of markers for specific-transmitter systems. We think that these multidisciplinary approaches may have important implications for the understanding of facets of Alzheimer's disease.

DR. TERRY: I think it is worth pointing out that in regard to both neuropathology and the clinical study of elderly patients we find three groups, not two. That is, one finds specimens with many plaques, and they correlate well with dementia. One finds other specimens that are essentially free of plaques or have very few, and again that correlates with real normality. In between, there are numbers of elderly patients coming to autopsy with small numbers of plaques per unit area in the neocortex. (When you see any significant numbers of neocortical tangles that patient was demented). Clinically there are many people who have numbers of errors on mental status tests, and these persons are demented. There are other people in large numbers who have fewer errors on mental status tests, and they are accepted as normal, but they are not. There are also supernormals, and some of them are famous, like Picasso, Casals, Rebecca West and others. These are the normals even though they are not as common as the mild cases. The problem, I think, is also relevant to monkeys. No one has done a very careful correlation of those supernormals with either the CAT levels or with plaque counts. That is the clinical state at which we should aim, not at the state where there are a few errors on a mental status test and only a few plaques per unit area.

DR. PRICE: I agree with Dr. Terry. In the first group are (super) normal individuals like Sophocles and Titian. In a second group are many old people who show some cognitive decline with age; some of these individuals, like the old monkeys, have plaques in low density. It is not clear if these individuals show focal cholinergic deficits, particularly in regions with relatively high plaque densities. This hypothesis could be tested by directly relating regional choline acetyltransferase activities and regional plaque densities. The third group, i.e. patients with Alzheimer's disease, are really quite different in that they show major reductions in certain groups of nerve cells, including cholinergic neurons in the medial septum, diagonal band, nucleus basalis, as well as plaques and tangles in the telencephalon.

Comparative Pathobiology of Major Age-Related Diseases:
Current Status and Research Frontiers, pages 401–410

AGING AND THE SEROTONERGIC SYNAPSE IN HUMAN BRAIN: A PRELIMINARY REPORT

David G. Morgan, Ph.D., James A. Severson, Ph.D., Jan O. Marcusson, Ph.D., and Caleb E. Finch, Ph.D.

Andrus Gerontology Center, Departments of Psychiatry and Biological Sciences, University of Southern California, Los Angeles, CA 90007 and Department of Pathology, University of Umea, Umea, Sweden

Brain serotonin neurons, located in the raphe nuclei of the brainstem, project to most forebrain regions and the spinal cord (Steinbusch 1981). Recent studies indicate that this neurotransmitter system has multiple high affinity recognition sites which may serve to transduce the serotonin signal postsynaptically (Peroutka, Snyder 1983; Nelson 1982). In addition, there are presynaptic recognition sites on serotonergic terminals which bind antidepressant drugs and regulate serotonin uptake (Raisman et al 1979). The studies described here examine human aging changes in serotonergic binding site components and the levels of serotonin (5-HT) and its major metabolite, 5-hydroxyindolacetic acid (5-HIAA), in frontal cortex and hippocampus. The data indicate a complex series of changes, the sum of which may contribute to the enhanced risk of depressive illness in old age.

Our theoretical framework for the central serotonergic synapse is depicted in Figure 1. This working model assumes that the serotonergic terminal is adjacent to several postsynaptic recognition sites which may mediate the diverse electrophysiological responses to serotonin and its agonists (Jacobs 1983).

The S-1 site has high affinity for ^{3}H-serotonin and other agonists, but low affinity for most putative serotonin antagonists. This site is regulated by guanine nucleotides and appears to stimulate adenylate cyclase (Peroutka, Snyder 1983). Recently, the S-1 binding site was resolved into two

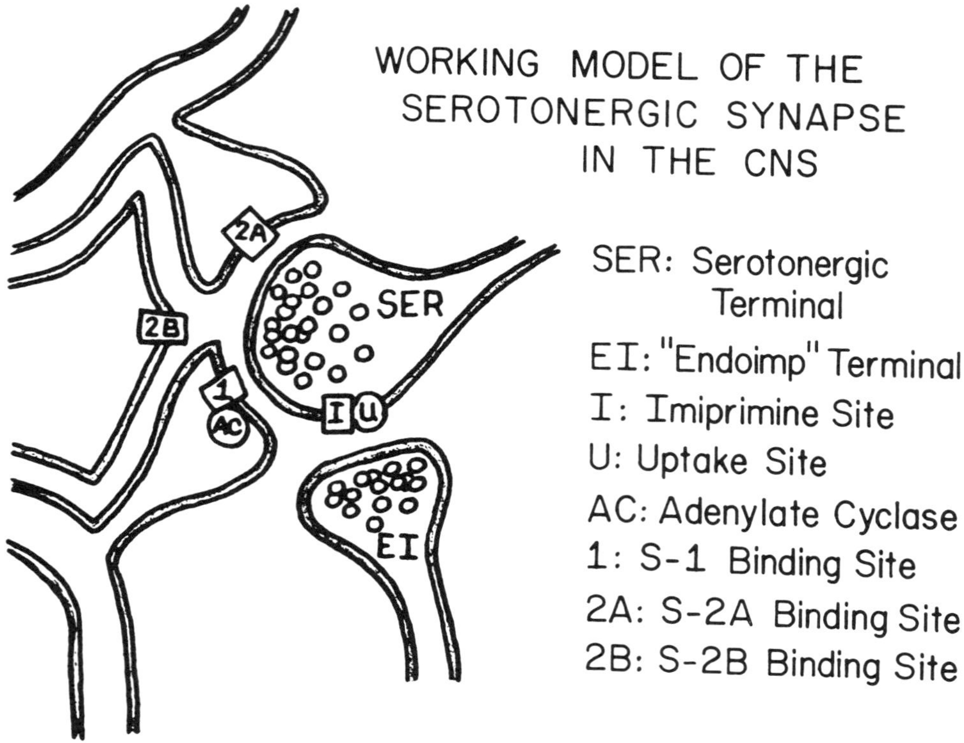
WORKING MODEL OF THE
SEROTONERGIC SYNAPSE
IN THE CNS
SER: Serotonergic Terminal
EI: "Endoimp" Terminal
I: Imiprimine Site
U: Uptake Site
AC: Adenylate Cyclase
1: S-1 Binding Site
2A: S-2A Binding Site
2B: S-2B Binding Site
SER
EI
2A
2B
1
AC
I
U

Fig. 1.

subtypes, S-1A and S-2B (Nelson 1982). However, the results presented here with ^{3}H-serotonin were obtained prior to the publication of these findings, and represent the aggregate, or total S-1 binding site.

The S-2 site displays high affinity for serotonin antagonists (ketanserin, cyproheptadine, cinanserin) and neuroleptics (spiperone, haloperidol), but low affinity for serotonin and most agonists. In recent studies of this binding site with ^{3}H-spiperone, we were able to discriminate two S-2 binding components with the serotonin antagonist methysergide (Morgan et al 1983). These binding sites are referred to as S-2A and S-2B, and do not appear to be linked to adenylate cyclase.

The serotonin terminal contains recognition sites for ^{3}H-imipramine, an antidepressant drug. These binding sites can regulate serotonin uptake, but are distinct from the uptake site itself (Barbaccia et al 1983). We propose the term "endoimp" to designate a hypothetical endogenous imipramine-like substance which acts as the *in vivo* ligand for the ^{3}H-imipramine recognition site. While not yet reported, several laboratories have found column fractions of brain extracts which modulate ^{3}H-imipramine binding (Severson, Marcusson 1983). These fractions may contain a novel transmitter substance, or a putative transmitter already identified.

We stress that the details of this working model are tentative. The various binding components are indicated as residing on separate anatomical entities, but may indeed be on the same cells and perhaps at the same synapses. The postulated transmitter, endoimp, may reside in serotonin terminals as a cotransmitter, or may not even exist. The model is intended as a framework within which to interpret the results presented here. While it represents our best approximation given the available evidence, future data will undoubtedly modify aspects of this model.

METHODS

Postmortem human brains from donors with no evidence of neurologic or psychiatric disease were obtained at the University Hospital, Umea, Sweden. The twenty-six subjects ranged from 17 to 100 years of age with a mean age of 57 years and a median age of 59. Fifteen separate brain regions were dissected, including frontal cortex, and hippocampus.

Portions of these brain regions were analyzed for serotonergic binding sites and for levels of 5-HT and 5-HIAA. S-1 sites were measured with ^{3}H-serotonin using 1 mM nonradioactive serotonin to define nonspecific binding (Marcusson et al 1983b). ^{3}H-Spiperone binding was used to measure the total S-2 sites; 0.5 μM ketanserin determined nonspecific binding. Characterization studies of S-2 binding confirmed the presence of two S-2 subtypes in human brain similar to those in mouse brain (Marcusson et al 1983a). Hence, the aggregate S-2 site was further resolved into S-2A and S-2B components using methysergide displacement curves to discriminate the two sites. Specific binding of ^{3}H-imipramine was defined as that binding displaced by 100 μM desipramine (Severson, Marcusson, 1983). Imipramine binding was determined in frontal cortex, parietal cortex, and hypothalamus, but not hippocampus. All ligand binding studies were performed using the filtration method to separate bound and free radioisotope.

5-HT and 5-HIAA were measured by high pressure liquid chromatography with electrochemical detection (HH Osterburg, JA Severson, J Marcusson, CE Finch, unpublished observations.)

RESULTS AND DISCUSSION

Ligand binding studies are summarized in Table 1. The density of S-1 sites declined in both frontal cortex and hippocampus by about 30% between 20 and 100 years. The mean B_{max} and K_d in frontal cortex were 465 fmoles/mg protein and 3.73 nM, while those in hippocampus were 475 fmoles/mg protein and 3.63 nM. No correlation was detected for the S-1 B_{max} values between the two regions. No age related change in K_d was observed.

The total S-2 site B_{max} decreased with age in the frontal cortex, but not in the hippocampus. The average B_{max} for total S-2 binding was 357 fmoles/mg protein in frontal cortex, and 162 fmoles/mg protein in hippocampus. No correlation was found between the two regions. The K_d for ^{3}H-spiperone was approximately 1 nM in both brain regions, but K_d was not affected by age.

Table 1

Site	r	n	% Change[a] 20-100 Y	p
		FRONTAL CORTEX		
S-1	-0.49	20	-29%	0.05
S-2	-0.73	24	-41%	0.01
S-2A	-0.65	19	-52%	0.01
S-2B	-0.32	19	-	N.S.
Imip	0.63	23	+130%	0.01
		HIPPOCAMPUS		
S-1	-0.62	14	-36%	0.02
S-2	-0.01	21	-	N.S.
S-2A	-0.46	21	-35%	0.05
S-2B	-0.18	21	-	N.S.

[a] "% change" refers to the difference between 20 and 100 years using 20 as the 100% value. Values were obtained from the linear regression analysis. Where linear regression analysis was not significant, no values are presented.

In the frontal cortex, S-2A sites decreased in density with age, while S-2B sites did not change. The S-2A site was the predominant subtype in this brain region with 60% more sites on the average than the S-2B subtype. Within the frontal cortex, total S-2, S-2A, and S-2B binding correlated significantly with the S-1 density (*r* = 0.472, 0.514, and 0.504 respectively).

In the hippocampus, the S-2A sites also declined with age, and as in cortex, there was no change in S-2B binding. However, the hippocampus contains twice as many S-2B sites as S-2A. This preponderance of the age stable S-2B subtype in the hippocampus may explain why the total S-2 site fails to change with age in this region. No correlation with S-1 binding density was obtained for the hippocampal S-2 site or its subtypes. In addition, hippocampal S-2 binding was not correlated with frontal cortical S-2 sites.

On the presynaptic side, the density of ^{3}H-imipramine binding in frontal cortex more than doubled between 20 and 100 years of age. A similar increase was detected in hypothalamus (r = 0.76, p = 0.0001) and parietal cortex (r = 0.60, p = 0.01). Age did not affect the affinity of ^{3}H-imipramine for its recognition site (mean K_d = 6.03 nM). ^{3}H-Imipramine B_{max} was inversely correlated with the S-2 B_{max} in the frontal cortex (r = -0.476). The levels of 5-HT and 5-HIAA did not show any age related trends in either frontal cortex or hypothalamus. Although some caution should be exercised when evaluating neurotransmitter levels from human samples due to the considerable postmortem period preceding dissection, most studies suggest maintenance of serotonin concentrations across the life span (Rogers, Bloom 1983). Thus, there is no indication of serotonergic terminal loss with age.

To summarize, a decline in S-1 and S-2A binding sites was observed in individuals of advanced age. Concurrently, the same individuals presented an increased density of ^{3}H-imipramine binding sites. No change in the density of S-2B binding sites or the level of 5-HT or 5-HIAA were seen with age.

We tentatively conclude from these data that the S-1 and S-2B binding may decline due to an age associated neuron or synapse loss, or due to a decline in the synthesis rate of these binding sites. While the positive correlation between these two measures suggests some common anatomic loci, the differences in the extent of the age decline indicates independent loci as well. The lack of change in S-2B binding suggests a different anatomical location for this putative receptor, perhaps on structures which do not decline with age such as glia, or on the serotonin terminal as the autoreceptor.

The dramatic, progressive increase in ^{3}H-imipramine binding contrasts with the absence of a change in 5-HT or 5-HIAA levels. Our working hypothesis is that serotonin terminal number is stable with age, but that a hypothetical endogenous imipramine-like substance (endoimp) declines with age. In turn, increased imipramine binding could result as a compensatory up-regulation response to the loss of endoimp by analogy with the well known effects of deafferentation on dopamine binding sites.

The elderly are reported to be at 2-3 fold greater risk for the development of depression than the general population. The two major pharmacologic agents used to treat depression are monoamine oxidase inhibitors, and tricyclic antidepressants, such as imipramine. Since monoamine oxidase inhibitors prevent degradation of serotonin (and catecholamines), and imipramine reduces serotonin uptake, an increased serotonergic activity or tone is one common action of these drugs.

Monoamine oxidase-A activity (selective for serotonin over catecholamines) is generally reported to increase with age (Rogers, Bloom 1983). The potential for increased degradation of serotonin combined with the predicted increase in serotonin uptake (due to loss of endoimp) would tend to reduce the duration of serotonin's action in old age. These events, together with the reduction in postsynaptic sensitivity (due to loss of the putative receptors S-1 and S-2A) may predispose the elderly to depressive illness. Conversely, the increase in ^{3}H-imipramine binding sites with age may explain the anecdotal accounts of enhanced sensitivity to imipramine in older individuals being treated for depression.

One should be cautious in assuming that enhanced serotonergic tone is the simple mechanism by which antidepressant therapy works. The enhanced serotonergic tone is of rapid onset following delivery of the drug (minutes) while the reduction of clinical symptoms requires 1-2 weeks of therapy. Thus some chronic effect of these drugs, most likely downstream from their site of action, mediates the therapeutic effect. Nonetheless, the common action of these agents in enhancing serotonergic tone may be the requisite trigger for the sequence of events which eventually alleviates the depressive symptomology.

Ongoing studies of dopaminergic sites in these same brains will explore the possible relationship of dopaminergic and serotonergic sites. In previous studies, we found progressive loss of dopaminergic sites in the caudate nucleus and substantia nigra with age (Severson et al 1982). These declines roughly parallel the decreased S-1 and S-2A binding described here.

ACKNOWLEDGEMENTS

We are grateful to Heinz Osterburg for his technical assistance. This work was supported in part by grants to CEF from the NIA (AG-00117; AG-00446; AG-03272). DM was supported by grants from the Glenn foundation and the NIA (AG-00093).

REFERENCES

Barbaccia ML, Brunello N, Chuang DM, Costa E (1983). On the mode of action of imipramine: Relationship between serotonergic axon terminal function and down regulation by beta-adrenergic receptors. Neuropharmacology 22:373.

Jacobs BL (1983). Mechanism of action of hallucinogenic drugs: Focus upon postsynaptic serotonergic receptors. In Cowen PJ (ed): "Psychopharmacology 1: Preclinical Psychopharmacology," Amsterdam: Excerpta Medica, p 344.

Marcusson JM, Morgan DG, Winblad B, Finch CE (1983a). Serotonin-2 receptor binding in human frontal cortex and hippocampus. Selective loss of S-2A receptors with age. Abstr Soc Neurosci 9.

Marcusson J, Oreland L, Winblad B (1983b). ^{3}H-5-Hydroxytryptamine binding in samples of human brain throughout the lifespan. Brain Res (in press).

Morgan DG, Marcusson J, Finch CE (1983). Serotonin receptors in mouse brain: Two S-2 binding sites discriminated by methysergide. Abstr Soc Neurosci 9.

Nelson DL (1982). Central serotonergic receptors: Evidence for heterogeneity and characterization by ligand binding. Neurosci Biobehav Rev 6:499.

Peroutka SJ, Snyder SH (1983). Multiple serotonin receptors and their physiological significance. Fed Proc 42:213.

Raisman R, Briley M, Langer SZ (1979). Specific tricyclic antidepressant binding sites in rat brain. Nature 281:148.

Rogers J, Bloom F (1983). Aging and neurotransmitter systems in the mammalian CNS. In Finch CE (ed): "Handbook of the Biology of Aging," Vol 2 New York: Van Nostrand Reinhold. In press.

Severson JA, Marcusson J (1983). ^{3}H-Imipramine binding sites in human hypothalamus and cerebral cortex increase with age. Abstr Soc Neurosci 9.

Severson JA, Marcusson J, Winblad B, Finch CE (1982). Age correlated loss of dopaminergic binding sites in human basal ganglia. J Neurochem 39:1623.

Steinbusch HWM (1981). Distribution of serotonin immunoreactivity in the central nervous system of rat cell bodies and terminals. Neuroscience 6:557.

DISCUSSION

DR. TERRY: This has been a very important demonstration that many fundamental studies of a neurobiological nature can indeed be carried out on human postmortem tissue. I would plead that such tissue be very carefully screened, prior to such use, for such subtle changes as anoxia, Parkinson's disease, mild changes of Alzheimer's and so on, which might significantly change the conclusions one would draw.

DR. REGELSON: Ketanserin is now going into the phase I study by Janssen Pharmaceutica Inc., for the treatment of thromboangiitis, peripheral vascular disease, hypertension, platelet aggregation and cardiac failure with some good clinical studies indicating it may have clinical value. At least in the population that they are reporting they are not encountering much in the way of CNS toxicity alterations. Do you have any experience with clinical information about ketanserin?

DR. MORGAN: No, I don't. One thing that is often a problem, as I am sure you are well aware, is that if you administer a drug peripherally it is not guaranteed to get into the central nervous system. That may be why they are not seeing any CNS toxicity. Other pure serotonin antagonists do not have a strong behavioral effect. However, binding to this S-2 receptor site is correlated well with the ability of drugs to regulate vascular constriction. It is also correlated well with what is called the serotonin behavioral syndrome, which is induced by serotonin agonists. These are not hallucinogenic drugs, but serotonin agonists which are nonhallucinogenic such as 5-hydroxytryptophan. I would be surprised, if it was getting into the CNS, that it would not be having some sort of central effect, but, again, it may be that only very small amounts are getting in, and it is not crossing the blood-brain barrier as well as many other drugs do.

DR. REGELSON: Do you have any thoughts about tetrahydrobiopterin (BH4), the tyrosine tryptophan hydroxylase cofactor as a factor in what you are describing here? You have a unique opportunity to sample tissue and to correlate it with the BH4 cofactor, and I wonder whether you have thought of looking at this.

DR. MORGAN: We haven't thought about it. Is it stable postmortem?

DR. REGELSON: I don't know whether anybody has ever really checked this point. Walter Lovenberg and Bob Levine, the group at the National Heart Institute are studying this with the National Institute of Neurological and Communicative Disorders and Stroke. They are using it to treat Parkinson's disease. The Japanese, and Curtius in Zurich are reporting clinical results with it. And, very recently there was a letter to the editor of Lancet by Bob Levine and the group from Switzerland reporting a dramatic response in the manic depression of aging in one or two cases, very anecdotal, but it represents a very promising cofactor which is supposedly decreased in Parkinson's patients.

DR. MORGAN: I would expect that BH4 would be decreased in Parkinsonism since it is a cofactor for tyrosine hydroxylase as well as trytophan hydroxylase. If there is no tyrosine hydroxylase there to bind BH4 or if there are no terminals there to take it up, it could well be that this explains the reduction. Parkinson's disease is characterized, as we heard earlier, by absence of dopaminergic cells, so there are no terminals; there is no tyrosine hydroxylase, so you just don't have any cofactor.

DR. REGELSON: But they are reporting some clinical success with it, so the hope is that there may be another possibility.

DR. MORGAN: The reason for clinical success is possibly due to the fact that BH4 is rate limiting for the enzyme tyrosine hydroxylase. However, I don't know of any *in vivo* data one way or the other on this subject.

DR. TURTURRO: You did give some indication of the physiological effects of the S-2 receptor. Do you have any idea of the functional effects of the S-2A and S-2B receptors?

DR. MORGAN: Not yet, but we are quite interested in that.

Comparative Pathobiology of Major Age-Related Diseases: Current Status and Research Frontiers, pages 411–423

NEUROTROPHIC FACTORS AND DISEASES OF AGING: AN APPROACH TO ALS, PARKINSONISM, AND ALZHEIMER'S DISEASE

Stanley H. Appel, M.D.

Baylor College of Medicine, Houston, TX 77030

INTRODUCTION

Amyotrophic lateral sclerosis, Parkinsonism, and Alzheimer's disease represent three of the most common and most devastating diseases of the nervous system. Each of these conditions is a degenerative disorder of unknown origin. In each, multiple etiologies including viral or immunological causes have been implicated, but never proven. All three diseases reflect pathologic changes in a relatively limited pathway within the peripheral or central nervous system. In all three the changes in the disease state resemble alterations known to occur in older individuals. Thus, all three disorders may represent accelerated aging of specific neuronal pathways.

Our thesis is that each of these disorders results from the lack of a neurotrophic hormone which is elaborated or stored in the synaptic target of the affected neurons and exerts a specific retrograde effect (Appel 1981). These neurotrophic hormones would be of vital importance to survival of neurons during development, to their sprouting during regeneration, and to their maintenance throughout the life cycle. Any process which depletes neurotrophic hormones, or interferes with their retrograde action on presynaptic receptors may result in gradual neuronal failure. This failure of specific neuronal pathways would be due to premature aging which, in turn, resulted from many different etiological factors. The common denominator would be a diminution in retrograde trophic effects.

TROPHIC FACTORS

Recent advances in developmental neurobiology have documented the importance of target cell trophic factors for the survival, growth, and differentiation of innervating neurons. This principle is most convincingly documented in the peripheral autonomic nervous system where nerve growth factor (NGF) can be demonstrated to influence neuronal viability and maturation _in vivo_ and _in vitro_ (Bradshaw 1978). Although _in vivo_ demonstrations of the retrograde effects of muscle factors on motor survival are not available, the experiments of Hamburger on the chick lumbar cord motor neuron survival are plausibly explained by the availability of muscle-derived retrograde neurotrophic effects (Hollyday, Hamburger 1976). If the chick limb is removed _in ovo_, motor neuron death is enhanced; if a limb is added, diminution in cell death results. Studies by Oppenheim and his colleagues suggest that diminution in muscle activity or blockade of the muscle nicotonic acetylcholine receptor would also decrease motor neuron cell death (Pittmann, Oppenheim 1978). The literature on sprouting of motor axons also supports the hypothesis that a neurotrophic hormone released from muscle may enhance motor neuronal growth. In fact, the same agents which enhance cell viability in the chick spinal cord also seem to promote motor neuron sprouting (Holland, Brown 1980).

RETROGRADE TRANSNEURONAL DEGENERATION

Further evidence supporting the potential role of neurotrophic factors acting in a retrograde fashion is the phenomenon of retrograde transneuronal degeneration (RTND) (Torch et al 1977). Such retrograde transneuronal degeneration has been noted in the limbic system; that is, in the medial mamillary nucleus or the ventral tegmental nucleus following lesions in the limbic cortex or cerebral cortex (Cowan 1970). It has also been demonstrated in pyramidal cells of precentral cortex following limb amputation, or in the inferior olivary nucleus following cerebellar or Purkinje cell damage. Lesions of anterior thalamic nucleus or medial mamillary nucleus result in retrograde transneuronal degeneration in ventral tegmental nucleus. Lesions of the occipital visual cortex have been noted to give rise to changes in retinal ganglion cells, optic nerve, and lateral geniculate body presumably secondary to retrograde transneuronal degeneration. In experimental animals this process may take from seventeen days to two months, while in the visual system it may take up to two years (Cowan 1970). Within the pathways involved in ALS, Parkinson's disease, and Alzheimer's disease, changes of retrograde transneuronal degeneration may take even longer periods of time, and may be due to a depletion of neurotrophic factors.

AMYOTROPHIC LATERAL SCLEROSIS

Amyotrophic lateral sclerosis is the name given to a complex of disorders that compromise function of upper and lower motor neurons. When only one form of motor neuron disease is present, it is commonly the lower motor neuron type, and may occur at any age. Lower motor neuron involvement may result from genetic disorders, drug toxicity, malignant paraproteinemia with macroglobulinemia, multiple myeloma or cryoglobulinemia, hexosaminidase A deficiency, or in conjunction with involvement of other systems such as Jakob-Creutzfeldt disease or Roussy-Levy cerebellar degeneration. Thus, a wide range of conditions and possibly a wide range of etiologies may be responsible for lower motor neuron dysfunction.

The majority of patients with ALS have manifestations of lower motor neuron as well as upper motor neuron involvement. The same toxic, hormonal, and immunologic abnormalities noted in lower motor neuron disease must be ruled out. The pathological changes in ALS are present in Betz cells, cranial motor neurons, and anterior horn cells. Chromatolysis is noted in the cell bodies; spheroids and neurofilamentous changes have been described in the axons as well as in the cell bodies, and Bunina eosinophilic bodies have been noted. None of these changes provide definitive clues as to the etiology.

Our own hypothesis is that motor neuron disease may be due to a lack of specific neurotrophic hormones (Appel 1981). In the lower motor neuron syndromes, the dysfunction may be secondary to the lack of a neurotrophic hormone synthesized in skeletal muscle and released from muscle into the synaptic cleft where it interacts with receptors on motor nerve terminals and exerts a trophic effect in a retrograde fashion.

According to this theory in ALS, both upper and lower motor neurons would undergo an age-related deterioration primarily due to the absence of important extrinsic neurotrophic effects. Degeneration of the motor pathway could be explained by diminished availability of motor neurotrophic hormones which are normally released by muscle, interact with the presynaptic axon terminal, and exert their action in a retrograde fashion. Involvement of the upper motor neuron would be due to a similar failure of neurotrophic maintenance of the upper motor neuron by factors released from lower motor neurons and/or muscle.

TISSUE CULTURE ASSAYS OF TROPHIC FACTORS

Assays for neurotrophic factors for the motor system can be provided by tissue culture. Studies from several laboratories have demonstrated that addition of skeletal muscle to cultured spinal cord enhances long-term survival of neurons, promotes outgrowth of neurites, and increases CAT activity (Giller et al 1977). Furthermore, media conditioned on muscle myotubes can reproduce some of these effects of co-culture (Dribin, Barrett 1980; Henderson et al 1981).

In our own laboratory proteins derived from rat, calf, and human skeletal muscle can promote neuron survival, neuritic outgrowth, and enhance acetylcholine synthesis (Smith, Appel 1983). Our assay system consists of dissociated ventral spinal cord cultured in Dulbecco's modified Eagle's medium supplemented with 10 percent horse serum. Within three days after the muscle extracts are added, the cultured neuronal and glia cells begin to associate into clusters. Concomitant with this change is a fourfold increase in the average number of neurites per neuron and a 3.5-fold increase in the average neurite length.

The muscle extract appears to have specific effects on ventral horn cells, since no morphologic changes are induced when extract is added to cultured dorsal spinal cord neurons. Furthermore, increases in acetylcholine synthesis and choline acetyltransferase of approximately 2.4-fold are observed only in ventral horn motor neurons, and not in dorsal horn cells. The relevant protein is not nerve growth factor since neither nerve growth factor nor antibody to nerve growth factor have significant effects on dissociated ventral cord cultures in the presence or absence of muscle extract.

Recent experiments from our laboratory have separated the morphologic and cholinergic activity. The ability to enhance neurite outgrowth appears to be specific for skeletal muscle extracts. Extracts from other tissues including cardiac muscle, brain, liver, spleen and kidney have no effect either on process outgrowth or process density in ventral horn cells. However, the ability to enhance acetylcholine synthesis is present not only in extract of skeletal muscle but also in extracts of cardiac muscle and brain cortical tissue. In addition, as a function of age, morphologic activity drops off whereas cholinergic activity is retained. By gel chromatography and isoelectric focusing, the morphologic activity can be totally separated from cholinergic activity. Both activities appear to reside in proteins as evidenced by their lability to heat and to tryptic digestion. However, they differ with respect to molecular weight. Thus, extracts prepared from skeletal muscle enhance the survival, development, and cholinergic differentiation of dissociated ventral cord cells *in vitro*, and may exert similar effects *in vivo*.

PARKINSONISM

Parkinson's disease is a disorder of older individuals with a mean age of onset of 67. It is characterized by tremor, bradykinesia, and rigidity as well as a loss of postural reflexes. The primary pathologic abnormality appears to be a loss of neurons in the substantia nigra. Pathologically, eosinophilic inclusions termed Lewy-bodies are present in nigral neurons. In cases of postencephalitic parkinsonism, neurofibrillary alterations are noted in nigral neurons. The loss of nigral cells leads to marked impairment in the nigral-striatal pathway, and a diminution in the dopaminergic synaptic input to the caudate and putamen. Of importance is the fact that no diminution is noted in the dopaminergic receptors within the striatum. Thus, the presynaptic neuron is impaired and the postsynaptic neuron is intact.

Our hypothesis of retrograde neurotrophic factors suggests that Parkinson's disease is due to the absence or impairment of neurotrophic factors normally supplied by the striatum to nigral neurons. With the failure of neurotrophic effects in this system, nigral cells would gradually die.

NEUROTROPHIC EFFECTS IN THE NIGRO-STRIATAL PATHWAY

Tissue culture provides the only available assay for such trophic factors. When rat substantia nigra explants are co-cultured with striatum, neuron survival, neuritic fluorescence, and specific dopaminergic uptake are enhanced in cultured nigral neurons (Prochiantz et al 1979; Hemmendinger et al 1981). In our own laboratory proteins extracted from newborn rat striatum enhanced neurite extension, catecholamine fluorescence, and dopamine uptake in nigral explants (Appel 1981). Extracts of muscle and occipital cortex do not provide the same neurotrophic effect. Evidence that protein is involved is based in the demonstration that the extract is heat labile and sensitive to tryptic digestion (K Ojika and SH Appel, unpublished observations). Furthermore, the specificity of this system is documented by the ability of benztropine to block the uptake of dopamine under control circumstances, as well as in the presence of striatal extracts.

ALZHEIMER'S DISEASE

Alzheimer's disease is a disorder characterized clinically by diffuse deterioration of mental function primarily in thought and memory and secondarily in feeling and conduct. It is a disorder of the later decades of life which is diagnosed primarily by exclusion. Secondary causes of loss of memory and impaired cognitive function by multiple infarcts, intracranial mass lesions, infections, or toxic and metabolic disorders must be ruled out.

The etiology of Alzheimer's disease is unknown. Although viral and immunologic causes have been suggested, no convincing reproducible data support the presence of an infectious agent or a cell-mediated or humoral immune factor. However, despite the paucity of data regarding the etiology, there has been substantial clarification of the pathology of this syndrome as noted in the present symposium. For purposes of our argument, the most striking changes are the loss of neurons in the nucleus basalis of Meynert (Whitehouse et al 1982). These cells are known to convey cholinergic input to cortical tissues, in the same way that medial septal projections provide cholinergic input to hippocampus (Johnston et al 1979).

This new insight into the pathophysiology of Alzheimer's disease has permitted a refocusing of attention from previous notions of widespread cellular damage, to the present notions of more limited network structural defects. In this framework, Alzheimer's disease becomes similar to ALS and Parkinson's disease, in which there is impairment of the presynaptic neuron with the postsynaptic cell remaining relatively intact. Thus, the lack of a specific neurotrophic hormone elaborated or released from the hippocampus and cortical cells may result in impairment of medial septal and nucleus basalis neurons respectively. In this system as well as in the motor system and the nigral striatal pathway, tissue culture may be employed to document the importance of neurotrophic factors.

NEUROTROPHIC EFFECTS IN THE SEPTAL-HIPPOCAMPAL SYSTEM

Medial septal tissues are obtained from the brains of 16-day embryonic albino Sprague-Dawley rats by dissection of whole septal region fragments. When grown in Sato's media (Bottenstein, Sato 1979) process growth and cell viability are maintained for at least eight days _in vitro_. The addition of hippocampal extract at three days _in vitro_ results in a gradual increase in the length and density of fiber outgrowth compared to control cultures. These effects begin within one to two days and can be monitored between six and eight days _in vitro_.

As an assay for cholinergic neurons, acetylcholine synthesis is monitored over this six-day period. After application of the hippocampal extract at day three _in vitro_, acetylcholine synthesis increases significantly and by day six, is more than twice control value. By day eight synthesis is increased to an average of three to fourfold. Other tissues such as cortex, striatum, cerebellum, spinal cord, muscle, liver, and kidney do not give the same effect. Several of these tissues do give some enhancement over control, but this increase is related to the fact that explants are being cultured in defined media. In addition, there is some effect of the extract on survival since in the absence of hippocampal extract, there is a diminution of acetylcholine synthesis between days six and eight. Thus, the effects of the extract from day three to day eight are a combination of increased survival as well as enhancement of acetylcholine synthesis independent of survival.

Nerve growth factor has been reported to enhance cortical cholinergic activity, but there is no evidence that it is responsible for our observed neurotrophic effects or morphology or acetylcholine synthesis. NGF produces no morphologic nor cholinergic effects in our cultured septal tissue, whereas it has a quite marked effect on rat dorsal root ganglia and superior cervical ganglia. Furthermore, antibodies to NGF have no effect on the enhancement noted in the presence of hippocampal extract or medial septal nucleus morphology in acetylcholine synthesis. The neurotrophic effect of hippocampal tissue is present both in soluble and particulate components. The particulate activity is present in synaptic membranes as well as those from myelin and microsomal fractions. It is absent in mitochondrial fractions. The supernatant activity resides primarily in a peptide fraction less than 2,000 daltons.

DISCUSSION

In the systems under discussion, it is clear that neurotrophic proteins can enhance neuron survival, promote neuritic extension, and increase the activity of the neurotransmitter synthetic enzymes *in vitro*. Muscle possesses neurotrophic factors which enhance morphologic and cholinergic function in cultured ventral spinal cord neurons. Striatal tissues possess neurotrophic factors which enhance neuritic outgrowth and specific dopaminergic differentiation of cultured nigral cells. Hippocampal extracts possess neurotrophic factors which enhance neuritic outgrowth and specific cholinergic differentiation in cultured medial septal neurons. The same factors responsible for neuritic outgrowth, survival, and neurotransmitted differentiation *in vitro* may also be responsible for development *in vivo*. The same factors may also be responsible for maintenance of neurons throughout the life cycle *in vivo*. They may decrease to a limited extent during aging, or undergo a marked diminution in the disease states under discussion.

Thus, the primary manifestations of ALS, Parkinson's disease, and Alzheimer's disease may reflect the failure of the target tissue to supply the necessary hormones, or they may reflect the presence of substances which interfere with the neurotrophic effects upon the presynaptic target neurons.

One of the advantages of this theory is its ability to

explain how many different causes, such as lead, trauma, viruses, infections, as well as inborn errors of metabolism could lead to similar results. In the motor system, these insults could compromise the production, release, neuronal uptake, intracellular transport, or neuronal regulatory function of motor neurotrophic hormones and thereby lead to motor neuron disease. If the defect is in the production or release of neurotrophic hormones, muscle would be the primary target of the insult and the motor nerve the secondary target. If the defect is in the uptake, transport, or regulatory functions of the motor neuron, then supplying an external source of motor neurotrophic hormone would not be expected to be of much benefit.

It is of interest that proteins which are transported in a retrograde fashion such as tetanus toxin, interact with specific nerve terminal receptors, such as gangliosides. Therefore, it is possible that the motor neuron involvement in hexosaminidase A deficiency (Yaffe et al 1979; Johnson 1981) might be due to an alteration in the ganglioside or lack of protein receptor of the motor neurotrophic hormone. The common denominator in all such conditions would be a deficiency in either the amount or the function of the motor neurotrophic hormones. Such factors can be clearly documented to exist in tissue culture assays. It remains to be determined whether they play a significant role in mammalian motor neuron development and maintenance *in vivo*, and whether they are deficient in lower motor neuron disorders such as Werdnig-Hoffmann disease, and in upper and lower motor neuron syndromes such as ALS.

Similarly, in Alzheimer's disease the primary failure could be in the inability of hippocampus or cortical cells to supply the relevant cholinergic neurotrophic hormone. Either the lack of appropriate neurotrophic hormones, or interference with its action, would impair the viability of the innervating septal and basal cells and result in gradual cell death.

Such a theory suggests the existence of neurotrophic hormones which are specific for a particular neuronal network or a specific neurotransmitter (e.g., cholinergic or dopaminergic). These neurotrophic factors may aid in maintenance as well as regeneration of these particular systems. Classic neuronal interactions have emphasized the importance of neurotransmitters such as acetylcholine, dopamine, norepinephrine, gamma immunobutyric acid, glutamate, and others.

Within the last decade it has become increasingly clear that another group of compounds, namely the neuropeptides may function both as modulators of neurotransmitter release and as neurotransmitters themselves. As modulators these neuropeptides may act over a longer period of time than do the neurotransmitters. The neurotrophic hormones may in fact be neuropeptides or larger proteins which would be expected to exert their effects over months to years rather than over the shorter time periods of neurotransmitters. Our hypothesis also suggests that neurotrophic hormone has specificity analogous to that of nerve growth factor for the development of the sensory and sympathetic systems. Such specificity may depend upon the particular neurotransmitters employed.

Clearly, no direct evidence presently exists to implicate deficiency of neurotrophic hormones in any of these diseases of premature aging. Nevertheless, such neurotrophic hormones can be documented in tissue culture, and exert their effects primarily on neurons known to innervate these target tissues *in vivo*. Purification of such hormones and clarification of their mechanism of action may not only shed light on long-term cell-cell interaction, but it may also provide a basis for understanding the pathophysiology of these devastating clinical disorders.

ACKNOWLEDGEMENTS

We are grateful to the John A. Hartford Foundation and the Robert J. Kleberg, Jr. and Helen C. Kleberg Foundation for their support of these investigations.

REFERENCES

Appel SH (1981). A unifying hypothesis for the cause of amyotrophic lateral sclerosis, parkinsonism, and Alzheimer's disease. Ann Neurol 10:499.

Bottenstein JE, Sato GH (1979). Growth of a rat neuroblastoma cell line in serum-free supplemented medium. Proc Natl Acad Sci USA 76:514.

Bradshaw RA (1978). Nerve growth factor. Annu Rev Biochem 47:191.

Cowan WM (1970). Anterograde and retrograde transneuronal degeneration in the central and peripheral nervous system. In Nauta WJ, Ebbson SD (eds.): "Contemporary Research Methods in Neuroanatomy," New York: Springer, p 217.

Dribin LB, Barrett JN (1980). Conditioned medium enhances neuritic outgrowth from rat spinal cord explants. Dev Biol 74:184.

Giller EL, Neale JN, Bullock PN, Schrier BK, Nelson PC (1977). Choline acetyltransferase activity of spinal cord cell cultures increased by co-culture with muscle and by muscle-conditioned medium. J Cell Biol 74:16.

Hemmendinger LM, Garber BB, Hoffmann PC, Heller A (1981). Target neuron-specific process formation by embryonic mesencephalic dopamine neurons in vitro. Proc Natl Acad Sci USA 78:1264.

Henderson CE, Hachet M, Changura JP (1981). Neurite outgrowth from embryonic chicken spinal neurons is promoted by media conditioned by muscle cells. Proc Natl Acad Sci USA 78:2625.

Holland RL, Brown MC (1980). Postsynaptic transmission block can cause terminal sprouting of a motor nerve. Science 207:699.

Hollyday M, Hamburger V (1976). Reduction of the naturally occurring motor neuron loss by enlargement of the periphery. J Comp Neurol 170:311.

Johnson WG (1981). The clinical spectrum of hexosaminidase deficiency diseases. Neurology 31:1453.

Johnston MV, McKinney M, Coyle JT (1979). Evidence for a cholinergic projection to neocortex from neurons in basal forebrain. Proc Natl Acad Sci USA 76:5392.

Pittmann R, Oppenheim R (1978). Neuromuscular blockade increases motor neuron survival during normal cell death in the chick embryo. Nature 271:364.

Prochiantz A, DiParzio N, Kato A, Berger B, Glowinski J (1979). In vitro maturation of mesencephalic dopaminergic neurons from mouse embryos is enhanced in the presence of their striatal target cells. Proc Natl Acad Sci USA 76:5387.

Smith RG, Appel SH (1983). Extracts of skeletal muscle increase neurite outgrowth and cholinergic activity of fetal rat spinal motor neurons. Science 219:1079.

Torch WC, Hirano A, Solomon S (1977). Anterograde transneuronal degeneration in the limbic system: Clinical-anatomic correlation. Neurology 27:1157.

Whitehouse PJ, Price DL, Clark AW, Coyle JT, DeLong MR (1982). Alzheimer's disease and senile dementia: Loss of neurons in the basal forebrain. Science 215:1237.

Yaffe MC, Kaback M, Goldberg M, Miles J, Itabashi H, McIntyre H, Mohandes T (1979). An amyotrophic lateral sclerosis-like syndrome with hexosaminidase A deficiency: A new type of GM_2 gangliosidosis. Neurology 29:611.

DISCUSSION

DR. KOSIK: The cultures you describe in the ALS model are not exclusively anterior horn cells. If your hypothesis is correct, one would think that the anterior horn cells would respond with neuritic outgrowth much more than non-anterior horn cells. Have you looked at that distinction? Also, would you repeat for me how you knew that any given cell was an anterior horn cell?

DR. APPEL: The answer to both questions can be answered by the same experiment. The question is, what percentage of the total neuronal population are classical motor neurons? The answer to that is probably no better than 3-5%. So, how are you going to know from the neuritic outgrowth whether you are dealing with motor neurons?

There is only one way that we thought of doing it, and that was to copy other investigators who injected muscles *in ovo* or *in utero* and maintained the cells in the spinal cord which possessed the particular dye. When you inject muscle with a dye like horseradish peroxidase or Lucifer yellow attached to wheat germ agglutinin, the material will be transported retrogradely and will be taken up into motor neurons of the anterior horn. Then you take out the ventral spinal cord, dissociate the cells, and culture the cells. You can monitor the outgrowth of the cells and determine whether motor neurons respond to trophic influences. Results from these experiments suggest that anterior horn motor neurons do respond to trophic influences, but it is quite clear that they cannot be the only cells participating in this process. Whether, in fact, the morphologic factors are working directly on the anterior horn motor neurons which in turn cause glial changes, or whether glial cells influence motor neurons cannot be deduced from the data I have given you.

DR. REGELSON: Do your factors cross species, and do they affect amphibian regeneration or some other species like the fish that show central nerve regenerative capacity?

DR. APPEL: We have not tested it with fish. We have analyzed chick, calf, rabbit, and human material. The nicest thing, I must tell you, is that human material is an elegant source for such factors. Of interest is the fact that human material behaves comparably to rat material. In the adult 70-year-old human we find high cholinergic and low morphologic effects, whereas in the newborn human we have both high morphologic and cholinergic effects.

Index